Functional Surgery of the Larynx and Pharynx

Functional Surgery of the Larynx and Pharynx

Waryam Singh F.R.C.S. (Ed), D.L.O. (Lond)
Consultant Otolaryngologist, Head and Neck Surgeon, Director Voice Research Laboratory, St John's Hospital, Livingston; Consultant Otolaryngologist, Head and Neck Surgeon, Western General Hospital, Edinburgh; Honorary Senior Lecturer, University of Edinburgh.

David S. Soutar Ch.M., F.R.C.S. (Ed), F.R.C.S. (Glas), M.B. Ch. B.
Consultant Plastic Surgeon, West of Scotland Regional Plastic and Oral Surgery Unit, Canniesburn Hospital, Glasgow; Honorary Clinical Senior Lecturer, University of Glasgow.

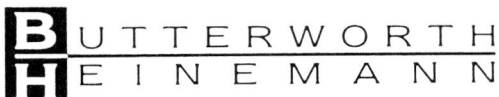

Butterworth-Heinemann Ltd
Linacre House, Jordan Hill, Oxford OX2 8DP

A member of the Reed Elsevier group

OXFORD   LONDON   BOSTON
MUNICH   NEW DELHI   SINGAPORE   SYDNEY
TOKYO   TORONTO   WELLINGTON

First published 1993

© Butterworth–Heinemann Ltd 1993

All rights reserved. No part of this publication
may be reproduced in any material form (including
photocopying or storing in any medium by electronic
means and whether or not transiently or incidentally
to some other use of this publication) without the
written permission of the copyright holder except in
accordance with the provisions of the Copyright,
Designs and Patents Act 1988 or under the terms of a
licence issued by the Copyright Licensing Agency Ltd,
90 Tottenham Court Road, London, England W1P 9HE.
Applications for the copyright holder's written permission
to reproduce any part of this publication should be addressed
to the publishers.

British Library Cataloguing in Publication Data

Singh, Waryam
　Functional Surgery of the Larynx and Pharynx
　I. Title.　II. Soutar, David S.
　617.5

ISBN 0 7506 0612 6

Library of Congress Cataloguing in Publication Data

Functional surgery of the larynx and pharynx/
　[edited by] Waryam Singh, David S. Soutar.
　　p.　cm.
　Includes bibliographical references and index.
　ISBN 0 7506 0612 6
　1. Voice disorders – Surgery.　2. Voice
　disorders.　3. Larynx – Surgery.　4. Pharynx –
　Surgery.　I. Singh, Waryam.　II. Soutar, David S.
　[DNLM: 1. Laryngectomy.　2. Pharyngectomy.
　3. Voice Disorders – therapy.　WV 540 F979]
　RF516.F86
　617.5′33059–dc20
　　　　　　　　　　　　　　　　　　　　　　　92–49424
　　　　　　　　　　　　　　　　　　　　　　　　CIP

Printed and bound in Great Britain by
Redwood Press Ltd, Melksham

Contents

Preface vii

Acknowledgements ix

List of Contributors xi

Part One – Voice Production

1 Surgical and pathophysiological considerations 3
   P. H. Rhys Evans, N. Stafford and J. Waldron

2 Aerodynamics of voice production 18
   H. K. Schutte

3 Normal and pathological speech: phonetic, acoustic and 31
   laryngographic aspects
   A. J. Fourcin

Part Two – Investigation of Voice Problems

4 Aids to diagnosis 55
   E. Loebell

5 The role of computers 60
   W. A. Ainsworth

6 The voice research laboratory in clinical practice 70
   W. Singh and G. McKenna

Part Three – Surgery of the Larynx and Pharynx

7 Laryngeal and pharyngeal surgery: past, present and future 97
   D. A. Shumrick and L. W. Savoury

8 Pharyngo-oesophageal reconstruction and rehabilitation   101
   D. S. Soutar

9 Near-total or parsimonious laryngectomy   116
   W. Singh

10 The carbon dioxide laser in laryngeal and pharyngeal surgery   147
   **G. Motta, G. Villari, G. Salerno, F. A. Salzano, L. D'Angelo,
   E. Esposito and S. Motta**

11 Nursing care of the patient undergoing laryngectomy   157
   J. M. Muir

Part Four – Voice Rehabilitation

12 Oesophageal speech   165
   P. H. Damsté

13 Fistula speech   171
   W. Singh

Index   204

Preface

Voice is a basic human attribute and a psychosocial and physiological necessity. It is therefore not surprising that many clinical disciplines have an interest in the science of voice, including otolaryngologists, phoniatricians, plastic surgeons, head and neck surgeons, neurologists, speech therapists, physicians, psychiatrists and psychologists.

Recently considerable progress has been made in the fields of phoniatry, laryngology and logopedics, in the form of improved investigative techniques for the diagnosis of voice problems, improved conservative laryngeal surgical techniques based on a better understanding of tumour type, invasion and pattern of spread, and an increased realization of the important contribution of voice rehabilitation and the development of various voice prostheses.

Dissemination of knowledge and further progress in voice research and clinical practice have been hampered, however, by the lack of an interdisciplinary approach. With this in mind, the editors have invited experts from various disciplines to contribute to this book which is aimed at the various surgical specialities involved in the management of voice problems.

Part One deals with the normal mechanisms of voice production and how these can be altered in certain pathological conditions. Part Two outlines important advances in clinical and research techniques which provide an aid to diagnosis. Part Three is concerned with surgery and hopefully points the way towards improved surgical techniques based on our knowledge of essential anatomy and our increased understanding of the mechanisms of voice production. Finally, Part Four deals with voice rehabilitation following ablative surgery and highlights the problems that remain in obtaining satisfactory intelligible voice.

The interaction of experts in various specialities is essential if improvements in diagnosis and surgical techniques are to be achieved. Such an approach should stimulate further research and development which will eventually result in improved quality of life for our patients.

Waryam Singh
David S. Soutar

Acknowledgements

As editors of this multidisciplinary book we wish to acknowledge our special thanks to the contributors for sharing their expertise with us and our readers. The fact that this book appears at all is due largely to the hard work and ability of our secretary, Margaret Stephenson. She showed great diplomatic skill in dealing with various contributors who were late with their promised manuscripts. We owe special thanks to our former secretary, Betty Morrison, who worked hard in the initial stages in managing the preparation of the manuscripts. Our other secretary, Maureen Howley, has been a tremendous help, both in keeping our morale high with her great sense of humour and by working extremely hard in the preparation of this book, spending many hours of extra time on it. It is also our pleasure to thank Eleanor Swan for taking a keen interest in typing parts of the manuscripts. We also express our thanks to Bob Yorston for beautiful line drawings, and to the Medical Illustration Department, St John's Hospital, for some of the photographs. Lastly, we thank the publishers, especially Charles Fry and later Geoffrey Smaldon, who have been very patient and helpful during the preparation of this book.

Contributors

W. A. Ainsworth B.Sc. Hons., Ph.D., Reader, Department of Communication and Neuroscience, University of Keele, Keele.

P. H. Damsté M.D., Ph.D., Professor of Phoniatrics, Medical School, University of Utrecht, Utrecht.

L. D'Angelo M.D., Professor, Department of Otolaryngology, University of Naples, Naples.

E. Esposito M.D., Department of Otolaryngology, University of Naples, Naples.

A. J. Fourcin Ph.D., Professor of Experimental Phonetics, Centre for Speech and Hearing Sciences, University College, London.

E. Loebell M.D., Professor and Head of Department of Phoniatrics, Hanover Medical School, Hanover.

G. McKenna, Research Assistant, Department of Otolaryngology, St John's Hospital, Livingston.

G. Motta M.D., Professor and Head of Department of Otolaryngology, Medical School, University of Naples, Naples.

S. Motta M.D., Department of Otolaryngology, University of Naples, Naples.

J. M. Muir R.G.N., J.B.C.N.S. Cert. E.N.T., Sister, Department of Otolaryngology, St John's Hospital, Livingston.

P. H. Rhys Evans D.C.C., F.R.C.S., Consultant Surgeon (Head & Neck/ENT), Royal Marsden Hospital, London.

G. Salerno M.D., Department of Otolaryngology, University of Naples, Naples.

F. A. Salzano M.D., Department of Otolaryngology, University of Naples, Naples.

L. W. Savoury M.D., Otolaryngologist Head and Neck Surgeon, Department of Otolaryngology, Saudi Aramco Health Centre, Dhahran, Saudi Arabia.

H. K. Schutte M.D., Ph.D., Professor of Voice and Speech Disorders, Voice Research Laboratory, Groningen State University and Centre for Voice Speech and Language Disorders, ENT Clinic, University Hospital, Groningen.

D. A. Shumrick M.D., Professor and Chairman, Department of Otolaryngology & Maxillofacial Surgery, University of Cincinnati Medical Center, Cincinnati, Ohio.

W. Singh F.R.C.S. (Ed), D.L.O. (Lond), Consultant Otolaryngologist, Head and Neck Surgeon, Director Voice Research Laboratory, St John's Hospital, Livingston.

Consultant Otolaryngologist, Head and Neck Surgeon, Western General Hospital, Edinburgh.

Honorary Senior Lecturer, University of Edinburgh.

D. S. Soutar Ch.M., F.R.C.S. (Ed), F.R.C.S. (Glas), M.B. Ch.B., Consultant Plastic Surgeon, West of Scotland Regional Plastic and Oral Surgery Unit, Canniesburn Hospital, Glasgow.

Honorary Clinical Senior Lecturer, University of Glasgow.

N. Stafford F.R.C.S., Consultant ENT Surgeon, St Mary's Hospital, London.

G. Villari M.D., Department of Otolaryngology, University of Naples, Naples.

J. Waldron F.R.C.S., Senior ENT Registrar, St Mary's Hospital, London.

Part One

Voice Production

Chapter 1

Surgical and pathophysiological considerations

P. H. Rhys Evans, N. Stafford and J. Waldron

Surgical anatomy of the larynx

During the third week of human embryonic growth the respiratory system starts developing as an endodermal outgrowth from the ventral wall of the foregut (Langman, 1969). Initially in open connection with the foregut lumen, this respiratory diverticulum is soon separated from it by the oesophagotracheal septum, which remains deficient at the laryngeal orifice.

Over the following 2 weeks, five pairs of branchial arches develop in the mesoderm surrounding the pharynx. The upper part of the body of the hyoid bone and its lesser horns are derived from second arch tissue, while the lower part of the body and the greater horns develop from third arch mesenchyme. The fourth and sixth arches (the fifth arch is rudimentary in the human) give rise to the thyroid, cricoid and arytenoid cartilages of the larynx. The fourth arch musculature (cricothyroid and the pharyngeal constrictors) are innervated by the superior laryngeal branches of the vagus nerve; the other intrinsic muscles of the larynx derived from the sixth arch mesenchyme are supplied by the recurrent branches of the vagus nerves.

The tongue develops from two lateral lingual swellings and a median swelling, the tuberculum impar. A second median swelling, the hypobranchial eminence, is formed by mesoderm derived from the second, third and fourth branchial arches.

The epiglottis develops from a third median swelling of fourth arch origin. Immediately behind this is the laryngeal orifice, which is flanked by the two arytenoid swellings. Although the orifice is temporarily closed off by the adherence of the two lateral walls to each other, luminal continuity is restored by 3 months.

The skeleton of the larynx is made up by the hyoid bone, single thyroid, cricoid and epiglottic cartilages and paired arytenoid, corniculate and cuneiform cartilages. These form a framework which is held together by a combination of ligaments, membranes and muscles. The corniculate, cuneiform and epiglottic cartilages are elastic fibrocartilage and do not ossify.

Cricoid cartilage

The cricoid cartilage narrows down from a broad, almost square, posterior lamina into an anterior arch. On each lateral aspect, at the junction of the lamina and the arch, is a facet for its articulation with the inferior horn of the thyroid cartilage. The upper edge of the cricoid lamina slopes inferolaterally and carries articular facets for the two arytenoid cartilages. All four joints are synovial, with capsular ligaments.

The cartilage starts to calcify in adulthood, usually in a posteroanterior direction.

Apart from the two cricothyroid joints and their associated ligaments, the cricoid is attached to the thyroid cartilage by three muscles, the cricothyroid ligament and the conus elasticus.

The conus elasticus, or cricovocal ligament, is a thick fibroelastic membrane which extends from the superior margin of the cricoid arch to the inner aspect of the laryngeal prominence of the thyroid cartilage in the midline anteriorly. Posteriorly, it is attached to the vocal process of the arytenoid cartilage on each side. Between these 'fixed' points, its free upper margins are thickened to form the two vocal ligaments. Anteriorly, the conus elasticus thickens to form the midline cricothyroid ligament. The cricothyroid membrane is attached to the inferior edge of each thyroid lamina, immediately lateral to the ligament.

The cricothyroid muscle arises from the outer lateral aspect of the cricoid arch on each side, effectively covering much of the cricothyroid membrane. It fans out in two parts: the posterior portion inserts into the anterior edge of the inferior cornu of the thyroid cartilage, while the anterior part inserts into the inferior border of the thyroid lamina, behind the insertion of the cricothyroid ligament. Contraction of the muscle results in rotation and forward tilting of the thyroid on the cricoid cartilage, with consequent lengthening of the vocal ligaments.

The paired posterior cricoarytenoid muscle is the only muscle that opens the glottis. It arises from the medial part of the posterior aspect of the cricoid lamina and inserts into the back of the muscular process of the ipsilateral arytenoid cartilage. The upper fibres, running almost horizontally, cause lateral rotation of the arytenoid on the cricoid cartilage. The lower, more lateral fibres run obliquely and their contraction causes the arytenoid to slide down the slope of the articular facet on the cricoid lamina. Both sets of fibres produce a widening of the glottic aperture; the horizontal fibres tending to form a diamond-shaped rima glottidis and the oblique fibres a triangular one.

The lateral cricoarytenoid muscle, which is also paired, runs superomedially from the superior margin of the lateral part of the cricoid arch, to insert into the muscular process of the arytenoid. Its contraction results in medial rotation of the arytenoid and closure of the glottis.

Thyroid cartilage

The thyroid cartilage is comprised of two laminae which are fused in the midline anteriorly, below the thyroid notch. In men the internal angle between the two laminae is 90 degrees; in women it is 120 degrees. The posterior border of each lamina is extended to produce superior and inferior cornua, the inferior cornua articulating with the cricoid cartilage.

The lateral aspect of each lamina is marked by an oblique line, where the thyrohyoid, sternothyroid and thyropharyngeal muscles are attached. The anterior commissure tendon inserts into the midline of the cartilage, just below the point where the epiglottis takes origin. The thyroepiglottic ligament connects the base of the epiglottis with the back of the thyroid cartilage, up to the level of the thyroid notch. A median and two lateral thyrohyoid ligaments form strong attachments between the hyoid bone and the thyroid cartilage. The intervening thyrohyoid membrane provides an anterior and lateral wall to the piriform fossa on each side. Triticeal cartilages lie within the lateral thyrohyoid ligaments.

The thyroarytenoid muscle is a broad sheet of muscle running between the thyroid lamina and the arytenoid cartilage on each side, immediately lateral to the conus elasticus. Each muscle arises from the posterior aspect of the junction of the two thyroid laminae, immediately below the level of the vocal cord, and the adjacent cricothyroid ligament. It runs posteriorly to insert into the anterolateral surface of the ipsilateral arytenoid cartilage. The free superior edge of the muscle is thickened to form the vocalis muscle. Whether some fibres of the vocalis muscle arise from the vocal ligament remains an unsettled issue. Some fibres of the thyroarytenoid muscle run in the ipsilateral aryepiglottic fold. The uppermost of these run from the thyroid cartilage to the free edge of the epiglottis on each side. Contraction of the thyroepiglottic muscle produces a slight widening of the laryngeal inlet.

Epiglottis

The epiglottis is held in position by attachments to the hyoid bone (the midline hyoepiglottic ligament), the thyroid cartilage (the thyroepiglottic ligament) and the arytenoid cartilages (the paired quadrilateral membranes). Each quadrilateral membrane can be regarded as a continuation of the ipsilateral cricovocal membrane. It extends from the anterior surface of the arytenoid cartilage to the lower half of the free lateral border of the epiglottis. The vestigial corniculate and cuneiform cartilages lie in the posterior part of its free upper border. The corniculate cartilage may make contact with its adjacent arytenoid cartilage. The lower free margin of the membrane is thickened to form the vestibular ligament; the upper free margin provides the framework for the aryepiglottic fold.

Arytenoid cartilages

Each arytenoid cartilage is an irregular three-sided pyramid, the base of which articulates with the upper edge of the cricoid lamina. An anterior vocal process is attached to the vocal ligament and a lateral muscular process provides attachment for the posterior and lateral cricoarytenoid muscles. In between these two processes are two fossae on the anterolateral face of the cartilage. The vestibular ligament inserts into the upper fossa, and the vocalis and lateral cricoarytenoid muscles insert into the lower fossa.

The transverse arytenoid muscle runs from the posterior surface of one muscular process to the same site on the contralateral cartilage. It is the only unpaired muscle in the larynx, and lies deep to the oblique arytenoid muscles which arise from the same site on the posterior aspect of each muscular process. Some of the fibres from each oblique arytenoid muscle insert into the apex of the contralateral arytenoid cartilage. The remaining fibres, passing around the apex into the aryepiglottic fold, constitute the aryepiglottic muscle.

Hyoid bone

The hyoid bone develops from mesenchyme derived from the second and third branchial arches. Four centres of ossification develop shortly before birth, another two appearing during the first year of life. The two centres in the body soon unite, fusing with those in the greater horns in middle age. The lesser horns only unite with the central mass in old age.

The bone is suspended in position by membranous and ligamentous attachments to the larynx, the strap muscles, the stylohyoid apparatus, the extrinsic tongue muscles and the middle pharyngeal constrictor.

Extrinsic muscles of the larynx

The extrinsic muscles of the larynx fall into three groups: muscles that elevate the larynx, those that depress it, and muscles that constrict the pharynx.

Laryngeal elevators
The mylohyoid, digastric, stylohyoid and geniohyoid muscles all elevate the hyoid bone and, therefore, the larynx.

The thyrohyoid muscle arises from the oblique line of the thyroid lamina and inserts into the inferior border of the greater cornu of the hyoid. It is supplied by C1 efferents running in the hypoglossal nerve, and only elevates the larynx when the hyoid bone is fixed. The stylopharyngeus muscle arises from the medial surface of the base of the styloid process and passes between the superior and middle pharyngeal constrictors, blending with fibres of the inferior constrictor and palatopharyngeal muscle. Some fibres insert directly into the posterior border of the thyroid cartilage, and are supplied by the accessory nerve via the pharyngeal plexus.

Laryngeal depressors
The sternohyoid, sternothyroid and omohyoid muscles are all supplied by the ansa cervicalis, which carries second and third cervical root efferents.

Pharyngeal constrictors
Despite having no direct effect on movement of the larynx, the middle and inferior pharyngeal constrictors have important attachments to its bony and cartilaginous framework.

The middle constrictor arises from the lower part of the stylohyoid ligament and from the greater and lesser horns of the hyoid bone. It inserts into the median raphe of the pharynx. The superior laryngeal vessels and the internal branch of the superior laryngeal nerve pierce the posterior part of the thyrohyoid membrane in the triangular gap defined by the middle constrictor above, the inferior constrictor below, and the thyrohyoid muscle anteriorly.

The inferior constrictor is made up of two parts. The thyropharyngeal muscle arises from the oblique line of the thyroid cartilage, the side of the cricoid cartilage and from the fascia on the lateral aspect of the cricothyroid membrane. It inserts into the posterior median raphe, where its upper fibres overlap the lower part of the middle constrictor. The cricopharyngeal muscle, arising between the origin of the cricothyroid muscle anteriorly and the articular facet for the inferior horn of the thyroid cartilage posteriorly, runs more horizontally. It does not insert into the raphe, but encircles the outlet of the hypopharynx, inserting into the same site on the opposite side of the cricoid cartilage. Inferiorly, it is in continuity with the circular muscle of the oesophagus.

The motor nerve supply to the pharyngeal constrictors is derived from the glossopharyngeal and vagus nerves, by way of the pharyngeal plexus. The cricopharyngeal muscle is also supplied by fibres from the external and recurrent laryngeal nerves on both sides.

Laryngeal epithelium

Morphological studies of epithelial distribution in larynges taken from non-smokers at postmortem have been carried out by Stell et al. (1978, 1980, 1981). They based their work on the selective uptake of alcian blue and phloxine by respiratory and squamous epithelium respectively. Macroscopic study of the stained hemilarynx allows the distribution of the two epithelial types to be mapped.

The glottis is lined by a circumferential rim of squamous epithelium, which may be broken by a narrow, vertical band of ciliated respiratory epithelium at the anterior commissure. In the subglottis, the epithelium changes to being predominantly respiratory in type. Electronmicroscopic study of the human fetal larynx demonstrates a transition zone between the two regions, where both types of epithelium are found together (Stafford and Davies, 1988). Both the site and the size of this zone are variable, but the observation of squamous epithelium in the fetal subglottis casts a question over the concept of 'pathological' as opposed to 'physiological' squamous metaplasia in this region (Heymann, 1889). Indeed, in one study of the larynges of non-smoking adults, squamous metaplasia was observed in the subglottis of as many as 40 of the specimens (Stell and Watt, 1984). The lower subglottis is covered entirely by respiratory epithelium.

The supraglottic epithelium is predominantly ciliated, respiratory in type. However, the lingual surface of the epiglottis and the free edge of the epiglottis and aryepiglottic folds are covered by squamous epithelium. Small islands of the latter can also be found on the laryngeal surface of the epiglottis. Mucus-secreting glands are particularly numerous in this area. Although absent from the squamous epithelium of the glottis, glands in the saccules provide lubrication for the vocal folds.

Blood supply of the larynx

The larynx has superior and inferior vascular pedicles. The superior pedicle contains the superior laryngeal artery, a branch of the superior thyroid artery, and the superior laryngeal veins, which drain via the superior thyroid or facial veins into the internal jugular vein. Running deep to the thyrohyoid muscle, the vessels pierce the thyrohyoid membrane and enter the framework of the larynx. They supply the larynx down to the level of the glottis.

The inferior pedicle contains the inferior laryngeal artery, a branch of the inferior thyroid artery, and its accompanying veins, which drain into the brachiocephalic veins. The inferior pedicle enters the larynx beneath the lower border of the cricopharyngeal muscle, having run up in the tracheo-oesophageal groove. The middle thyroid veins drain some blood from the larynx into the internal jugular veins.

The cricothyroid artery is also a branch of the superior thyroid artery. It runs down the lateral wall of the larynx, crossing the upper part of the cricothyroid ligament to anastomose with its counterpart on the other side.

Lymphatic drainage of the larynx

Above the level of the glottis, the laryngeal lymphatics drain — via vessels running in the superior vascular pedicle — into the upper deep cervical chain nodes. Below the glottis, the lymphatics run in the inferior vascular pedicle and drain, either directly or via the prelaryngeal or pretracheal nodes, into the lower deep cervical chain nodes.

The glottis is devoid of lymphatics.

Nerve supply of the larynx

The internal branch of the superior laryngeal nerve is a branch of the vagus nerve. It pierces the thyrohyoid membrane above the superior vascular pedicle and carries sensory afferents from the mucosa of the supraglottis and adjacent piriform fossa. The nerve also carries proprioceptor afferents from muscle spindles in the larynx. The external branch of the superior laryngeal nerve descends, alongside the cricothyroid artery, to supply the cricothyroid muscle. All other intrinsic muscles of the larynx are supplied by the recurrent laryngeal nerve. This nerve enters the larynx deep to the cricopharyngeal muscle and also carries sensory afferents from the glottis and subglottis.

Stretch receptor afferents from the larynx run in both the internal branch of the superior laryngeal nerve and the recurrent laryngeal nerve.

The laryngeal spaces

Reinke's space
Reinke's space is a submucosal space which extends along the full length of the free edge of each vocal fold.

Pre-epiglottic space
The fat-filled pre-epiglottic 'space' is bounded by the hyoepiglottic ligament superiorly, the thyroid cartilage and thyrohyoid membrane anteriorly, and the epiglottis and thyroepiglottic ligament posteriorly. Laterally it contains the saccule of the larynx and becomes continuous with the paraglottic space, lateral to the quadrilateral membrane and superior to the ventricle. The space is important in the spread of supraglottic tumours.

Paraglottic space
The medial extent of the paraglottic space is formed by the quadrilateral membrane superiorly and the conus elasticus inferiorly. The thyroid cartilage forms the lateral boundary and the piriform fossa mucosa the posterior boundary. Above the level of the ventricle, the space is separated from the supraglottic space by the quadrilateral membrane.

Inferolaterally, the paraglottic space is continuous with the cartilaginous defect between the thyroid and cricoid cartilages (the cricothyroid space).

This space is important in the spread of laryngeal carcinomas, and explains how involvement of the space by a ventricular tumour can result in transglottic spread. The relatively common occurrence of cord fixation in association with an adjacent piriform fossa tumour, even when direct invasion of the larynx is not macroscopically apparent, may be explained by tumour invasion of the space.

Anatomical levels
For the purposes of clinical description, the larynx can be subdivided into three levels. The supraglottis includes the ventricles, the false cords, the laryngeal surface of the epiglottis and the aryepiglottic folds, back to and including the mucosa overlying the arytenoid cartilages. The glottis consists of the true vocal cords, the anterior commissure and the posterior commissure. Its anterior two-thirds is membranous, the posterior third being cartilaginous.

It is more difficult to be dogmatic about where the glottis ends and the subglottis begins. Variations in the site of the transition from squamous to respiratory epithelium make this an anatomically and clinically unreliable indicator of the boundary. Most laryngologists take the subglottis as commencing 5 mm below the free edge of the vocal fold, at the level of the conus elasticus. It extends to the lower border of the cricoid cartilage.

Physiology of the larynx

The human larynx has four major physiological functions and its structure has evolved to integrate these vital but largely incompatible roles: airway control (opening for respiration and closure for protection of the lower airway); swallowing; phonation; and effort closure during strenuous activity and coughing. The conflicting requirements of these diverse functions have demanded a three-tier valve structure consisting of the aryepiglottic folds and epiglottis, the false cords and the true vocal folds.

The position of the vocal folds is altered during each of these functional states: they may be tightly closed, as in effort fixation when both true and false cords are closely sealed, or they may be fully abducted during maximal inspiration. During phonation the true cords alone are delicately opposed, whereas in swallowing closure of the laryngeal inlet is accomplished by a combination of elevation of the larynx under the tongue base, sphincteric contraction of the aryepiglottic muscles and caudal rotation of the epiglottis.

Respiratory function

Although the larynx as a whole acts as a conduit for passage of air during respiration, it is the posterior glottis that is primarily concerned with the respiratory function of the larynx. This is evident from the presence of respiratory epithelial lining in the posterior glottis which is histologically continuous with that of the subglottis and trachea. The squamous epithelium found in most adult smokers is a result of metaplastic change, but this is reversible on cessation of smoking when the epithelium reverts back to the respiratory type.

Further evidence of the respiratory function of the posterior glottis can be seen from measurements of laryngeal dimensions. The posterior glottis increases dramatically in size during inspiration as compared with the anterior glottis: in the cadaveric position of the vocal cords the posterior glottis constitutes 40% of the total glottic area, but this increases to 60% of the total area during maximal inspiration (full vocal cord abduction). This is achieved by an enlargement of 400%, whereas the anterior glottis only increases in size by 160% (McIlwain, 1988).

During quiet respiration movement of the vocal cords is minimal, but in deep inspiration the larynx is pulled caudally by the sternohyoid and sternothyroid muscles, stabilized superiorly by fixation of the hyoid. Opening of the posterior glottis and lateralization of the true and false cords is brought about by abduction and outward rotation of the arytenoid cartilages from contraction of the posterior cricoarytenoid muscle. In maximal inspiration the lateral cricoarytenoid and cricothyroid muscles probably also assist in abduction of the arytenoids (Suzuki et al., 1970; Fink, 1975; Sellars and Sellars, 1983). On completion of inspiration the natural recoil of these tensed structures allows the vocal folds to return to their resting respiratory position (Graney, 1986).

Desiccation of the laryngeal mucosa, particularly the squamous epithelium of the true vocal cords, is a potential problem during respiratory effort. Mucous glands are freely distributed throughout the mucous membrane, especially on the posterior surface of the epiglottis and the lower borders of the false cords and ventricles. Lubrication of the true cords, which themselves do not possess any glands, is from secretions of the mucous glands in the ventricles.

Swallowing

Aspiration of food and liquid into the lower respiratory tract in swallowing is prevented by involuntary closure of the laryngeal inlet during the pharyngeal stage of deglutition. The swallowing reflex is mediated in the reticular formation of the brain stem adjacent to and coordinating closely with the respiratory centre, so that respiration ceases for a brief moment during this phase. Airway protection involves two components: closure of the laryngeal sphincters and elevation of the larynx.

Closure of the laryngeal inlet is thought to involve contraction of all three sphincters, although the relative importance of each is still a matter of debate (Ardran and Kemp, 1967; Fink and Demarest, 1978). This is brought about by anteromedial rotation of the arytenoids and contraction of the aryepiglottic muscles, causing narrowing of the glottis, inward bulging of the vestibular folds, forward movement of the cartilages of Wrisberg and obliteration of the interarytenoid space. Most authors agree that the glottic sphincter plays the major role in this protective function.

With passage of the food bolus from the oral cavity into the pharynx to the level of the tongue base, there is usually a brief moment when its descent is checked, the phase of vallecular arrest, during which the hyoid and larynx are elevated by contraction of the geniohyoid, mylohyoid and digastric muscles. Retroversion of the epiglottis is further assisted by downward rotation of the greater cornua of the hyoid bone. As the mass of the bolus increases, the epiglottis folds backwards over the laryngeal inlet, its midline arch accentuated by the hyoepiglottic ligament. This helps to direct the bolus into the piriform fossae and past the laryngeal entrance. Forward elevation of the laryngeal complex further assists deglutition by drawing the cricoid cartilage upwards and anteriorly so that opening of the cricopharyngeal sphincter is effectively increased.

Phonation

During phonation the true vocal cords are approximated so that the glottic airway is reduced to a thin, linear chink. Crude adduction of the vocal folds is brought about by contraction of the lateral cricoarytenoid and cricothyroid muscles, and fine adjustments of tension of the cords are controlled by the thyroarytenoid muscles. Closure of the posterior glottis is further assisted by the action of the interarytenoid muscle which pulls the arytenoid cartilages together. Table 1.1 shows the main functions of the five major intrinsic muscles of the larynx and their actions (Figure 1.1). The laryngeal muscles are also of great importance in regulating the mechanical properties of the vocal cords, controlling not only their position and shape, but also the elasticity and viscosity of each layer of the vocal fold.

Voice sound is produced by the passage of air under pressure through the adducted cords in their phonatory position, about 3 mm apart. The vocal folds are brought into contact with each other by a combination of forces: first, the Bernoulli effect which sucks the folds together as air escapes through the glottis; second, the tension of the cords; and third, the decreasing subglottic air pressure. As soon as the cords are in contact, the subglottic air pressure rises and forces them apart again and the cycle is repeated.

The characteristics of voice sound depend on variations in the vibratory cycle of the vocal cords. The basic pitch of the voice is determined by the frequency of vibration depending on changes in length and tension. The vocal intensity depends on the amplitude of vibration, and the timbre and other finer qualities which give the

Table 1.1 Characteristic functions of laryngeal muscles in vocal fold adjustments

	CT	VOC	LCA	IA	PCA
Position	Parallel	Adduct	Adduct	Adduct	Abduct
Level	Lower	Lower	Lower	0	Elevate
Length	Elongate	Shorten	Elongate	(Shorten)	Elongate
Thickness	Thin	Thicken	Thin	(Thicken)	Thin
Edge	Sharpen	Round	Sharpen	0	Round
Muscle (body)	Stiffen	Stiffen	Stiffen	(Slacken)	Stiffen
Mucosa (cover and transition)	Stiffen	Slacken	Stiffen	(Slacken)	Stiffen

CT, cricothyroid; VOC, vocalis; LCA, lateral cricoarytenoid; IA, interarytenoid; PCA, postcricoarytenoid.

voice its particular sound 'colour' are regulated by changes in the duration of the opening and closing phases of the vibration cycle. In males the basic pitch of the complex voice sound is in the region of 65 Hz to 500 Hz with a frequency of vibration of 100–260 cycles per second. A higher frequency in females gives a basic pitch of 130–1000 Hz.

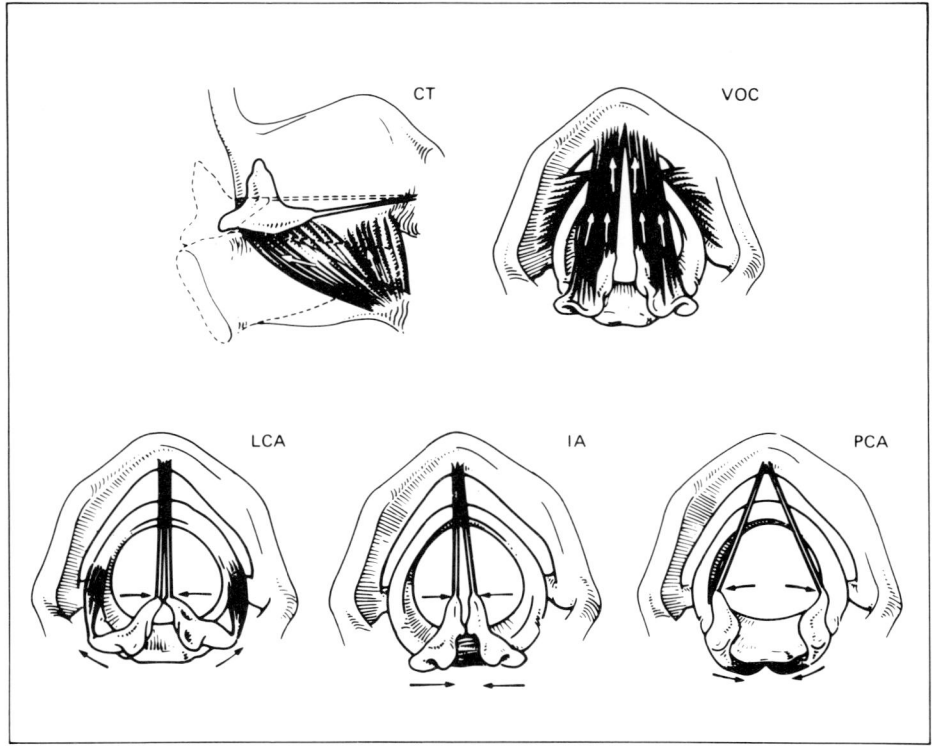

Figure 1.1 Action of intrinsic laryngeal muscles. CT, cricothyroid; VOC, vocalis; LCA, lateral cricoarytenoid; IA, interarytenoid; PCA, postcricoarytenoid

Effort closure

Forced closure of the larynx is an important function which is essential for protection of the lower airway and fixation of the trunk during strenuous effort. It enables the intrathoracic and intra-abdominal pressure to be raised significantly during coughing, weightlifting, defecation, micturition and parturition. Tomographic and myographic studies have shown that this closure is brought about by forced adduction of both the vocal and vestibular folds with collapse of the laryngeal ventricle. Closure of the supraglottis is also assisted by elevation of the thyroid cartilage towards the hyoid bone.

Surgical pathology of the larynx

Congenital and developmental abnormalities

Laryngeal webs and atresia
A series of developmental abnormalities may occur, ranging from a thin membranous web across the anterior glottis to complete atresia of the larynx. These conditions appear to represent failure of the larynx to recanalize during development. Severe defects may result in asphyxiation at birth; less severe abnormalities may require a tracheostomy and subsequent laryngeal surgery.

Laryngeal cysts
Cysts in the larynx may be congenital or developmental; they are most common in the supraglottis. Cystic lymphangiomas may occasionally present in the larynx. Most laryngeal cysts are, however, developmental in origin and are due to obstruction of the lumen of a mucous gland in the laryngeal mucosa. They may be lined with columnar or squamous epithelium.

Obstruction of the lumen of the saccule produces a saccular cyst. The cyst does not communicate with the laryngeal lumen. Saccular cysts may be congenital or acquired; in the latter case a carcinoma may be the cause of the obstruction.

Laryngoceles
A laryngocele is a dilatation of the saccule, which is filled with air and is in communication with the laryngeal lumen. It is more common in men. Laryngoceles may be *internal*, where the swelling is confined to the larynx; *external*, where the swelling protrudes through the thyrohyoid membrane into the neck at the point of entry of the superior laryngeal pedicle; or *mixed* — a combination of the two.

Laryngoceles may be congenital or acquired, although there is dispute as to whether wind-blowing activities contribute to their development.

Subglottic stenosis
Subglottic stenosis may be congenital or acquired (usually as a result of trauma due to prolonged intubation). The congenital stenoses can be of two types: cartilaginous stenosis, due to abnormal development of the cricoid cartilage; and soft tissue stenosis, due to overdevelopment of the glandular mucosa and connective tissue of the subglottis and upper trachea.

Acquired stenosis is caused by circumferential fibrosis following mechanical trauma to the subglottis. This is most frequently the result of prolonged intubation.

Conditions associated with abnormal laryngeal function

There are a series of conditions, distinguishable clinically, which present with hoarseness, and in which similar pathological changes are seen. They are frequently associated with vocal abuse, smoking and in some cases chronic nasal and sinus disease.

Vocal cord nodules (singer's or screamer's nodes) are small, bilateral swellings arising at the junction of the anterior one-third and posterior two-thirds of the vocal cords. They are usually associated with vocal abuse.

Reinke's oedema is bilateral oedema of Reinke's space affecting the anterior two-thirds of both vocal cords and is more common in women. A similar clinical appearance may be seen in hypothyroid patients; in these cases histological examination usually shows myxoid changes.

Vocal cord polyps are usually unilateral and are more common in men. They arise from the anterior two-thirds of the vocal cord.

Histological examination of these lesions shows a combination of the following features: deposition of fibrin and other blood products in Reinke's space; proliferation of fibroblasts and new blood vessels; and reactive changes in the overlying squamous epithelium.

Inflammatory conditions of the larynx

Sarcoidosis
Sarcoidosis is an inflammatory condition of uncertain aetiology, characterized histologically by non-caseating granulomas. It may affect any area of the respiratory tract. The larynx is involved in 3–5% of cases, the supraglottis being the most common site within the larynx. The symptoms are usually those of airway obstruction.

Wegener's granulomatosis
This systemic disorder may affect the subglottis and upper trachea, producing airway obstruction. The classic histological picture of a vasculitis is often not seen, the findings being those of acute and chronic inflammation. The diagnosis is usually made from the clinical picture of an inflammatory subglottic stenosis in a patient with known Wegener's disease.

Amyloidosis
Amyloid deposits may occur anywhere in the upper respiratory tract. The most common site in the larynx is the false cord. Macroscopically, submucosal swellings are visible and these may compromise the airway or affect the voice. Histological examination reveals infiltration of the lamina propria by an acellular material which stains positively with Congo red.

Specific infections of the larynx

Tuberculosis
Tuberculosis of the larynx is now rare in Europe and North America, and when seen it occurs in association with pulmonary tuberculosis. The most common macroscopic

appearance is of a localized lesion (or lesions), most commonly on the false or true vocal cords, which may be ulcerated, raised or nodular.

Scleroma
Scleroma is due to infection by *Klebsiella rhinoscleromatis*. Its manifestations are most common in the nose, but are seen in the larynx in a minority of cases. Macroscopically, submucosal deposits are seen which may result in significant reduction of the airway. The histological picture is that of infiltration of chronic inflammatory cells including Mikulicz cells which contain bacillus.

Benign tumours

Squamous cell papilloma
Squamous cell papilloma is seen in adults and children. The lesions appear as exophytic, fronded structures which may be up to 2 cm in diameter. They may be single or multiple, and in extensive cases may arise from large areas of the laryngeal epithelium. The most common sites of origin are the true and false vocal cords and the ventricle. The colour of the lesions varies from white to red. Recurrence after surgical removal is common and appears to be more frequent in those cases with more florid disease at presentation (Capper et al., 1983).

Histological examination reveals projecting fronds of squamous epithelium, usually non-keratinizing, arising from the epithelium. There may be several orders of branching of these fronds.

It is thought that these lesions are caused by human papilloma virus, although it is difficult to detect virus particles in many biopsy specimens.

Haemangioma
True haemangiomas are rare in the adult larynx, although vascular vocal cord polyps and granulomas of the vocal cord may have a similar histological appearance.

Haemangiomas are more common in infants, where they occur in the subglottis. They may be associated with cutaneous haemangiomata. They usually present with stridor and voice change, and may require a tracheostomy. Macroscopically they appear as a blue or purple swelling, usually unilateral, in the subglottis. They tend to regress as the child ages.

Chondroma
Chondroma of the larynx is a rare tumour; the majority arise from the lamina of the cricoid cartilage. It appears as a smooth submucosal swelling which presents with airway obstruction and voice change.

Premalignant conditions

A spectrum of changes occur in the laryngeal mucosa which are known to be associated with subsequent development of squamous cell carcinoma. These changes are similar to those seen at other sites, such as the cervix and oral cavity. The term *leukoplakia*, which is sometimes used to describe these lesions, is a clinical description of a white patch on the mucosa and has no greater pathological significance. The most common site within the larynx for the development of these changes is the mucosa of the true cords; however, other areas, particularly the false cords, may be involved.

Dysplasia is a premalignant condition of the epithelium. It is characterized by the presence of individual cells with malignant features in the epithelium. The basement membrane is intact, and the malignant cells are seen in the basal layers in the early stages of the condition. The severity of the dysplasia may be graded by the pathologist. Hellquist et al. (1982) showed subsequent development of squamous carcinoma in 2% of cases of mild dysplasia, 12% of moderate dysplasia and 25% of severe dysplasia.

Carcinoma in situ is the term used to describe cellular dysplasia involving the entire thickness of the mucosa, without invasion through the basement membrane. The macroscopic appearance of these changes is not a reliable guide to the microscopic findings; the lesion may be localized or widespread, the colour may vary from white to red, and the texture may be smooth or granular. It is therefore vital that representative areas are taken for histological examination in these cases.

Malignant tumours

Squamous cell carcinoma
The vast majority of malignant tumours of the larynx are squamous cell carcinomas. They account for approximately 1% of malignancies in men in the UK, where carcinoma of the larynx is between six and eight times more common in men than in women. The mean age at presentation is in the fifth decade. The aetiological factors of importance appear to be smoking, alcohol consumption, local irradiation and urban living. The glottis is the most common site of origin within the larynx, followed by the supraglottis; the subglottis is the site of origin in approximately 5% of cases.

The macroscopic appearance can vary from a raised plaque to an exophytic or ulcerated lesion, or may be a combination of these. Destruction of the cartilaginous framework of the larynx and extralaryngeal spread is not uncommon. A feature of tumours that destroy cartilage is the presence of osteoclasts at the edge of the tumour (Carter and Tanner, 1979).

Spread of tumour supraglottic lesions may spread across the midline or downwards to involve the vocal cords. Direct upward spread may involve the valleculae or tongue base. Epiglottic tumours, particularly those arising from the laryngeal surface of the epiglottis, may invade through the cartilage of the epiglottis into the pre-epiglottic space, thus escaping from the larynx (Olofsson and van Nostrand, 1973).

Tumours arising from the aryepiglottic fold may invade the arytenoid, or the cricoarytenoid joint, and may involve the medial wall of the adjacent piriform fossa.

Glottic tumours arise most commonly from the anterior part of the vocal cords, and may spread into the supraglottis or subglottis, or across the midline. The anterior commissure is only a few millimetres from the thyroid cartilage, and the most common route for extralaryngeal spread with these tumours is by cartilage destruction at this point. Limitation of vocal cord movement may be produced by a spread of vocal cord tumour into the underlying thyroarytenoid muscle, which does not preclude partial laryngeal surgery. Fixation of the vocal cord, however, is frequently associated with invasion of the cartilaginous framework of the larynx or with extralaryngeal spread of the tumour, and may contraindicate partial surgery.

Subglottic tumours often spread circumferentially, and may extend to involve the vocal cord. Anterior lesions may penetrate the cricothyroid membrane; other routes of extralaryngeal spread are via the cricothyroid joint and the cricotracheal membrane.

Metastases to cervical lymph nodes are most common with supraglottic tumours, and are rare with tumours that are confined to the glottis. The nodes most commonly involved are those of the jugular chain. Posterior triangle nodes are much less frequently involved. Distant metastases are most common in the lung and are seen in a significant proportion of patients at postmortem (O'Brien et al., 1971). However, they are uncommon in patients who do not have cervical nodal metastases.

Verrucous carcinoma

Verrucous carcinoma is a variant of squamous carcinoma. It is highly differentiated, and rarely invades the cartilaginous framework or metastasizes. It most commonly arises from the glottis and has a pale colour and papilliferous appearance. On histological appearance it may be difficult to distinguish from laryngeal papillomatosis (Michaels, 1987).

Spindle cell carcinoma

Spindle cell carcinoma (carcinosarcoma) is a rare tumour containing both squamous and spindle cell elements. The majority arise from the vocal cord and are polypoid. The spindle cell component is usually predominant and the squamous component may be difficult to find. Metastases to cervical lymph nodes may occur, and may consist of either the squamous or spindle cell components, or both. There is some evidence of improved survival in cases treated with primary surgery (Tucker, 1987).

Other malignant tumours

Adenocarcinoma represents less than 1% of laryngeal malignancies. It is more common in men and arises most frequently from the subglottis. Metastases are common and the treatment of choice is primary surgery.

Adenoid cystic carcinomas also arise most commonly in the subglottis, but are more common in women (Fechner, 1975). These tumours frequently show evidence of perineural invasion and have a tendency to recur locally after a long time interval, despite apparently adequate local excision.

Chondrosarcomas usually arise from the posterior lamina of the cricoid cartilage and impinge on the subglottic airway, presenting with hoarseness and respiratory obstruction. Most of them are low grade and can be difficult to differentiate from a benign chondroma. Treatment is most commonly by surgical excision. Local recurrence and even distant metastases are reported with the high-grade tumours.

A number of other tumours are rarely encountered arising in the larynx, such as malignant melanoma, synovial sarcoma and rhabdomyosarcoma.

References

Ardran J., Kemp F. (1967). The mechanism of the larynx. II. The epiglottis and closure of the larynx. *Br. J. Radiol.*, **40**, 372.

Capper J.W.R., Bailey C.M., Michaels L. (1983). Squamous papillomas of the larynx in adults. A review of 63 cases. *Clin. Otolaryngol.*, **8**, 109–19.

Carter R.L., Tanner N.S.B., Clifford P., Shaw N.S. (1979). Perineural spread in squamous carcinomas of the head and neck; A clinicopathological study. *Clin. Otolaryngol.* **4**, 271–81.

Fechner R.E. (1975). Adenocarcinoma of the larynx. *Can. J. Otolaryngol.*, **4**, 284–9.

Fink B.R. (1975). The human larynx: a functional study. New York: Raven Press.
Fink R., Demarest R. (1978). Laryngeal biomechanics. Cambridge, Mass: Howard University Press.
Graney D.O. (1986). Anatomy of the larynx. *J. Otolaryngol*. Head and Neck Surgery, **94**, 1737.
Hellquist H., Lundren J., Olgasson V. (1982). Hyperplasia, keratosis, dysplasia and carcinoma in situ of the vocal cords. A follow-up study. *Clin. Otolaryngol*., **7**, 11–27.
Heymann R. (1889). Beitrag zur Kenntnis des Epithels und der Drüsen des menschliches Kehlkopfes im gesunden und kranken Zusande. *Virchows Arch.*, **118**, 320–48.
Langman J. (1969). In *Medical Embryology*, 2nd edn. Baltimore: Williams & Wilkins, pp. 247–50.
McIlwain J.C. (1988). The posterior glottis. Thesis, University of Belfast.
Michaels L. (1987). *Ear, Nose and Throat Histopathology*. Berlin: Springer, pp. 409–12.
O'Brien P.H., Carlson R., Stubner E.A. et al. (1971). Distant metastases in epidermoid cell carcinoma of the head and neck. *Cancer*, **27**, 304–7.
Olofsson J., van Nostrand A.W.P. (1973). Growth and spread of laryngeal and hypopharyngeal carcinoma with reflections on the effect of preoperative irradiation. 139 cases studied by whole organ sectioning. *Acta Otolaryngol.*, (suppl.) **308**, 1–84.
Sellars I., Sellars S. (1983). Cricoarytenoid joint structure and function. *J. Laryngol. Otol.*, **97**, 1027.
Stafford N., Davies S., (1988). Epithelial distribution in the human fetal larynx. *Ann. Otol. Rhinol. Laryngol*. **97**, 302–7.
Stell P.M., Watt J. (1984). Squamous metaplasia of the subglottic space and its relation to smoking. *Ann. Otol. Rhinol. Laryngol.*, **93**, 124–6.
Stell P.M., Gregory I., Watt J. (1978). Morphometry of the epithelial lining of the human larynx. I. The glottis. *Clin. Otolaryngol.*, **3**, 13–20.
Stell P.M., Gregory I., Watt J. (1980). Morphology of the human larynx. II. The subglottis. *Clin. Otolaryngol.*, **5**, 389–95.
Stell P.M., Gudrun R., Watt J. (1981). Morphology of the human larynx. III. The supraglottis. *Clin. Otolaryngol.*, **6**, 389–93.
Suzuki M., Kirchner J.A., Murakami Y. (1970). The cricothyroid as a respiratory muscle; its characteristics in bilateral recurrent laryngeal nerve paralysis. *Ann. Otol. Rhinol. Laryngol.*, **79**, 976.
Tucker H.M. (1987). *The Larynx*. New York: Thieme, pp. 65–6.

Chapter 2

Aerodynamics of voice production

H. K. Schutte

Voice production is a process of making air particles vibrate. The sound source itself is located in the larynx, the voice organ. In this organ vibrating air at audible frequencies is generated by the opening and closing action of the vocal folds. This action is based on an ingenious counterplay of aerodynamic and myoelastic forces, working together under the government of aerodynamic, biomechanic and acoustic laws (van den Berg, 1958; Miller and Schutte, 1984).

The actuator system: lung and breathing mechanism

The aerodynamic driving system for sound production is also used for breathing. Inspired air is used for gas exchange within the lungs; on expiration, in a coordinated action it is used to make the vocal folds vibrate. For voicing, the vocal folds become adducted under the control of the intrinsic laryngeal muscles, creating resistance to the outgoing air. This airway resistance is not constant but changes repeatedly over time, with a repeating frequency which correlates with the frequency of the produced sound.

The breath stream is controlled by a subtle balance between the inspiratory and expiratory muscles of respiration. In this process the diaphragm muscle plays an important role, known to singers as 'breath support'.

Pulmonologists and lung physiologists divide the lung into a number of functional compartments: residual volume, tidal volume, vital capacity, total lung capacity and so on. For clinical studies on voice these subdivisions are less important. It is true that a certain amount of air is necessary to drive the larynx, but if the breathing mechanism is so weak that it cannot bring up enough air for voicing, the patient must be in a physically bad condition. The fact that the patient cannot speak loudly is ignored and the physical condition takes all the attention.

The generator: the larynx

The sound is generated at the vocal folds and the tone is modified by the configuration of the vocal tract. In voicing, the outgoing air column from the lungs is counteracted by the vocal folds, building up a subglottal pressure under the vocal folds which causes them to separate. The open glottis slightly reduces the differential pressure and, helped by elastic tissue forces and the Bernoulli effect, the vocal folds close again and the vibratory cycle repeats. In this way a vibratory source is set up which sends a harmonically rich signal into the supraglottal tract. In the supraglottal vocal tract this basic sound is modified. The dimensions of the supraglottal tract are manipulated to attenuate or amplify parts of the harmonic structure. In speech and singing this action is used to define vowel tone. In singing the resonant resources are used to create tonal quality which makes the voice heard over the classical sound environment of an orchestra.

The vocal folds consists of a muscular body covered by epithelium. Between the epithelium and body is a transitional layer of loose connective tissue which permits the epithelium to slide freely over the body. This freedom of movement enables the epithelium to act as a separate centre of mass during fold vibration which is fundamental to the quality of the voice.

In one vibratory cycle the glottis opens and closes. In modal register, also called 'chest voice', the glottis remains closed for about 50–55% of the total cycle duration. This closed phase is reduced to about 30% in another mode of vibration called 'falsetto voice'. Air escapes during the open phase of the total cycle duration, and consequently the amount of escaping air depends, among other factors, on the vibrational mode used.

The momentum for the acoustic longitudinal wave propagation stems from the abrupt closing action of the glottis. There is a relationship between the abruptness of the glottis closure and the richness of harmonic overtones in the voice produced: the more abrupt the stop of the respiratory air column, the better the voice quality. This makes it understandable why complete glottis closure is an important factor for a good voice. Organic changes of the vocal folds, e.g. a polyp, influence glottis closure considerably.

It should be mentioned that apart from organic abnormalities (polyp, cyst, etc.), glottis closure is also a matter of geometry. There is a great variability in the geometry of the larynx which implies that there is also a great variability in completeness of glottis closure during phonation. Some people show complete glottis closure during phonation, while others with a differently shaped larynx show incomplete glottis closure. It is a matter of 'nature', like length of legs, hair colour and so on. This means that a good voice is partly a matter of nature: some people can become singers, others cannot.

Aerodynamic interactions: subglottal pressure and air flow

The adducted vocal folds constitute an airway resistance to the outgoing air. The height of resistance depends on the muscular tension in the adducting muscles. The muscular tension counterbalances the aerodynamic forces in such a way that a certain mean subglottal pressure is maintained. Around this mean subglottal pressure the momentary pressure changes in accordance with the acoustic laws that govern the subglottal tract (i.e. the pulmonary airway system). These fast pressure changes, superimposed on the mean subglottal pressure, may vary greatly in amplitude. Under specific circumstances the subglottal pressure may show momentary amplitude changes of 100% (Schutte and Miller, 1986). This fact has consequences for the definition of the efficiency of the voice organ.

The air flow rate or air usage during phonation depends on the duration of the open phase of the glottal cycle as well as on the height of the subglottal pressure. The mean air flow rate depends on other factors, such as effective closure time during a glottis cycle, subglottal air pressure, timbre related to registers and vibrational modes of the vocal folds, pitch and loudness. Because of all these factors the mean air flow rate is not useful as a measure of 'good' or 'bad' voice.

The concept of the efficiency of voice production can be used to study the energy conversion process of aerodynamic power into sound power. The aerodynamic power is determined by the product of the lung pressure or subglottal pressure and the mean air flow rate. The sound power can be derived from intensity measurements of the radiated acoustic power from the mouth (Bouhuys et al., 1968; Schutte, 1980). Glottal efficiency is then defined as the ratio of radiated output power to aerodynamic power; the efficiency ranges from 0.01% to 1% (Schutte, 1980). In this traditional definition of glottal efficiency as proposed by van den Berg (1956), one major problem is its strong dependence on fundamental frequency. High frequencies are radiated much more effectively than low frequencies, so efficiency calculations will generally favour high-pitched vocal productions. Likewise, loud productions will be favoured more than soft productions because glottal efficiency increases at a rate of about 3 decibels per doubling of subglottal pressure, regardless of the quality of the sound. Thus, if measurements before and after intervention include vocal efficiency, the pitch and loudness levels should be the same, otherwise an improvement in vocal efficiency may simply reflect a different choice of pitch and loudness by the subject (Titze, 1989). The first steps towards calculating the vocal efficiency of voice production are measurements of the aerodynamic power and radiated sound power. These can be assessed by (a) measurement of the mean air flow rate, (b) measurement of the mean subglottal pressure and (c) measurement of the sound power, which can be derived from sound intensity level measurements (Figure 2.1). These different methods are discussed in the following sections.

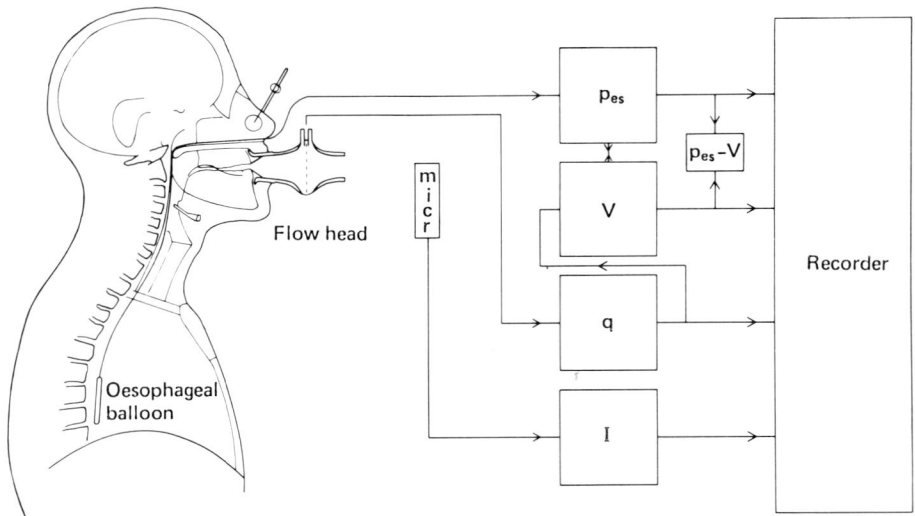

Figure 2.1 Schematic depiction of the experimental set-up for the simultaneous measurement of sound intensity I, air flow rate q, variation of lung volume V, and oesophageal pressure P_{es}, together with apparatus for registering $P_{es}-V$ diagrams

Measurement of mean air flow rate

The mean air flow rate can be derived or estimated from (a) measuring the maximal phonation time, (b) measuring the phonation volume divided by the phonation time, or (c) measurement using a pneumotachograph or hot-wire anemometer.

Maximal phonation time
Air flow rate is expressed as the volume of displaced air per unit of time. The total amount of available air for phonation equals the vital capacity, which ranges between about 3.5 litres and 5 litres. A simple method to measure the mean air usage during phonation is to measure the maximal phonation time of a sustained vowel. Waste of air is easily recognized if the maximum phonation time is reduced to about 10–12 seconds. This test is unreliable if patients do not have sufficient control over their breathing mechanism, for example if they do not inspire sufficiently or waste air just before the phonation starts. Many other factors may influence the maximal phonation time, as pointed out by Ptacek and Sander (1963a, b) and Hirano et al. (1968).

Phonation volume
The total amount of expired air during maximally sustained phonation can be measured with a spirometer or with a body plethysmograph. If the duration of the phonation is measured simultaneously the air usage can be expressed in volume per unit time. The test should be done after a maximum inspiration (Bouhuys et al., 1966; Isshiki et al., 1967; Sawashima et al., 1978; Moser and Kittel, 1979).

Pneumotachograph
A pneumotachograph based on the principles of Fleisch (1925) or Lilly (1950) gives a small pressure difference across an airway resistance. The pneumotachograph is connected to a mask or to a mouthpiece which is held between the teeth. The pressure difference is sensed by means of a differential pressure transducer which gives a signal related to the amount of air expired during phonation. This method has been used in many clinical studies as well as in research (Luchsinger, 1951; Vogelsanger, 1954; Isshiki, 1964; Yanagihara and Koike, 1966; Rubin et al., 1967; Yanagihara and von Leden, 1967; Hirano et al., 1968; Iwata et al., 1972; Stürzebecher et al., 1973; Seidner et al., 1976, 1978; Schutte and van den Berg, 1976; Bastian et al., 1978; Schutte, 1980; Dejonckere et al., 1985).

A pneumotachograph suitable for the range of the air flow rate during phonation (100–500 ml/s) is useful to measure the mean air flow rate. A disadvantage is the fact that an airtight connection with the vocal tract is necessary. The tubing to the spirometer, to the mouthpiece or to the mask connected to the pneumotachograph hinders the radiation of sound at the lips to the outer air (Figure 2.2). This influences the resonance characteristics of the vocal tract and alters the normal interaction between vocal tract and larynx. This is particularly a problem in voice research in professional singing; in research on speaking voice in patients this aspect becomes less important.

Hot-wire anemometers also have been used for registration of the mean air flow rate. The general interest in measuring mean air flow rate in phonation has diminished after the many studies on this topic in the 1960s and 1970s. Interest on air flow during phonation nowadays is more directed to the rapid changes of the flow patterns, e.g. glottal volume velocity waveforms; these can be measured by means of

22 Functional Surgery of the Larynx and Pharynx

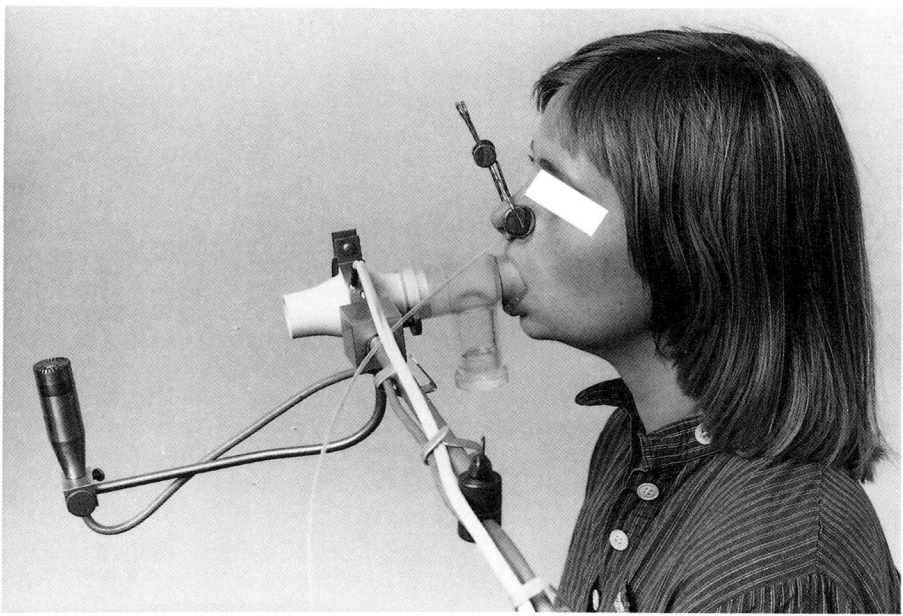

Figure 2.2 Detail of the measuring set: microphone, flow head (Lilly), connecting piece with fluid receptacle. A mouthpiece is kept between the teeth to maintain the same degree of mouth opening. The catheter of the oesophageal balloon is led through the nose. A nose clamp prevents air leakage through the nose, which would otherwise disturb the registration of the constantly changing lung volume

inverse filtering of the acoustic signal, with the help of the circumferential vented mask designed by Rothenberg (1973). Research on the usefulness for clinical evaluation is yet to come.

Measurement of mean subglottal pressure

The most reliable way to measure the mean subglottal pressure is by puncturing the subglottal space, but ethical and logical reasons restrict the application of this method. Moreover, the real value of measuring the subglottal pressure is not known, although the first measurements were made as early as 1900 by Roudet. Van den Berg (1956) developed and verified an indirect method to determine the subglottal pressure during phonation; this method is based on a proper use of lung mechanics and can be used routinely in patients as well as in professional voice users without any risk.

Direct measurement of the subglottal pressure can be done using a transcutaneous needle (Loebell, 1969; Schutte, 1980), or using a transglottally placed catheter (van den Berg, 1956) or miniature pressure transducer (Kitzing and Löfqvist, 1975; Schutte and Miller, 1986). With a transcutaneous needle, owing to the necessary tubing, only the mean subglottal pressure can be measured, whereas with miniature pressure transducers high-frequency resolution measurements may be carried out: this allows momentary pressure changes within one glottal cycle to be registered. Especially in singing voice research, these measurements help to elucidate phenomena well known in singing voice pedagogy, but still unexplained by research. Direct measurements with a needle have been recorded in a few studies (van den Berg, 1956; Isshiki, 1959; Kunze, 1962, 1964; Ladefoged, 1962; Lieberman, 1968; Loebell, 1969). The total number of subjects in all these studies is about 100, only a few of whom were patients.

Indirect measurement of the subglottal pressure using an oesophageal balloon was introduced by van den Berg (1956) (Figures 2.3, 2.4). Pressure changes in the oesophagus sensed with a pressure transducer coupled to the oesophageal balloon reflect the pressure changes in the intrapleural space, which in turn are closely related to elastic forces built up in lung tissue and the thoracic cage.

Owing to the positive subglottal pressure under the adducted vocal folds the intrathoracic pressure increases to the same value. At the end of the phonation the oesophageal pressure drops to an absolute value which, however, is not the same as before the phonation. During the phonation air escapes from the lungs and as a result the absolute value of the oesophageal pressure increases. The pressure drop itself can be used to determine the subglottal pressure, if some conditions have been fulfilled. These conditions are: abrupt stop of phonation, the glottis must be kept open and there should be no change in lung volume for about 0.5 sec. This so-called van den Berg manoeuvre requires some skill and training in breath management, as is found in singers. In voice patients, who mostly lack such skills, this method is not easy to use. In these cases the following indirect measuring method may be used to determine the mean subglottal pressure.

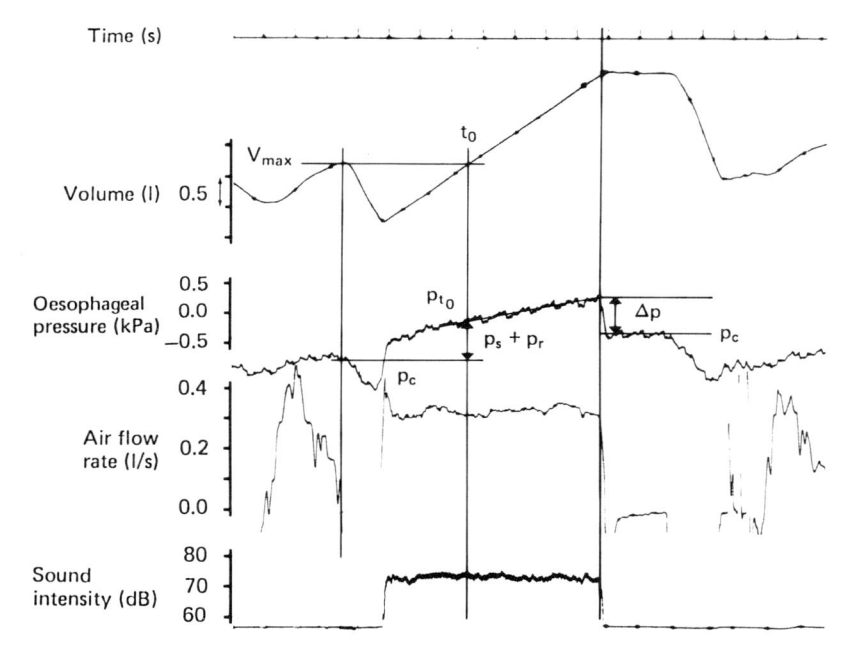

Figure 2.3 Two ways of deriving subglottal pressure using an oesophageal balloon; on the right-hand side, by abruptly stopping phonation (the van den Berg manoeuvre). For a short moment after phonation the lung volume is kept constant with an open glottis. The pressure in the oesophagus drops to a value P_c corresponding with that lung volume. The pressure drop $\triangle P$ equals the difference between the actual pressure at moment t_o and the reference oesophageal pressure, derived from the relation between lung volume and oesophageal pressure just before phonation (P_s is the subglottal pressure, P_r is the product of the viscous resistance and air flow rate during phonation; P_r is negligible in normal lungs)

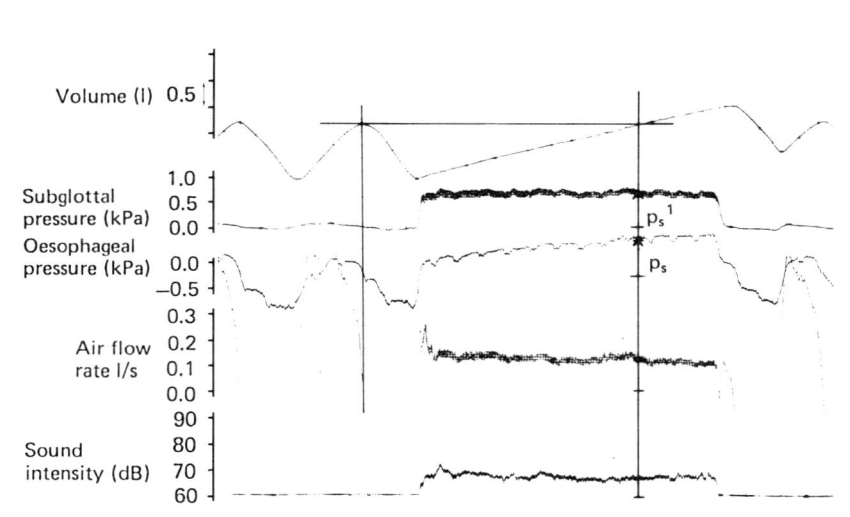

Figure 2.4 The indirect measuring method using an oesophageal balloon compared with simultaneous measurement of the subglottal pressure by a direct method. To measure the subglottal pressure directly, a hollow needle connected to a pressure transducer is inserted into the subglottal space. P_s^1 = oesophageal; P_s = direct

During quiet breathing the oesophageal pressure varies from about -4 cmH$_2$O (-400 Pa) at the end of the inspiration to -2 cmH$_2$O at the moment of change from expiration to inspiration. The absolute value of the oesophageal pressure is, within a great part of the vital capacity, linearly related to the lung volume. Keeping track of the lung volume makes it possible to determine a reference pressure value of what the oesophageal pressure would have been if no phonation occurred. The difference between the actual pressure and the reference pressure reflects the value of the subglottal pressure.

The inspired and expired air of the lungs can be measured by a pneumotachograph held between teeth and lips. The measured flow signal is integrated to a volume signal. In this procedure the physical differences between inspired and expired air should be considered (Schutte, 1980). This indirect measurement with an oesophageal balloon permits routine measurement of the subglottal pressure in a large number of research subjects and patients.

Normative values

Normative values are needed to evaluate pathologic processes during phonation. Measuring physiologic variables in voice patients will be helpful in diagnosis and therapy.

In physiologic research the measured variables are not subjected to special criteria for what constitutes useful data. The measurements, provided they are correct, may contribute to our knowledge of voice physiology. In clinical practice normative data are useful if they are specific for a typical disorder. In statistical terms this means an established mean value with a small standard deviation for each type of disorder. The

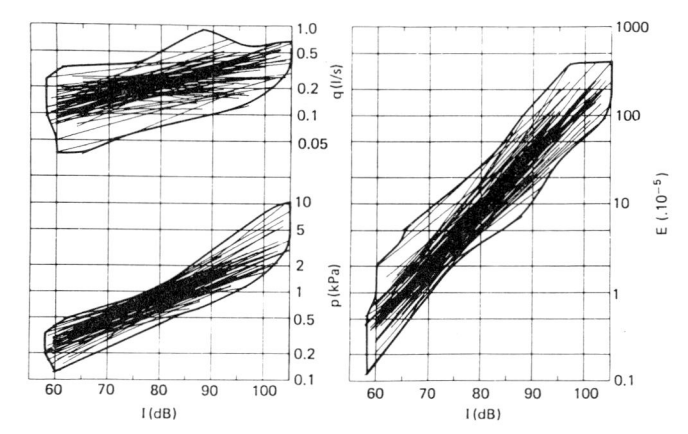

Figure 2.5 The set of all regression lines through the measuring values of the phonations of the test subjects. The regression lines from 72 measuring series in 45 subjects have been represented. Contour lines around the regression lines indicate the limits of the reference areas. E, efficiency; I, sound intensity, p, pressure; q, air flow rate

more specific the normative value, the more useful it is for diagnostic purposes. However, the physiologic variables of voice production that are usually measured show a considerable spread. This unfortunately reduces the usefulness of normative aerodynamic values for diagnostic purposes. Sometimes the limited usefulness of a single value can be improved by measuring simultaneously different physiologic variables, e.g. air flow rate, subglottal pressure, sound pressure level and pitch, at the same instance of phonation and thereafter trying to establish correlations between these variables.

In a study carried out in the Voice Research Laboratory at Groningen State University (Schutte, 1980), the efficiency was calculated from measurements of mean air flow rate, mean subglottal pressure and the resultant sound power. The latter was calculated from the measured sound pressure level 30 cm in front of the mouth. Data were taken from 72 measuring series, each consisting of at least 15 evaluated instances of phonation from 45 test subjects with no voice problems. There was no statistically significant difference between male and female subjects, except for the pitch range. The data were therefore lumped together. The aerodynamic variables and sound pressure levels were measured for different sound pressure levels. For each measuring series, after proper statistical data reduction, a regression line was obtained for flow and pressure as well as for efficiency (Figure 2.5). All regression lines of the normal subjects constitute a reference area. The normative data of flow and pressure appear to follow a statistically normal distribution pattern, but unfortunately show a wide spread. Table 2.1 summarizes the mean values and for each of the variables the established range, based on a 90% probability level.

Table 2.1 Normative aerodynamic values at a sound pressure level of 70 dB measured 30 cm in front of the mouth, modal voice

	Mean	Range
Subglottal pressure (cmH$_2$O)	4.4	2–7.5
Air flow rate (ml/s)	160	45–350
Efficiency (10^{-5})	2.1	1–10

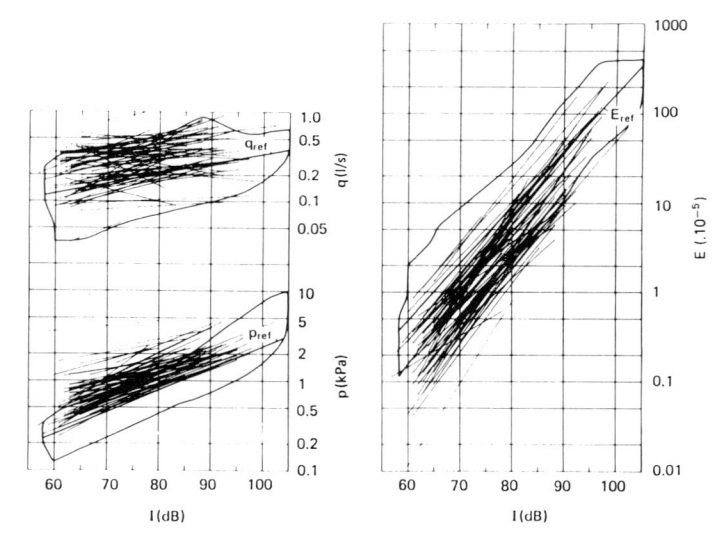

Figure 2.6 Set of regression lines for flow (q), subglottal pressure (p) and efficiency (E) from the first measuring series with 64 patients, together with the corresponding reference areas

Figure 2.6 shows the results which should be compared with the reference areas. It became clear that the efficiency did not enhance the diagnostic power of aerodynamic measurements. In other words, calculating efficiency does not help to distinguish normal subjects from patients. Patients generally use more air during phonation than normal subjects, and all patients showed subglottal pressures that were higher than the mean subglottal pressure of the normals, but most of the patients showed data that fell within the reference area; statistically, they cannot be considered to be aerodynamically pathological. The subglottal pressure appeared to have the greatest diagnostic value, but this measure is the most difficult value to obtain.

Normative aerodynamic data for 'normal' voices to compare with aerodynamic values of pathological voices did not lead to improvement of our diagnostic tools. The ranges of the data of healthy and pathological voices show too much overlap. There is, however, another approach in using the data, and this is to use them for intraindividual comparison, e.g. before and after treatment.

In 47 of the 64 patients investigated in the above-mentioned study, the efficacy of therapeutic measures, derived from the change in efficiency values before and after surgical therapy and/or voice training, was noticeable. However, the relative efficiency compared with the reference value nearly always remained negative. We discovered that in aerodynamic terms there is no difference between patients with or without bilateral vocal fold nodules. Both groups, generally speaking, have in common that the dorsal part of the glottis does not close completely (Morrison et al., 1983; Schutte, 1980, 1984). This incomplete glottis closure does not improve after surgical removal of the nodules, nor does it disappear after voice therapy. Based on intraindividual comparison of aerodynamic data from measurements before and after surgical therapy and/or training, it could be explained that the main improvement can be found in the use of muscular tension in the glottis region. The leakage of air through the glottal chink of the incompletely closed glottis remains the same or decreases only very little. A clear reduction of the subglottal pressure, however, can be measured and this is correlated with the muscular adduction forces of the muscles at glottis level.

Improvement in aerodynamic pattern of the flow can easily be established in patients with laryngeal paralysis after surgical treatment. After glottis closure using Teflon, collagen or thyroplastic techniques, the loss of air usually decreases. It was also found that the value of the subglottal pressure in patients with a unilateral or bilateral paralysis almost always lay outside the reference area. This is remarkable because the clearly incomplete closure of the glottis intuitively leads to the expectation of a low subglottal pressure. In these cases a high subglottal pressure can be explained by the fact that patients need to expire forcefully to create an audible basic sound, and that compensatory muscular actions are used synergistically in an attempt to obtain a better glottis closure.

Aerodynamics in patients after laryngectomy

Aerodynamic values can be used to evaluate alaryngeal voice in patients after laryngectomy: i.e. oesophageal voice, fistula (shunt) voice after tracheo-oesophageal fistula operation (Singh, 1988) or neoglottal voice in near-total laryngectomy with myomucosal valved neoglottis (Singh, 1989b). The voice source in oesophageal and fistula voice is the pharyngo-oesophageal segment, whereas in near-total laryngectomy it is the neoglottis. In oesophageal voice air needs to be injected into the oesophagus before sound can be produced. By proper use of certain consonants in speech the intake of air could be facilitated (Moolenaar-Bijl, 1953). The air supply for the vibratory action of the pharyngo-oesophageal segment can be improved by creating a fistula between the trachea and oesophagus. A silicone valve prosthesis is inserted in the fistula to prevent aspiration of liquid and saliva (Mahieu, 1988; Singh, 1988). The aerodynamics of oesophageal speech and shunt speech differ (Nieboer et al., 1989). Patients with oesophageal voice can only produce short sentences as they need to inject air into the oseophagus more often.

Laryngectomy patients with tracheo-oesophageal fistula (Singh, 1988) or tracheo-pharyngeal shunt (Singh, 1989b) are able to use most of the available pulmonary air for phonation by closing the tracheostoma with a finger or by a tracheostoma valve (Singh, 1985, 1987, 1989, 1990).

Nieboer et al. (1989) compared the acoustic, perceptual and aerodynamic variables observed in laryngectomy patients using the injection method with those in patients using the Groningen prosthesis. The values of subpseudoglottal pressure, intratracheal pressure, transpseudoglottal flow and efficiency for these patients are given in Table 2.2. The values of the intratracheal pressure appear to be high; this is partly caused by the pressure loss across the valve, which is the pressure needed to pass the air through the Groningen button. In the above study the Groningen prosthesis is responsible for about half of the total intratracheal pressure. This is partly due to the growth of *Candida* species in the silicone material. New valve prostheses usually need less air pressure.

Conclusion

The study of the aerodynamics of voice generation has given a useful insight into the working of the larynx. The diagnostic value of measuring the air flow rate, the subglottic pressure and the efficiency in relation to the produced sound, appears to

Table 2.2 Typical aerodynamic values in laryngectomy patients

	Injection	Valve prosthesis (Groningen button)
Subpseudoglottal pressure (cmH$_2$O)		
mean	26	41
range	5–125	10–108
Intratracheal pressure (cmH$_2$O)		
mean	–	93
range	–	30–175
Transpseudoglottal flow (ml/s)		
mean	82	131
range	10–360	20–800
Efficiency, based on subpseudoglottal pressure ($\times 10^{-5}$)		
mean	0.56	0.19
range	0.009–47.0	0.004–32.0

be low and is overestimated in the literature. However, in the individual patient, changes due to treatment can be easily followed by measuring air usage during phonation. For comparison, care should be taken to measure at comparable pitches, loudness and vibration mode or registers.

References

Bastian H.J., Sasama R., Unger E. (1978). Aerodynamische Leistungsprüfung und Funktionsdiagnostik der normalen Frauenstimme. *Folia Phoniatr.*, **30**, 85–93.
Bouhuys A., Proctor D.F., Mead J. (1966). Kinetic aspects of singing. *J. Appl. Physiol.* **21**, 483–95.
Bouhuys A., Mead J., Proctor D.F., Stevens K.N. (1968). Pressure-flow events during singing. *Ann. NY Acad. Sci.*, **155**, 165–76.
Dejonckere P.H., Greindl M., Sneppe R. (1985). Débitmétrie aérienne à paramètres phonatoires standardisés F. *Folia Phoniatr.*, **37**, 58–65.
Fleisch A. (1925). Der Pneumotachograph: Ein Apparat zur Geschwindigkeitsregistrierung der Atemluft. *Pflügers Arch. Gesamt. Physiol.*, **209**, 713–28.
Hirano M., Koike Y., Von Leden H. (1968). Maximum phonation time and air usage during phonation. *Folia Phoniatr.*, **20**, 185–201.
Isshiki N. (1959). Regulatory mechanism of the pitch and volume of voice. *Otorhinolaryngol. Clin. Kyoto*, **52**, 1065–94.
Isshiki N. (1964). Regulatory mechanism of voice intensity variation. *J. Speech Hear. Res.*, **7**, 17–29.
Isshiki N., Okamura H., Morimoto M. (1967). Maximum phonation time and air flow rate during phonation: simple clinical tests for vocal function. *Ann. Otol. Rhinol. Laryngol.*, **76**, 998–1007.
Iwata S., Von Leden H., Williams D. (1972). Air flow measurement during phonation. *J. Commun. Disord.*, **5**, 67–79.
Kitzing P., Löfqvist A. (1975). Subglottal and oral air pressure during phonation — preliminary investigation using a miniature transducer system. *Med. Biol. Eng.*, **13**, 644–8.

Kunze L.H. (1962). An investigation of the changes in subglottal air pressure and rate of air flow accompanying changes in fundamental frequency, intensity, vowels, and voice register in adult male speakers. Thesis, University of Iowa.

Kunze L.H. (1964). Evaluation of methods of estimating subglottal air pressure. *J. Speech Hear. Res.*, **7**, 151–64.

Ladefoged P. (1962). Subglottal activity during speech. In *Proceedings of the IVth International Congress on Phonetic Science* (Sovijärvi A., Aalto P., eds), Helsinki, 1961. The Hague: Mouton, pp. 73–91.

Lieberman P. (1968). Direct comparison of subglottal and esophageal pressure during speech. *J. Acoust. Soc. Am.*, **43**, 1157–64.

Lilly J.C. (1950). Flow meter for recording respiratory flow of human subjects. In *Methods in Medical Research* (Comroe J.H., ed.) Chicago: Yearbook, pp. 113–21.

Loebell E. (1969). Über die direkte Messung des subglottischen Luftdruckes. *Arch. Klin. Exp. Ohren Nasen Kehlkopfheilkd.*, **194**, 316–20.

Luchsinger R. (1951). Schalldruck- und Geschwindigkeitsregistrierung der Atemluft beim Singen. *Folia Phoniatr.*, **3**, 25–51.

Mahieu H.F. (1988). Voice and speech rehabilitation following laryngectomy. Thesis, University of Groningen.

Miller D. G., Schutte H.K. (1984). Characteristic patterns of sub- and supraglottal pressure variations within the glottal cycle. In *Trans XIIIth Symp Care Prof Voice* (Lawrence V.L., ed.) New York: Voice Found., pp. 70–5.

Moolenaar-Bijl A.J. (1953). The importance of certain consonants in esophageal voice after laryngectomy. *Ann. Otol. Rhinol. Laryngol.*, **62**, 979–88.

Morrison M.D., Rammage L.A., Belisle G.M. (1983). Muscular tension dysophonia. *J. Otolaryngol.*, **12**, 302–6.

Moser M., Kittel G. (1979). Automatisierte bodyplethysmographische Atemmessungen: der phonatorische Wirkungsgrad. *HNO*, **27**, 100–2.

Nieboer G.L.J., Schutte H.K., de Graaf T. (1989). Physiological and aerodynamic measurements in esophageal speakers with and without a Groningen valve prosthesis. *J. Speech Hear. Res.*, **32**.

Ptacek P.H., Sander E.K. (1963a). Breathiness and phonation length. *J. Speech Hear. Disord.*, **28**, 267–72.

Ptacek P.H., Sander E.K. (1963b). Maximum duration of phonation. *J. Speech Hear. Disord.*, **28**, 171–82.

Rothenberg M. (1973). A new inverse-filtering technique for deriving the glottal air flow waveform during voicing. *J. Acoust. Soc. Am.*, **53**, 1632–45.

Roudet L. (1900). Recherches sûr la rôle de la pression sous-glottique dans la parole. *La Parole*, **1**, 599–612.

Rubin H.J., LeCover C.M., Vennard W. (1967). Vocal intensity, subglottic pressure and air flow relationships in singers. *Folia Phoniatr.*, **19**, 393–413.

Sawashima M., Yoshioka H., Honda K. et al. (1978). Clinical evaluation of air usage during phonation. In *Proceedings of the XVIIth International Congress of the International Association of Logopedics and Phoniatrics*, Copenhagen, 1977 (Buch N.H., ed.). Copenhagen: Organizing Committee, pp. 419–22, 451–4.

Schutte H.K., van den Berg Jw. (1976). Determination of the subglottic pressure and the efficiency of sound production in patients with disturbed voice production. In *Proceedings of the XVIth International Congress of the International Association of Logopedics and Phoniatrics*, Interlaken, 1974 (Loebell E., ed.). Basel: Karger, pp. 415–20.

Schutte H.K. (1980). The efficiency of voice production. Thesis, University of Groningen.

Schutte H.K., Miller D.G. (1986). The effect of F0/F1 coincidence in soprano high notes on pressure at the glottis. *J. Phon.*, **14**, 385–92.

Schutte H.K. (1984). Zur Unterscheidung organischer und funktioneller Stimmstörungen bei leichten Adduktionsstörungen des Kehlkopfes. *HNO*, **32**, 21–3.

Seidner W., Stürzebecher E. (1978). Variabilität normaler Phono-Pneumotachogramme. In *Proceedings of the XVIIth International Congress of the International Association of*

Logopedics and Phoniatrics, Copenhagen, 1977 (Buch N.H., ed.). Copenhagen: Organizing Committe, pp. 563–9.

Seidner W., Wendler J., Stürzebecher E. (1976). Das normale Phono-Pneumotachogramme. In *Proceedings of the XVIth International Congress of the International Association of Logopedics and Phoniatrics*, Interlaken, 1974 (Loebell E., ed.). Basel: Karger, pp. 421–6.

Singh W. (1985). New tracheostoma flap valve for surgical speech reconstruction. In *New Dimensions in Otorhinolaryngology — Head and Neck Surgery*, vol. II (Myers E., ed.) Amsterdam: Elsevier, pp. 480–1.

Singh W. (1987). Tracheostoma valve for speech rehabilitation in laryngectomees. *J. Laryngol. Otol.*, **101**, 809–14.

Singh W. (1988). A simple surgical technique and a new prosthesis for voice rehabilitation after laryngectomy. *J. Laryngol. Otol.*, **102**, 332–4.

Singh W. (1989a). Singh tracheostoma valve. In *Proceedings of the International Voice Symposium*, Edinburgh (Singh W., ed.), pp. 81–2.

Singh W. (1989b). Near-total laryngectomy. In *Proceedings of the International Voice Symposium*, Edinburgh. (Singh W., ed.), pp. 53–8.

Singh W. (1990). Singh Tracheostoma Valve. In *Proceedings of the XXIst International Congress of the International Association of Logopedics and Phoniatrics*, Prague, pp. 435–7.

Stürzebecher E., Seidner W., Wagner H., Wendler J. (1973). Erfassung von Atemgrössen während der Phonation. *Monatsschr. Ohrenheilkd. Laryngorhinol.*, **107**, 271–8.

Titze I.R. (1989). Voice research: vocal efficiency. *NATS J.*, **45**, 31–4.

van den Berg Jw. (1956). Direct and indirect determination of the mean subglottic pressure. *Folia Phoniatr.*, **8**, 1–24.

van den Berg Jw. (1958). Myoelastic–aerodynamic theory of voice production. *J. Speech Hear. Res.*, **1**, 227–44.

Vogelsanger G.T. (1954). Experimentelle Prüfung der Stimmleistung beim Singen. *Folia Phoniatr.*, **6**, 193–227.

Yanagihara N., Koike Y. (1966). Phonation and respiration: function study in normal subjects. *Folia Phoniatr.*, **18**, 323–40.

Yanagihara N., Von Leden H. (1967). Respiration and phonation: the functional examination of laryngeal disease. *Folia Phoniatr.*, **19**, 153–66.

Chapter 3

Normal and pathological speech: phonetic, acoustic and laryngographic aspects

A. J. Fourcin

Work in speech sciences and technology is making a progressively more important contribution to the understanding of mechanisms and the management of rehabilitation in speech pathology. The aim of this chapter is to give a brief overview of some basic aspects of the phonetic and quantitative descriptions of speech which are readily clinically accessible, are in current use and have the potential to contribute to future developments.

Segmental descriptions

Although we perceive and produce speech sound sequences rather than separate sounds, writing conventions give a bias towards the description of the basic components of speech in terms of separate segments. The 'phone level' relates broadly to the nature of individual sounds, and the 'phoneme level' is concerned with the contrastive use of sounds to convey meaning. This distinction is an important one, since physically and phonetically the concern is not only with meaning but also with the nature of the utterance. Linguistically, however, the preoccupation is with the structures used for meaningful communication. Useful discussions of the phone and phoneme levels of representation are given by Gimson (1980), Ladefoged (1982) and Wells and Colson (1971). Table 3.1 gives a summary of the main sound groups used for communication in English, divided simply into vowel and consonant classes. In the first column the key words are written as in this text. The second column represents individual sounds using the conventions of the International Phonetic Association, which can be used at the phone level. The International Phonetic Alphabet (IPA) has recently been revised (International Phonetic Association, 1989) and now includes some descriptors of pathological speech. The third column uses another notation, the Speech Assessment Methods phonetic alphabet (SAMPA), which is based on the use of modern computer-compatible symbols in which only the characters available on a normal keyboard are employed. The SAM project in ESPRIT introduced this phonetic alphabet (Wells et al, 1989) which is designed to provide phonemic representations for the main European languages; its use of standard keyboard symbols could be of great practical value in the processing of phonetic case notes. The SAMPA notation provides the basis for a broad phonetic representation which is intermediate between the phone and phoneme levels. Its use simplifies the typed or printed discussion of problems in respect of the segmental

Table 3.1 Main sound groups used for communication

Keyword	IPA	SAMPA
Vowels		
1 bead	iː	iː
2 bid	ɪ	I
3 bed	e	e
4 bad	æ	{
5 card	ɑː	Aː
6 cod	ɒ	Q
7 cord	ɔː	Oː
8 good	u	U
9 food	Uː	uː
10 bud	ʌ	V
11 bird	ɜː	3ː
12 allow	ə	@
13 day	eɪ	eI
14 know	əu	@U
15 eye	aɪ	aI
16 cow	au	aU
17 boy	ɔɪ	OI
18 beer	ɪə	I@
19 bare	eə	e@
20 tour	uə	U@
Consonants		
sing	ŋ	N
thin	θ	T
then	ð	D
shed	ʃ	S
beige	ʒ	Z
etch	tʃ	tS
edge	dʒ	dZ

Those common to both IPA and SAMPA:
p t k b d g m n f v s z r l w j h

description of pathological forms of speech output, and can conveniently be incorporated in case notes; it is used in the following discussion.

Tables 3.2 and 3.3 give classifications of the vowels and consonants represented in Table 3.1, with reference to their vocal tract, articulatory, origin. For the vowels the classifications 'front', 'central' and 'back' simply refer to the position, between lips and pharyngeal wall, of the main body of the tongue; similarly, 'close' to 'open' refers to the degree to which the jaw and tongue are raised or lowered. These descriptors are widely employed in clinical phonetics to define speech sound contrasts in the immediately understandable terms of oral cavity shape. Speech training is often oriented towards the use of these dimensions, and displays have been designed to provide the patient with vocal tract targets. In practice, however, it is the sound rather than its precise source which is important — partial glossectomy provides an example where large departures from normal oral cavity shape can be accommodated by the patient to produce acceptable sound contrasts.

Table 3.2 Articulatory representation of English vowels using the case-note phonemic notation SAMPA

	Front	Central	Back
Close	i:		u:
Half-close	i		U
Half-open	e	3: @	O:
Open	{	V	A: Q

Figure 3.1 gives an approximate acoustic correlate of this articulatory classification for two single-accent groups of British English speakers. The men have a well-developed set of contrasts which is clearly reflected in their resonant frequency patterns (discussed below). The children's distribution is of special interest in two ways: first, in regard to the large difference in the physical values for their utterances compared with those for the men (although their vowels are perceived as being phonetically equivalent); second, in respect of the details of structure — that for the children is not as well defined as for the adults. In both cases there is a need for a basis for the flexible interpretation of sounds in context. This is often referred to as 'normalization'; it is a receptive process which is at the heart of speech communication and applies to disorder as well as normality. The use of differing systems of contrast is discussed for example by Grunwell (1987).

Vowels are characterized by the absence of any special constrictions of the vocal tract, apart from the control of the velar port for purely oral, as opposed to nasal,

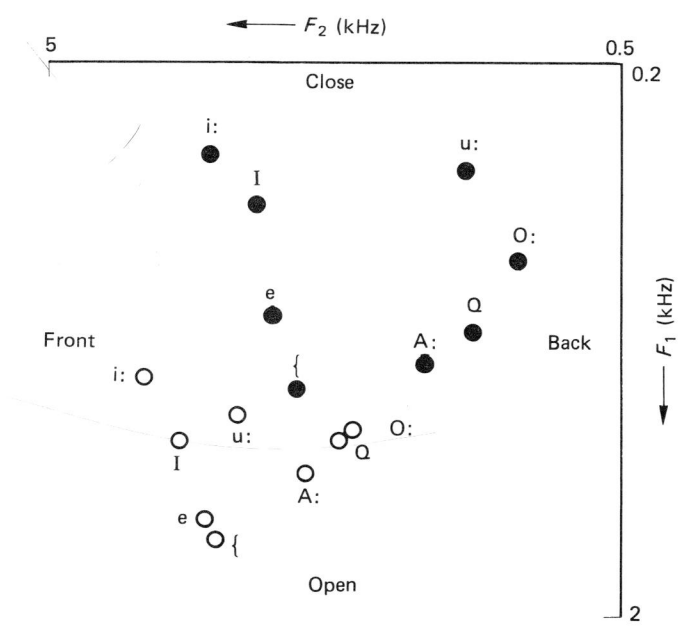

Figure 3.1 Articulatory and acoustic representations of English vowels using the case-note phonemic notation SAMPA. The formant frequencies for adult male speakers are shown by solid circles; open circles represent frequencies for 4-year-old children. From *Scott-Brown's Otolaryngology* (1987)

Table 3.3 Articulatory representation of English consonants using SAMPA. Voiced sounds are shown in bold

Manner	Place						
	Bilabial	Labiodental	Dental	Alveolar	Palatal	Velar	Glottal
Approximants	w			r	j		
Lateral				l			
Plosive	pb			td		kg	
Affricative				tS dZ			
				tr dr			
Fricative		fv	TD	sz		SZ	h
Nasal	m			n		N	

vowels. Consonant contrasts are always based upon the controlled evolution of a constriction or closure within the vocal tract. Table 3.3 shows the ways in which constrictions are normally defined phonetically in regard to position, or 'place', within the vocal tract and in regard to 'manner', the nature of control as a function of time in association with oral and nasal resonances. Table 3.3 also indicates whether the sound is purely voiced or voiceless. The purely voiced sounds owe their primary characteristics to their association with an acoustic excitation derived from the regular vibration of the vocal folds — discussed more quantitatively below — as well as to vocal tract shaping. The discussion which follows also touches on the non-periodic excitation associated with the turbulent flow of air which is basic to the pure fricative, voiced fricative and voiceless sounds. (At increasingly complete levels of physical description, these areas have been discussed by Pickett (1980), Linggard (1985) and Flanagan (1972); four basic descriptors are essential to a first level of understanding. *Intensity* relates to the energy per unit time that is associated with a sound. *Frequency* describes the number of events per unit time that occur. *Periodicity* is related to the repetition of the part of the sound sequence that is being observed — a particular aspect of frequency. *Turbulence* is the term used to describe the non-streamlined flow of air responsible for aperiodic sound transmission from the vocal tract — ordinarily referred to as friction, and when produced in isolation from voicing, at the origin of 'voiceless' sounds.)

Signals

Figure 3.2 relates these vocal tract, phonetic descriptors to the results of more objective approaches. The figure is based on different physical analyses of a single utterance 'a view on speech' spoken by a south-east British woman speaker using normal voice. The ordinary text representation of the speech is shown at the foot of the figure and the computer-compatible SAMPA representation, defined in Table 3.1, is shown immediately above. The acoustic pressure waveform, S_p, is shown in Figure 3.2a; the accompanying waveform of Figure 3.2b, L_x is derived from the speaker's vocal fold closures and monitors vocal fold vibration, which is basic to voice, throughout the utterance. The first sound [@] is voiced and this is clearly

Normal and pathological speech: phonetic, acoustic and laryngographic aspects 35

shown by the correspondence between S_p and L_x. From [j] to [n] the L_x waveform shows vocal fold vibration to be continuous. There is a break in vocal fold vibratory activity for [sp] before a final stretch of vibration for the vowel [i:]. Information of this type is of practical value in understanding the origin of production difficulties, and displays can help in interactive training. The L_x waveform is derived from the use of an electrolaryngograph in which electrodes are placed on the wings of the thyroid cartilage externally on the speaker's neck.

The electrical method of sensing vocal fold vibration basic to the L_x waveform, was

a view on speech

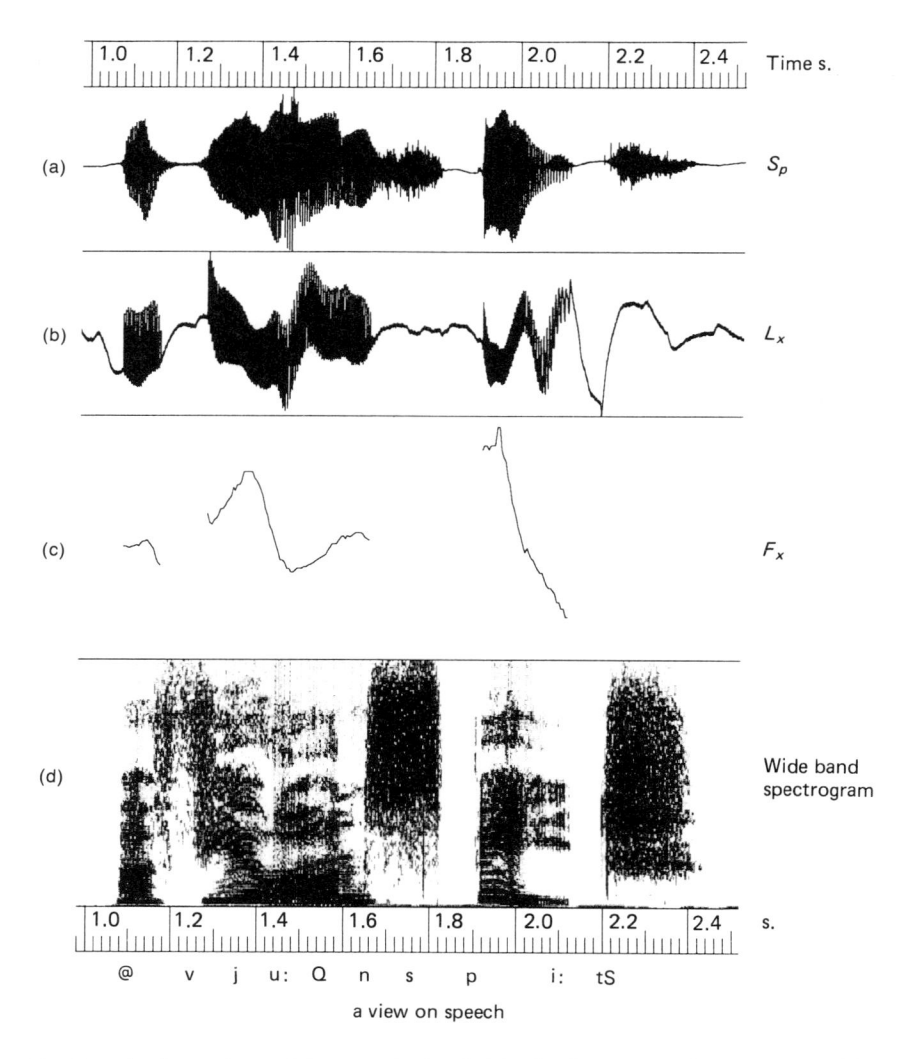

Figure 3.2 Quantitative analyses of the acoustic signal. (a) S_p, the pressure-time waveform; (b) L_x, the synchronous electrolaryngograph detection of vocal fold closure and supporting structure movement; (c) F_x, period by period larynx frequency measurement from L_x, log scale 100 to 300 Hz; (d) wide-band (200 Hz) frequency-time spectrogram: O–8 kHz

introduced by Fabre (1957); the electrolaryngograph (Laryngograph Ltd, 1 Tolmers Square, London NW1 2HE, UK) used here (Fourcin, 1981; Cotton and Conture, 1990) is based on the same principle but is a development using electrically isolated guard ring electrodes with conductance rather than impedance monitoring, with an automatic setting of the operating conditions from speaker to speaker, and moment to moment. The special value of this approach comes from the close relation between vocal fold closure and the interval of vocal tract excitation in voiced sounds, and the non-invasive nature of the examination.

Vocal fold activity is basic to the most salient physical aspects of the production of voice — the input to the vocal tract which gives speech its characteristic pitch and enables the contrasts of intonation to be produced. In all languages the voiced sounds are the most important in regard to the load that they carry in communication. A comprehensive phonetic description of the sound contrastive systems in a wide range of languages is given in Maddieson (1984).

The perceived pitch of voiced sounds (discussed for example by Moore, 1986) is directly related to the rate at which the speaker's vocal folds vibrate. In Figure 3.2c the rate of vocal fold vibration, F_x, has been derived directly from the L_x signal and is shown as an essentially smoothly varying curve interrupted only by periods of silence and voiceless activity. Although the curve of F_x appears smooth it is in fact made up from the individual contributions of each larynx period and may, as discussed below, be used as the basis of quantitative analyses leading to indications of normality and pathology. An excellent overview of established methods of estimating speech fundamental frequency is given by Hess (1983).

In Figure 3.2a the acoustic waveform S_p, obtained from the output of a simple pressure-sensitive microphone, shows the voiced sounds (from laryngeal excitation of the acoustic resonances of the vocal tract) to be the most prominent in regard to their amplitude. As well as being of greatest frequency of occurrence in all languages, these sounds are also first in order of developmental acquisition. The voiceless fricative sounds, which are not dependent upon laryngeal vibration, can be seen in this particular example for those situations where L_x is absent but the speech signal is present. In Figure 3.2d an analysis is shown of the complete speech signal in terms of its frequency range as a function of time — the spectrogram. The spectrogram is a method of displaying intensity as a function of time horizontally, and frequency vertically, to give a graphic illustration of these descriptors, as in Figure 3.2d. Within the spectrogram, the resonances of the vocal tract — formants — are shown as dark concentrations of marking, during intervals of voicing. These vary in position with the speech sequence and are more or less clearly defined, partly as a function of the sharpness of vocal fold closure and partly its relative duration. In Table 3.2 the front close vowel is described simply with reference to the position of the speaker's tongue within the oral cavity; in Figure 3.2d [i:] in the word 'speech' is associated with a pattern of resonances — formants — in which low-frequency energy is clearly separated from a higher-frequency grouping of formant resonances. For many practical purposes only the first three major peaks of energy concentration shown in an analysis of this sort determine the auditory nature of a sound. Formant patternings in time, frequency and amplitude characterize the sounds of speech. The vowels have well-defined slowly changing formant structures. In distinction to [i:], [u] in the word 'view' has its main energy concentration associated with formants having lower frequencies and this can be seen clearly at the beginning of the spectrogram (1.44 s). At the start of the word 'on' the back open vowel [Q] is intermediate between the two previous vowel examples in terms of the distribution of its energy. Although notionally the vowels are often associated with unchanging patterns in a frequency–time presentation of this spectrographic form, their real identity depends on the change in formant patterning induced by context. Another class of sound which comes into the consonantal grouping in Table 3.3, the semi-vowel, is intrinsically associated as for all consonants, with the changing pattern in time which reflects a changing articulatory origin. The [j] in 'view' is a particular example of this class of sound — at the top of the consonantal grouping in Table 3.3. The semivowels taken together with the liquids [r] and [l] are often referred to as 'approximants'. Other consonantal groupings exemplified in the sentence include the stop consonants; [p] is a particular example which is voiceless — involving a cessation of vocal fold vibration — and defined articulatorily by its bilabial closure. The affricate at the end of the word 'spee**ch**' [tS] is a combination of a voiceless stop consonant and a voiceless fricative. The example [p] in the spectrogram immediately follows a voiceless fricative [s] and this combination in English has removed an acoustic element ordinarily found in [p] — that of aspiration — which is associated with the noise excitation of the whole vocal tract prior to the beginning of the next voiced segment. (Speech sound sequences in any language are not simply made up of strings of physical events which, for a given phoneme, are the same from one context to another, and the lack of aspiration in [p] here is only one example of context-dependent variability.) At the very beginning of the sound sequence of Figure 3.2, following the neutral vowel [@], the consonant [v], a voiced fricative, is a sound that combines both the noise-like component of a voiceless fricative and a regular periodic component of voicing (see Figure 3.4b). Finally, in this brief sequence of illustrations of consonantal characteristics, the sound at the end of the word 'on' [n] illustrates an aspect of speech production in which the nasal resonances are coupled to those of the oral cavity to produce a further set of contrastive features.

Figure 3.3 illustrates a sequence of instants in the cycle of vibratory activity for a particular adult male speaker sustaining a neutral vowel sound [@]. The electrolaryngograph waveform L_x was obtained by the use of electrodes lightly placed in superficial contact with the speaker's neck at the level of the alae of the thyroid cartilage. An X-ray flash source has been synchronized with this laryngograph waveform so that any predetermined instant can be used to trigger a frontal irradiation of the speaker's vocal folds. Figure 3.3a shows the vocal folds in their position immediately before complete closure. The ventricular folds are clearly seen above and the superficial edges of the folds themselves are just visible as the result of their anterior tilt. In Figure 3.3b the closure cycle has been completed and the vocal folds are shown with their maximum contact. Maximum contact is typically associated with only a modest abuttal of the opposing vocal folds in normal phonation. In Figure 3.3c the vocal folds are beginning to separate after the peak of closure shown by the laryngograph waveform and the inferior edges are widely spaced. Figure 3.3d shows the attitude of the vocal folds when they are maximally separated. The glottal area is greatest and the output from the laryngograph electrodes is near to its minimum. This is the precursive shaping of the vocal folds prior to the beginning of a new oscillatory cycle in which the superior edges once more come rapidly into slight but intimate contact, and initiate a new acoustic excitation of the vocal tract.

Laryngographic aspects of normal voice production

In Figure 3.4, citation examples have been modelled on sounds taken from the sentence 'a view on speech' to illustrate different effects of vocal fold excitation in

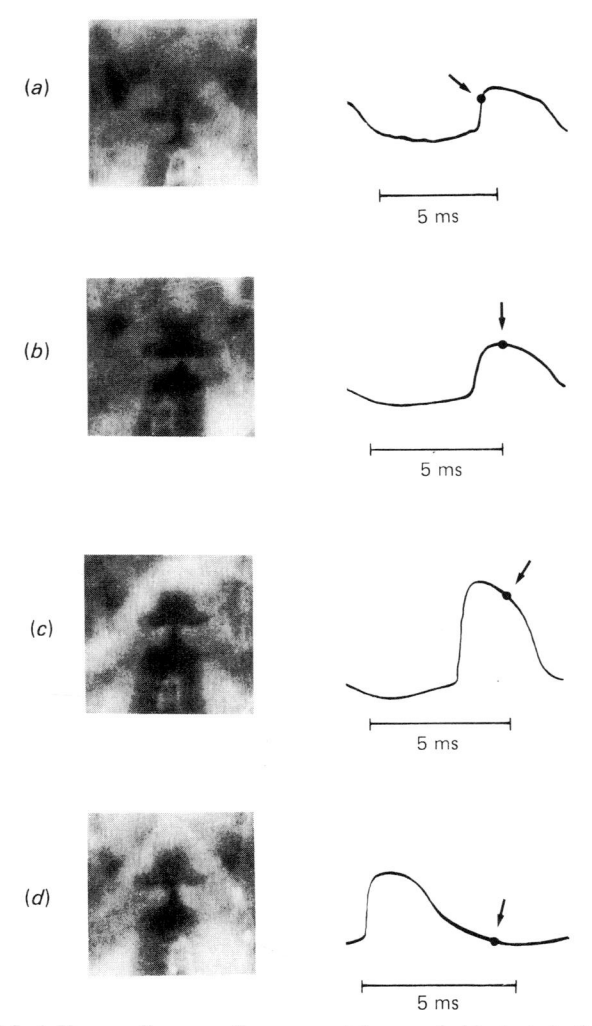

Figure 3.3 Frontal flash X-ray radiograms. Four separately recorded instants in the cycle of vocal fold vibratory activity for a sustained [A:] from an adult male speaker; the triggering instants are shown on the L_x waveform: (a) immediately prior to maximum vocal fold contact; (b) point of maximum closure; (c) beginning of separation (d) mid-open phase. From *Scott-Brown's Otolaryngology* (1987)

achieving acoustically contrastive outputs from the speaker's vocal tract. Figure 3.4a illustrates some physical correlates of the vocal tract setting for the vowel [@] taken from the beginning of the utterance. The upper waveform shows the speech pressure waveform S_p previously illustrated in Figure 3.2 but now substantially expanded in time; the corresponding synchronous expansion of the L_x waveform is shown below. In the pair of waveforms in Figure 3.4a the sequence of vocal fold vibratory activity clearly relates to what has just been described in Figure 3.3. Here, however, one can see that the closure of the vocal folds which produces a sharp upward rise in the L_x waveform is associated with the beginning of an oscillatory

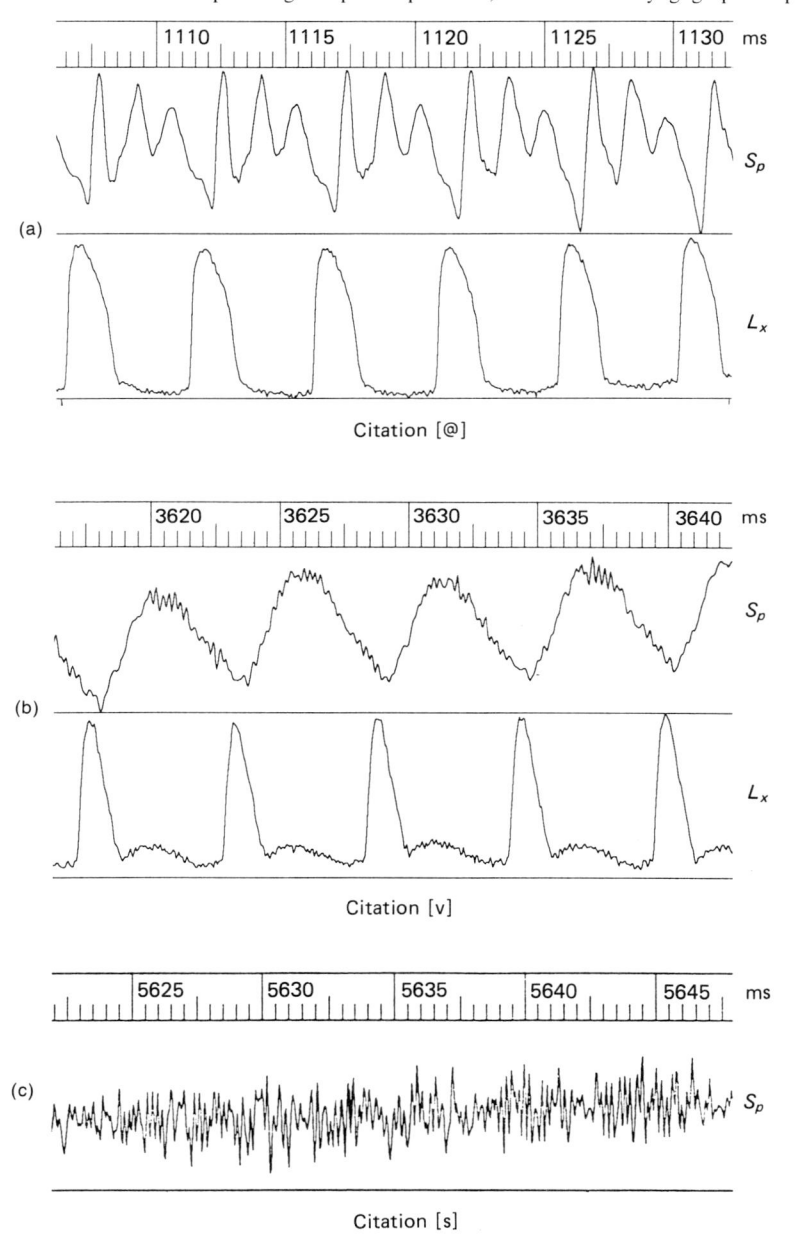

Figure 3.4 S_p and L_x waveforms for: (a) a purely voiced sound; (b) a voiced fricative; (c) a voiceless fricative

acoustic output from the speaker's vocal tract. The peak of acoustic activity follows the sharp closure of the vocal folds. The resonant responses of the vocal tract reduce in amplitude following excitation and during the open phase, when the vocal folds are maximally separated, there is the largest reduction in acoustic energy. The whole

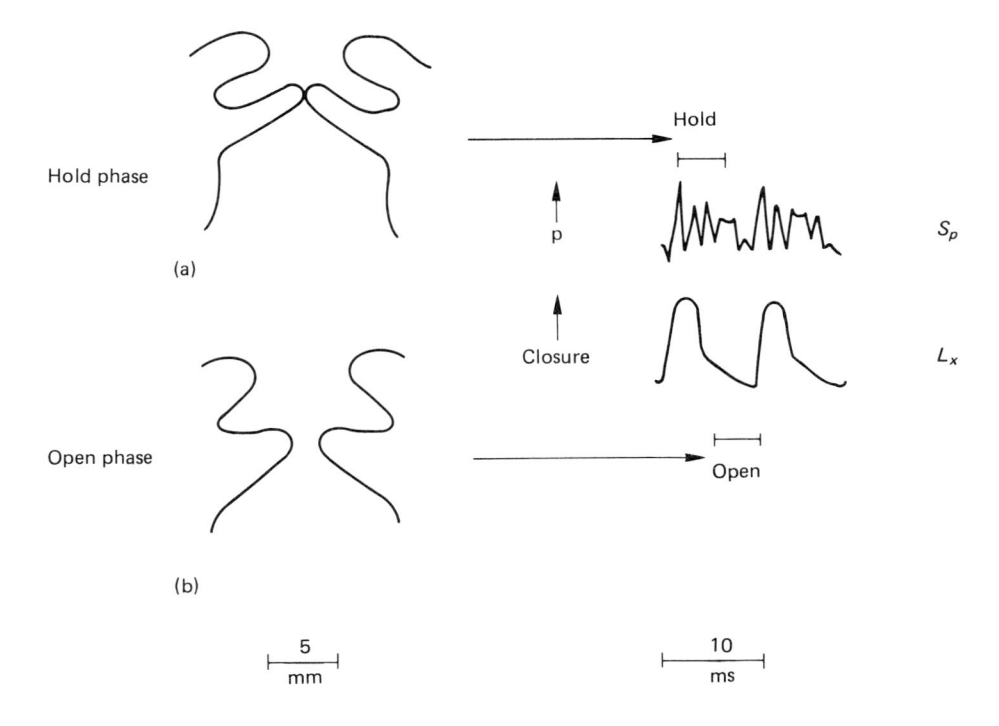

Figure 3.5 Acoustic and laryngographic waveform aspects of good voice: (a) the closed phase during which the supraglottal vocal tract is isolated from the trachea; (b) the open phase, during which there is an acoustic link

sequence begins again with the next sharp closure of the vocal folds. In Figure 3.4b a voiced fricative is illustrated with breathy larynx excitation and a correspondingly less well-defined acoustic set of resonances in the acoustic output. Once more the illustration is based on a citation example from the sequence 'a view on speech', and the expanded waveform is from the voiced fricative consonant [v]. A somewhat breathy voice is associated with this illustration and the characteristic small closure interval and relatively long open phase can be seen as well as the rather slower closure of the vocal folds. These two effects together tend to reduce the intensity of acoustic output as well as its spectral definition in terms of formant components. Friction is generated from the turbulence associated with large air flow in the open phase of each cycle. Finally, in the production of the voiceless fricative [s], in Figure 3.4c, there is no vocal fold vibration and the excitation of the vocal tract results entirely from the turbulent air flow at the point of vocal tract constriction which is associated with the place of articulation for this speech sound.

Aspects of normal and pathological voice quality

Figures 3.5 and 3.6 illustrate in more detail three of the salient factors which emerged from the discussions of Figures 3.3 and 3.4—regularity and frequency range of vocal fold vibration; rapidity of vocal fold closure; and closure effectiveness. In Figure

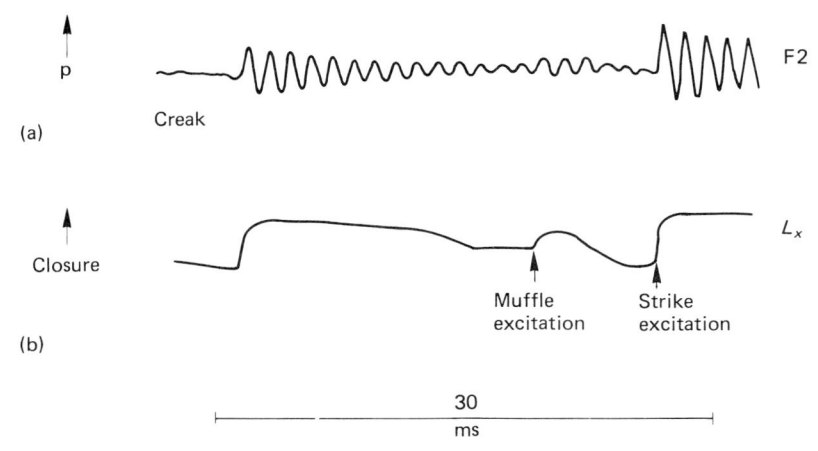

Figure 3.6 Characteristic waveform aspects of 'creaky' voice: (a) speech pressure waveform for the isolated second formant of [A:]; (b) the accompanying L_x waveform. (a) and (b) are, here, time aligned. From *Scott-Brown's Otolaryngology* (1987).

3.5a the vocal folds are shown in contact as for Figure 3.3b and the 'hold phase', which is shown above the speech pressure waveform S_p, relates to the period of time for which the vocal folds effectively isolate the subglottal from the supraglottal vocal tract cavities. During this interval the damping (reduction in intensity due to energy loss from the resonances of the vocal tract to the subglottal cavities) is least. In Figure 3.5b the vocal folds are shown separated, and for this period of time, when there is an effective link between the glottal and the subglottal cavities, energy can be lost from the resonances of the vocal tract so that they are less well defined. The open phase is, in consequence, associated in the speech pressure waveform with a marked reduction in amplitude and a change in the resonant structure. For good voice production the closed phase should be long compared with the total length of the laryngeal period. Although there are many other factors contributing to good voice, one above all is important in this context: vocal fold closure must be rapid as well as regular in order for the resonances of the vocal tract to be appropriately acoustically excited.

Figure 3.6 gives a brief qualitative indication of the way in which variation in the rapidity of vocal fold closure can substantially contribute to the intensity of response of vocal tract resonances. In this particular instance, Figure 3.6a shows not the complete speech waveform but, for the purposes of discussion, the isolated second resonance, F_2; this particular example of inverse filtering comes from the work of Melvin Hunt (1987). Figure 3.6b shows the associated L_x waveform defining the laryngographic nature of the vocal fold closures associated with the acoustic excitation leading to the response in Figure 3.6a. This excitation corresponds to 'creaky' voice, where the speaker's vocal folds are held in an untensed, flaccid adjustment so that their vibration is intrinsically associated with a degree of irregularity. There are two main types of creaky voice, each being characterized by very long closure to open phase ratios and a very long overall period of vibration of the vocal folds (Baken, 1987). The example here has two closures for each complete cycle of laryngeal vibratory events; this is a type which is often found in British English. The other type has one closure per period and it is convenient to refer to this as vocal 'fry'. In 'creak' large variations can take place in regard to the rapidity of closure and the length of

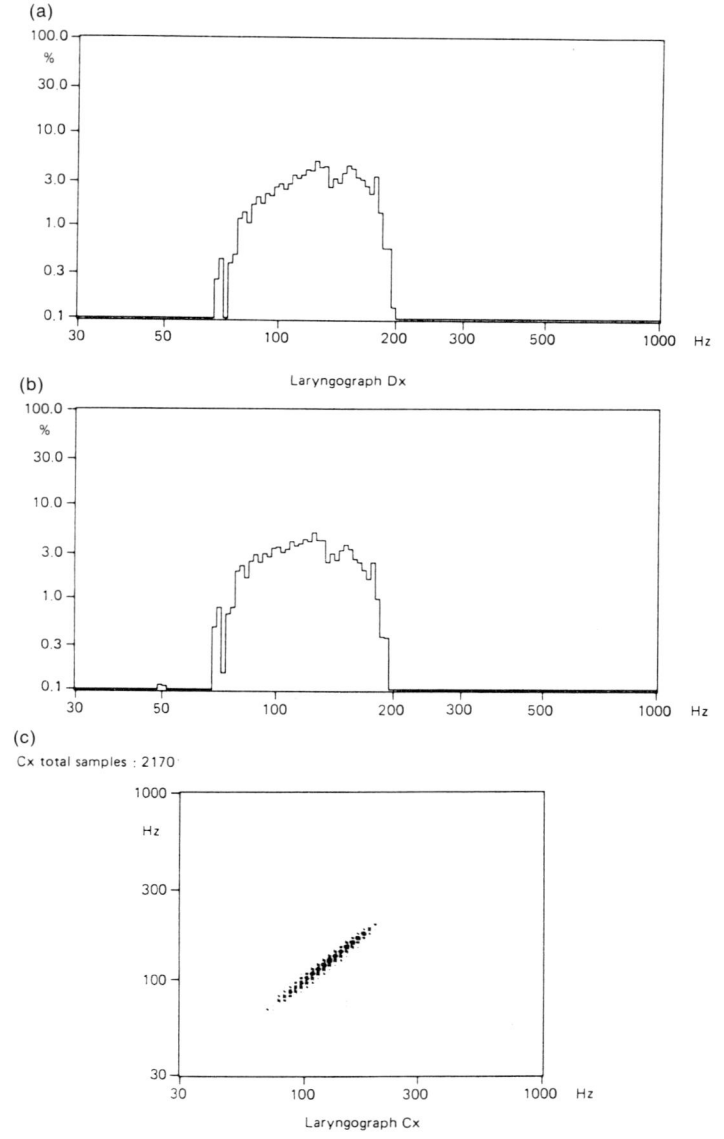

Figure 3.7 Voice frequency range and period to period scatter measurements using the PCLX suite of programs from Laryngograph Ltd. Normal voice: (a) D_x plot of frequency range based on number of larynx periods; (b) Frequency range based on time spent at any larynx frequency bin; (c) C_x scatter plot of adjacent larynx periods with a deviation from the diagonal of 4.6%. Profoundly deaf speaker:

the hold phase from one period to another. In the 'creak' example of Figure 3.6 the greatest rapidity of closure, here called strike excitation, is linked with the greatest intensity of F_2 response. The first closure of the vocal folds, shown to the left of the figure, is not nearly as effective in producing an acoustic output, and the subsidiary closure which has a very low rate of vocal fold contact, here called 'muffle excitation', has the smallest response of all. These are typical effects, found to different degrees

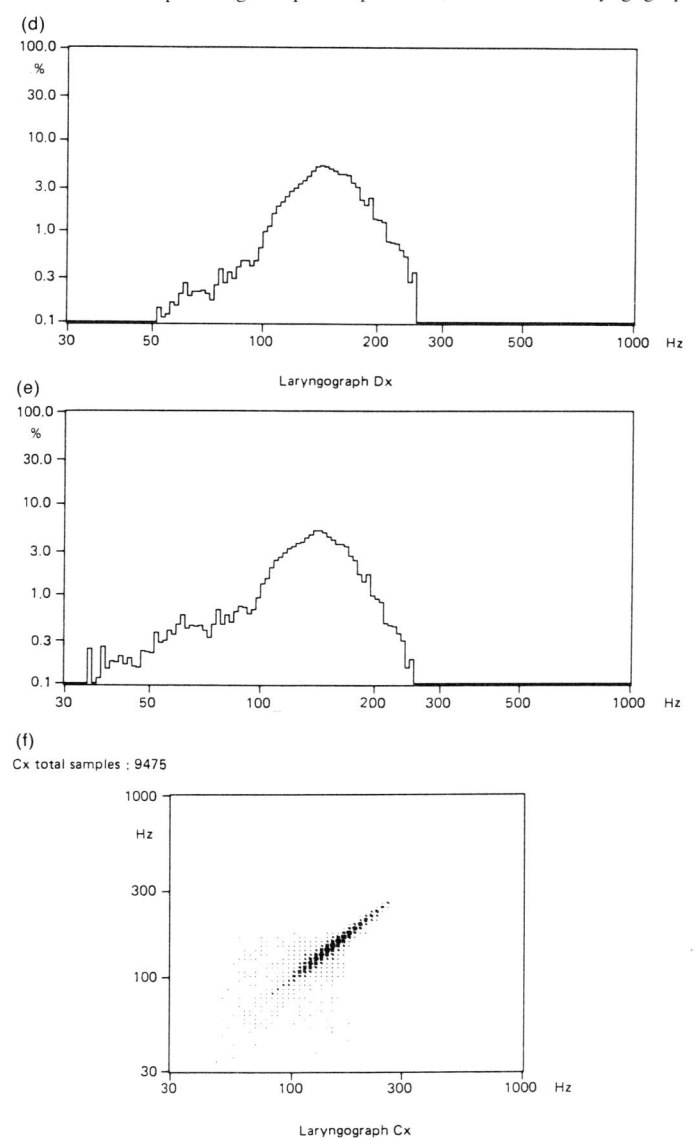

Figure 3.7 *contd.* (d) D_x of larynx period distribution; (e) D_x of time elapsed — note the increased emphasis on the lower frequencies of vocal fold vibration; (f) C_x scatter plot showing abnormal deviation from diagonal. The data for these observations are from the work of the EPI group (especially V. Ball) at UCL, working on speech pattern (SiVo) prostheses for the profoundly deaf

in all voiced sounds, normal as well as pathological. Strikingly important audible features of pathological speech which are not easily analysed physically are directly due to the way that the vocal folds vibrate. The three main factors contributing to these percepts are discussed below.

First, since the pitch of the speaking voice is dependent on the regularity of vibration of the vocal folds, one important characteristic of pathology is often to be found in some degree of departure from a well-defined pitch and, correspondingly, a departure from regular laryngeal periodicity. Many quantitative techniques have been evolved for the measurement of these deviations from normality. For example, 'jitter' was the term that originally referred to the perceptual correlate of laryngeal period-to-period variation; it is now coupled with 'shimmer', similarly referring to amptitude variation, to provide a pair of quantitative descriptors (Baken, 1987). Figure 3.7 illustrates particular examples of laryngograph signal-based analyses which have been developed for the purposes of both quantification and rapid clinical appraisal. The first three examples in Figure 3.7 come from electrolaryngograph recordings of normal voice; the others are derived from laryngograph recordings made in conjunction with routine clinical observations in work with a profoundly deaf patient — the considerable irregularity found here can often be substantially reduced by using a speech pattern element hearing aid (Si Vo). The D_x distributions shown (a, d) represent the range of larynx frequencies used by the speaker in terms of the number of larynx periods occurring in a sample of speech; Figure 3.7d and e relate to the actual time spent speaking at each larynx bin-frequency range, more emphasis is given here to the low frequencies in the speech signal. The C_x plot shows the correspondence between successive vocal fold periods; the greater the scatter the less appropriate is the speaker's voice pitch control. These types of D_x and C_x plots provide an effective basis for the rapid clinical appraisal of the voice features relating to regularity of vocal fold vibration. They have the further (and more important) advantage of being obtained directly from the source of excitation in the larynx, rather than being inferred from measurements of the acoustic output of the vocal tract.

The second factor, rapidity of closure, is of especial clinical importance if the closure of the vocal folds is not well defined in time, for example when the rapidity of vocal fold closure is reduced by oedematous vocal folds. The main result of this deficiency of laryngeal excitation is to impair the spectral definition of the resonances of the vocal tract — the higher formants are not adequately excited. The L_x waveform as in Figure 3.6 can be used directly to gain some insight into this condition in a relatively sensitive way by the direct measurement of the time from the onset of closure to its peak. In addition, L_x can be used in the acoustic analysis of S_p to provide a quantitative measure of spectral definition by the use, for instance, of inverse filtering of the acoustic signal (Hunt, 1987), on the basis of 'closed phase' information — the interval between the onset of vocal fold contact and vocal fold separation.

The nature of normal laryngeal excitation, as already discussed, has the vitally important feature that the subglottal cavities of the vocal tract are automatically isolated from the main vocal tract immediately following main acoustic excitation. When formant energy decay occurs substantially within the closed phase of each period of vocal fold vibration, good voice quality is produced because the resonant response of the vocal tract is then sharply defined with a minimum of internal energy loss. If, however, the closed phase is short, formant energy is prematurely lost by subglottal damping — and vocal tract resonances are less well defined.

The third factor, 'quality' of voice, is partly defined by the closed phase duration — to the extent that the closure is patent. The interarytenoid gap, for example, which is often associated with breathy voice production, will introduce damping in addition to that attributable to the low closed-to-open phase ratio which normally characterizes this condition. In many practical situations, however, the two effects are closely

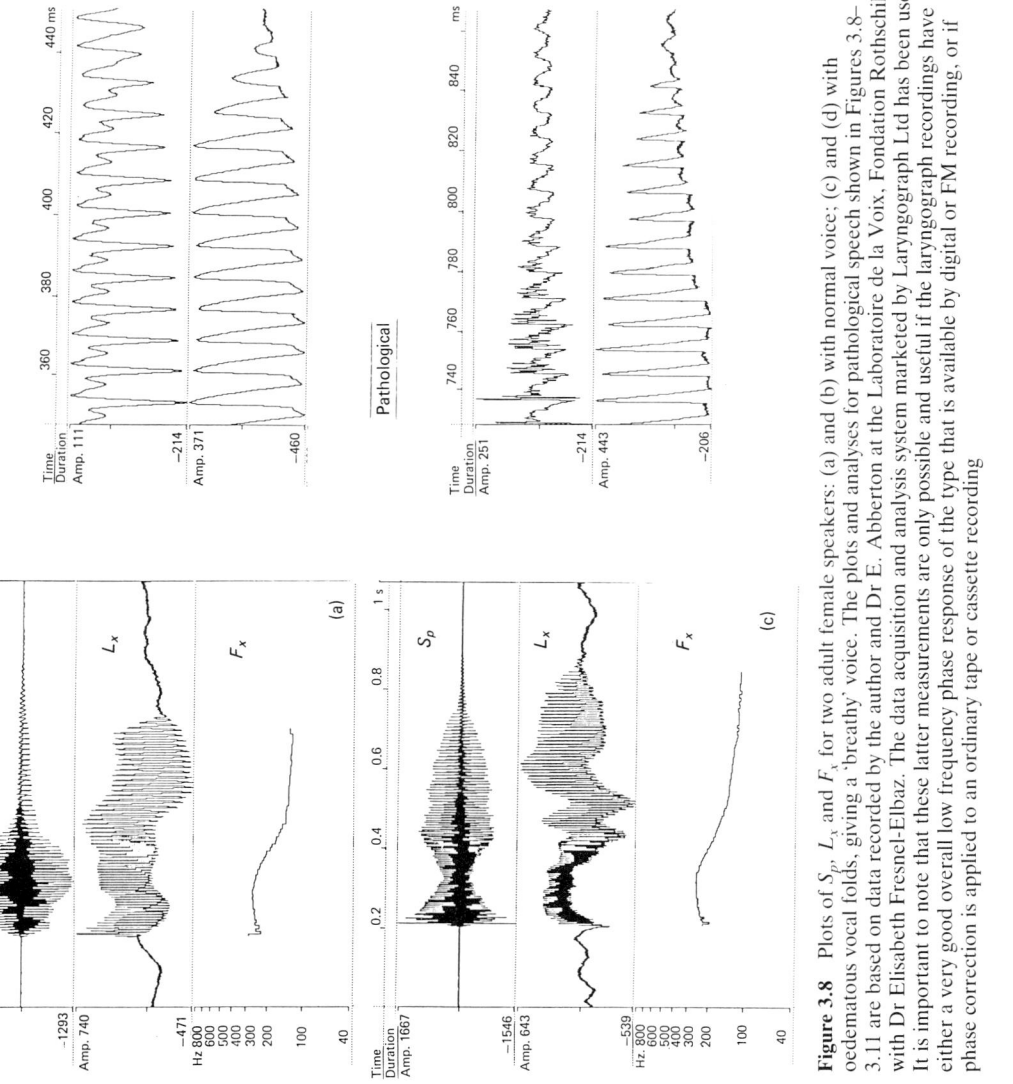

Figure 3.8 Plots of S_p, L_x and F_x for two adult female speakers: (a) and (b) with normal voice; (c) and (d) with oedematous vocal folds, giving a 'breathy' voice. The plots and analyses for pathological speech shown in Figures 3.8–3.11 are based on data recorded by the author and Dr E. Abberton at the Laboratoire de la Voix, Fondation Rothschild, with Dr Elisabeth Fresnel-Elbaz. The data acquisition and analysis system marketed by Laryngograph Ltd has been used. It is important to note that these latter measurements are only possible and useful if the laryngograph recordings have either a very good overall low frequency phase response of the type that is available by digital or FM recording, or if phase correction is applied to an ordinary tape or cassette recording

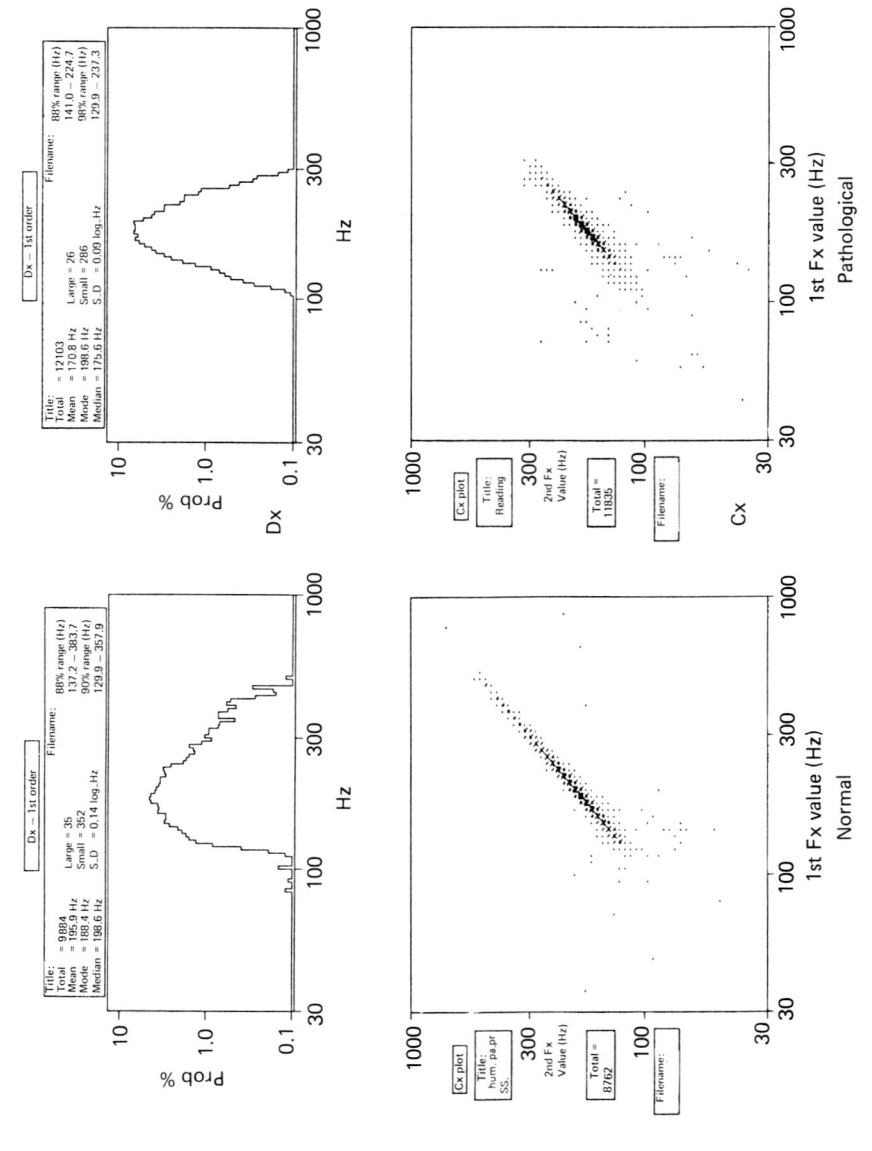

Figure 3.9 D_x and C_x distributions for the normal (left) and pathological speakers of Figure 3.8

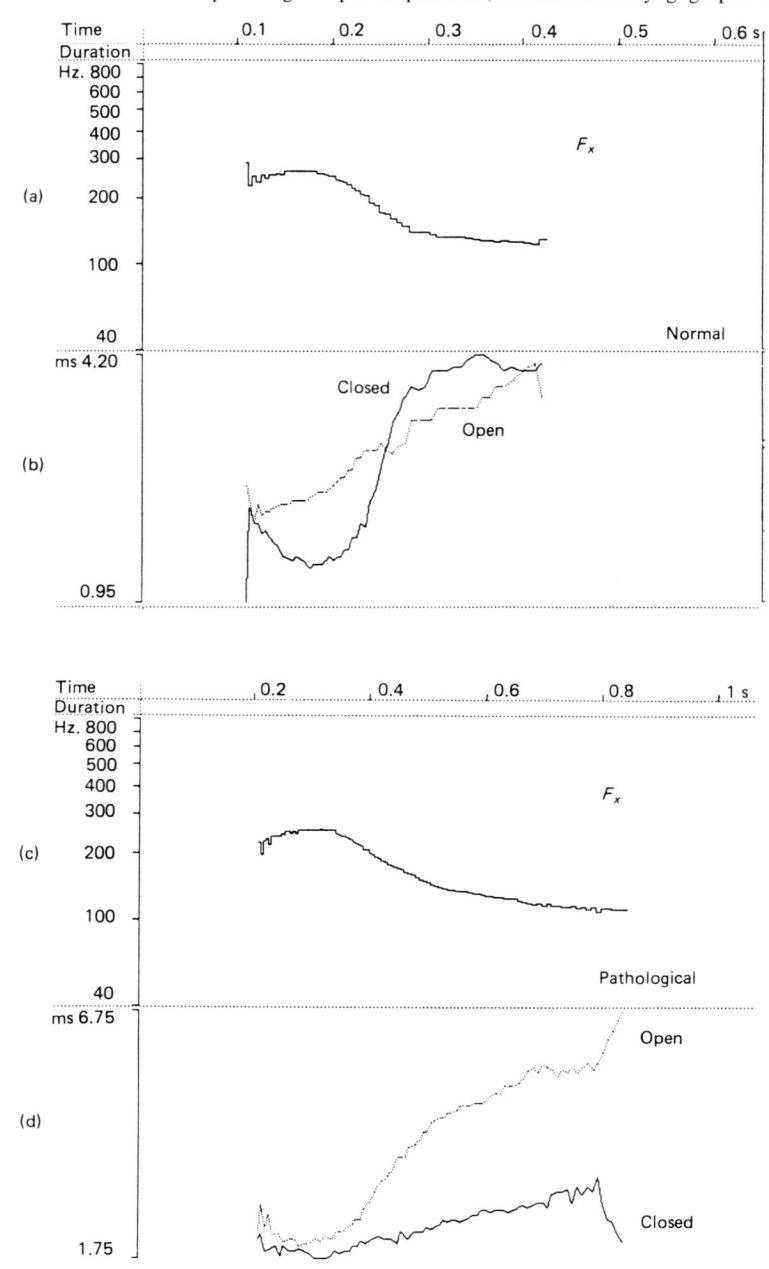

Figure 3.10 F_x contours and open and closed phase measurements for a falling intonation for the normal and pathological speakers of Figure 3.8

related, and a simple estimation of this third factor by considering closed phase measurements alone would facilitate clinical and more general assessment.

Figure 3.8 illustrates the basic problem: (a) shows a family of three traces derived from a normal speaker producing a falling intonation on a completely voiced utterance — S_p, speech acoustic; L_x, laryngograph; and F_x, period by period larynx frequency estimated from laryngograph closure onsets. Figure 3.8c gives the same family of analyses derived from a speaker with chronically oedematous vocal folds. Both speakers are women of about 45 years old. Although there are obvious visual (and gross auditory) differences between the utterances, perceived intonation and the F_x traces are essentially similar.

The D_x plots in Figure 3.9 for these two speakers are both based on the analysis of a read text. Although there is a difference in range, there is no evidence of abnormality in the pathological data. The C_x plots in Figure 3.9 also show that the normal speaker has a large range with some creak-dependent scatter, and that the pathological speaker has slightly larger than normal scatter, but only to a degree that is often seen with very mild laryngitis.

A clue to the perceptually evident voice quality differences between these two speakers can be seen in the contrast between Figure 3.8b and d, which are expanded versions of the ends of the complete utterances. The pathological L_x waveform has a distinctly smaller closed phase — although not an evidently smaller rapidity of closure in this particular example. The variation in closed phase is plotted together with the corresponding change in open phase and the previous F_x traces for each speaker in Figure 3.10. The contrast in dynamic control of the closed phase is now confirmed and clarified for this particular example. The patient has a comparatively low closed-to-open phase ratio for the whole of the utterance. This is a useful quantitative basis for the examination of her poor voice quality in general.

Although the plots of Figure 3.10 are of potential importance in the more detailed study of voice quality differences, they are not especially helpful in the clinical situation since they do not relate to a sufficiently representative sample. Speech characteristics can readily change from one utterance to another even in normality. Figure 3.11 illustrates an approach to the presentation of a closed phase analysis based on the use of much more material. In each case the analyses are of a complete text with a reading time of not less than 3 minutes. The closed phase ratio Q_x (Q_x is the ratio of closed phase to total larynx period) is plotted vertically while the same logarithmic scale for F_x is used horizontally as for the D_x and C_x plots. The same F_x range differences are evident as in Figure 3.9 for D_x and C_x. The closed phase contrast found in Figure 3.10 is confirmed, in the sense that the normal speaker is able to achieve appreciably greater closed phase values for much of her production. Any treatment of the disorder is open to a well-focused evaluation using this new analysis. The approach involves a simple extension of the previous laryngographic techniques, and the relation between the individual utterance closed phase plots of Figure 3.10 and these Q_x (quality of excitation) plots in Figure 3.11 is similar to that between individual F_x plots for a particular utterance and the long-term average plots of F_x distribution given by the D_x distributions.

In Figure 3.12 the results are given of a quite different analysis made on the whole acoustic signal. In each case a long-term average spectrum (LTAS) has been recorded so that an overall energy/frequency spectral distribution for a complete utterance is shown. Figure 3.12a relates to the utterance of Figure 3.2, which was produced with normal voicing. Figure 3.12b is based on the same sentence spoken by the same adult male but with 'breathy' voice quality; this analysis shows a greater

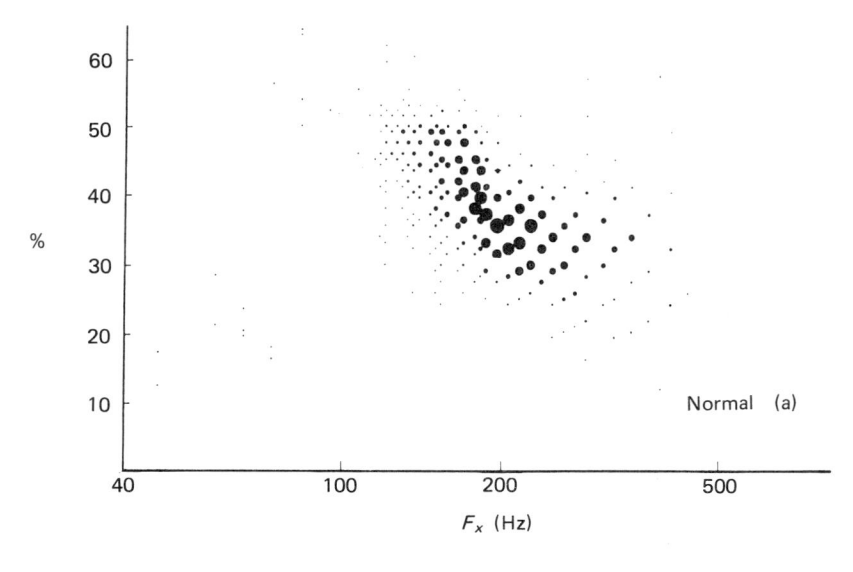

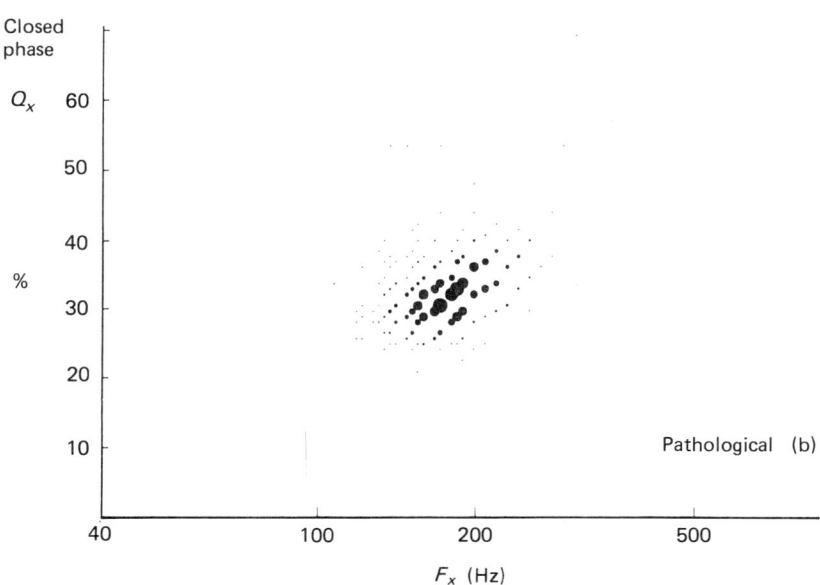

Figure 3.11 Q_x — closed phase as a percentage of larynx period versus larynx frequency, F_x for (a) the normal speaker of Figure 3.8, (b) the speaker with oedematous vocal folds

relative amount of low-frequency energy and less well-defined higher harmonics of the fundamental frequency. Phonetogram analyses (Schutte and Seidner, 1983) differ from this simple LTAS measurement, relating the range of vocal energy output as a function of laryngeal frequency to give a dynamic energy/frequency spectrum area representation of the limits to phonation. Global analyses like these have the special advantage of being based on the acoustic signal alone and of using readily

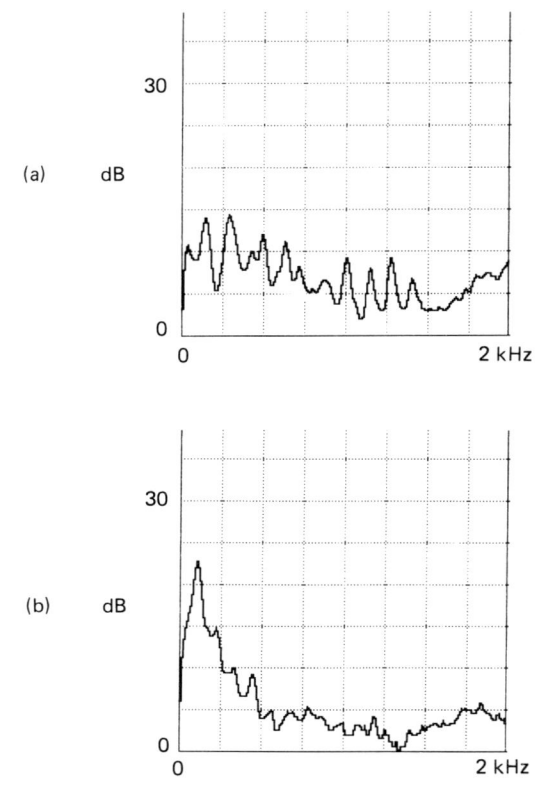

Figure 3.12 Long-term average spectra (200 Hz analysing filter) for the sentence of Figure 3.2 with a male adult speaker producing (a) normal voice; (b) breathy voice

available technology. Their disadvantage is that they are not sufficiently diagnostic. However, current work in speech technology is beginning to yield methods of analytic treatment which will be more specific in regard to the quantitative links between the origins of production and the perceptual quality of sounds in both normal and pathological speech. One approach is to link acoustic pattern-seeking techniques with laryngograph targets. The use of artificial 'neural nets' in speech analysis is likely to provide a major advance in the analysis of both normal and pathological speech, since it is now becoming possible to base quantitative measurement on pattern-seeking processes which can be trained relative to perceptually important factors (Howard and Huckvale, 1988) – as in the SiVo hearing aids.

Acknowledgements

This chapter makes use of material from the work of the author and his colleagues at University College London, Laryngograph Ltd and at the Fondation Rothschild in Paris. Special thanks are due to V. Ball at UCL, D. Miller at Laryngograph Ltd, Dr E. Fresnel-Elbaz in Paris and Dr Evelyn Abberton.

References

Baken R.J. (1987). *Clinical Measurements of Speech and Voice*. Taylor & Francis.
Colton R.H., Conture G.C. (1990). Problems and pitfalls of electro-glottography. *J. Voice*, **4**, 10–24.
Fabre P. (1957). Un procédé électrique percutané d'inscription de l'accolement glottique au cours de la phonation: glottographie de haute fréquence. Premiers résultats. *Bull. Acad. Nat. Méd.*, **141**, 66–9.
Flanagan J.L. (1972). *Speech Analysis Synthesis and Perception*. Berlin: Springer.
Fourcin A.J. (1981). Laryngographic assessment of phonatory function. In *Proceedings of the Conference on the Assessment of Vocal Pathology* (Ludlow C.L., Hart M.V., eds.) ASHA Reports, 11, pp. 116–27.
Gimson A.C. (1980). *An Introduction to the Pronunciation of English*, 3rd edn. London: Edward Arnold.
Grunwell P. (1987). *Clinical Phonology*. London: Croom Helm.
Hess W. (1983). *Pitch Determination of Speech Signals*. Berlin: Springer.
Howard I.S., Huckvale M.A. (1988). Speech fundamental period estimation using a trainable pattern classifier. *Proceedings of Speech '88* (7th FASE Symposium), Institute of Acoustics, Edinburgh, vol. 1, pp. 129–136.
Hunt M.J. (1987). Studies of glottal excitation using inverse filtering and glottography. *Proceedings of the XIth International Congress of Phonetic Sciences*, Taleinn, vol. 3, pp. 23–6.
International Phonetic Association (1989). Report on the 1989 Kiel Convention. *JIPA*, **19**, 67–80.
Ladefoged P.L. (1982). *A Course in Phonetics*, 2nd edn. London: Harcourt Brace Jovanovich.
Linggard R. (1985). *Electronic Synthesis of Speech*. Cambridge University Press.
Maddieson I. (1984). *Patterns of Sounds*. Cambridge University Press.
Moore B.C.J. (1986). *Frequency Selectivity in Hearing*. London: Academic Press.
Pickett M. (1980). *The Sounds of Speech Communication*. University Park Press.
Schutte H., Seidner W. (1983). Recommendation by the Union of European Phoniatricians (UEP): standardising voice area measurement/phonetography. *Folia Phoniatr.*, **35**, 286–8.
Scott-Brown's Otolaryngology, (1987) Vol. 1, ed. D. Wright. Butterworth-Heinemann.
Wells J.C., Colson G. (1971). *Practical Phonetics*. London: Pitman.
Wells J.C., Barry W., Fourcin A.J. (1989). Transcription, labelling and reference. In *Speech Input and Output Assessment, Multi-lingual Methods and Standards* (Fourcin A.J., Harland G., Barry W., Hazan V., eds.) Chichester: Ellis Horwood, pp. 141–188.

Part Two

Investigation of Voice Problems

Chapter 4

Aids to diagnosis

E. Loebell

The science of phoniatrics is comparatively new in the UK, although it is well established in Europe. Until recently phoniatricians depended mainly on subjective assessment as an aid to diagnosing diseases related to voice. It has been recognized in Europe for the last two decades and in the UK very recently that instrumental studies of speech and voice production allow a more objective and more precise quantification of many features of the process than is possible through purely auditory analysis by the phoniatrician (see Chapter 6). This chapter describes some well-known methods of diagnosing phoniatric problems. It is hoped that these objective techniques will be more commonly used in the 1990s.

Stroboscopy

Electrostroboscopy is useful for the examination of the movements of the vocal folds in the larynx. An electronic flashlight is used, and the fundamental frequency is controlled by use of a contact microphone in the area of the subject's larynx. Figure 4.1 shows the flashes as points in relation to the opening and closing phases of vocal fold movements during phonation. Phase shifting permits observation of the so-called 'still' picture (Figure 4.1a). Figure 4.1b shows the so-called 'moving' stroboscopy, representing a slow-motion version of the real movements.

Electrostroboscopy using a mirror or a microscope permits binocular observation of the larynx. The experienced laryngologist may use the monocular method of endostroboscopy. With the aid of a video camera all examination findings may be transferred to a video screen or videotaped.

Figure 4.2 represents one complete phase of opening and closing of the vocal folds during phonation. These movements are related to aerodynamic function during expiration. The flash points are shown on the right-hand side of the figure. Figure 4.3

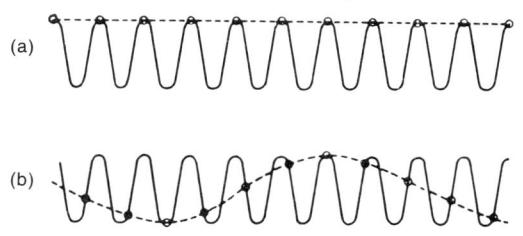

Figure 4.1 Electrostroboscopy: (a) still picture, (b) slow motion

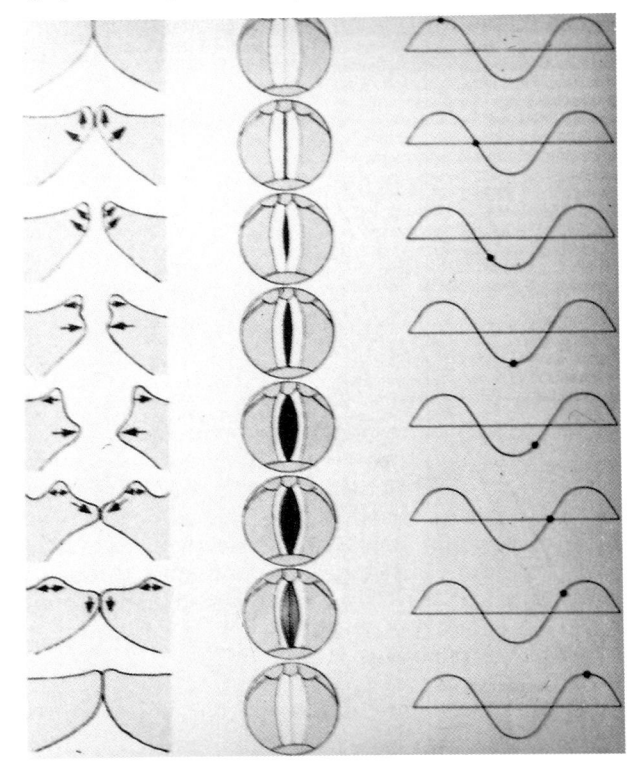

Figure 4.2 Electrostroboscopy showing opening and closing phases of vocal folds

shows, on the left side, the details of the motion of the surface layers superficial to the vocalis muscle. The drawings in the middle and on the right-hand side represent the stroboscopy findings in cases of superficial laryngitis and severe laryngitis respectively.

Electrostroboscopy is extremely important for detection of early carcinoma of the larynx and is useful for detecting organic voice disorders. It is also useful for observation of the vocal functions during or after surgery performed under local anaesthesia.

Electroglottography

The best measurement of the fundamental frequency of the voice is by electroglottography (EGG). Two electrodes are positioned on the neck one each side of the larynx, covering the larynx in an electrical field. The impedance changes may be watched and registered. Use of filters permits recording of both the phonatory changes and the slow movements of the vocal folds and the larynx. Electroglottography is non-invasive and is the only method that permits the simultaneous registration of changes in phonation and articulation. Furthermore, it is very useful for detection of early carcinoma of the vocal fold.

The Danish-made Froekjer-Jensen EGG equipment has an electronic design to

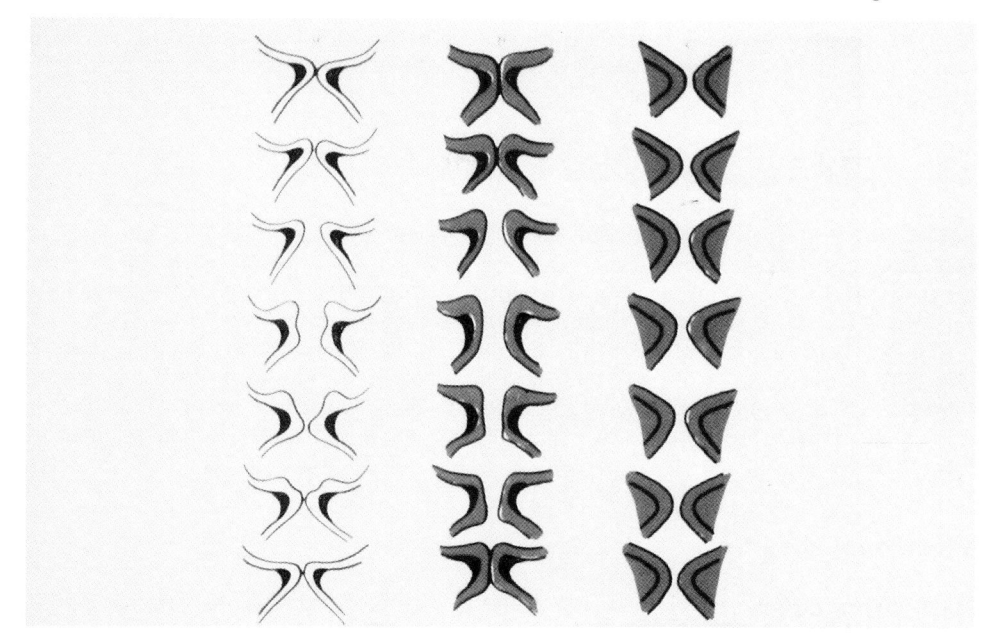

Figure 4.3 Vocal fold movements in health and disease

measure the time from opening to the glottal full wave by means of a quasi-opening quotient. This quotient has proved useful for classification of organic and functional voice disorders. As shown in Figure 4.4, it is possible to differentiate between hypofunctional and hyperfunctional voice disorders.

Objective EGG findings may be taken and documented before and after surgery or voice therapy; EGG may also be used for audiovisual feedback during voice therapy. This technique has proved to be a reliable method of detecting cancer

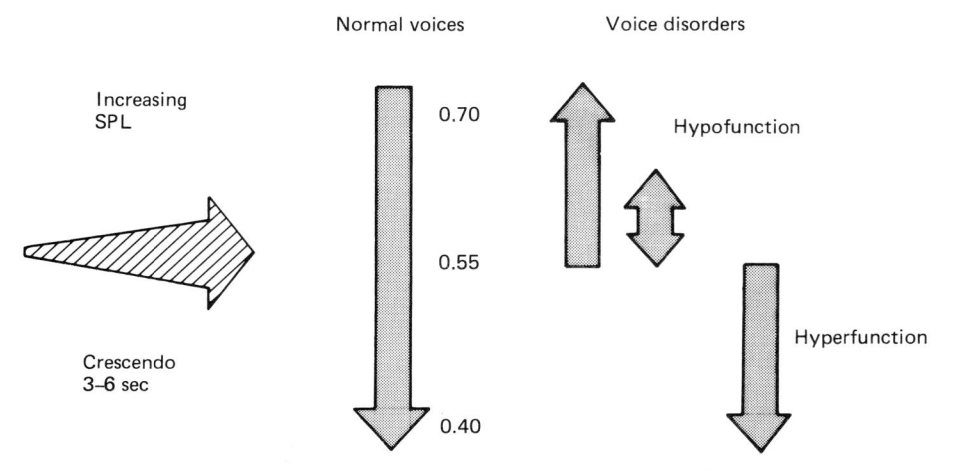

Figure 4.4 Electroglottography to differentiate normal from pathological voice (SPL, sound pressure level)

recurrence after surgery or radiotherapy treatment. In the presence of radiation scars in the larynx it may be the only way of ensuring a realistic follow-up of these patients.

Air pressure measurements

Air pressure measurements may be taken by means of an oesophageal balloon or by direct puncture of the subglottal region. An air pressure transducer is used to record air pressure levels during normal speech of 7–10 mmHg; in the head register or in falsetto voice there is a marked increase of the air pressure levels.

Air pressure measurements are helpful to classify functional voice disorders. A decrease of the air pressure will be found in hyperfunctional voice disorders and an increase in hypofunctional disorders. Organic voice disorders show a marked increase of air pressure in cases of vocal fold paralysis and laryngeal cancer with an immobile vocal fold.

Electromyography

Electromyography may help to determine the differential diagnosis of vocal folds paralysis and ankylosis by puncture of the vocalis or other intrinsic laryngeal muscles. In breathing disorders or stuttering a bipolar electrode can be used, which has to be swallowed into the oesophagus as far as the hiatus of the diaphragm.

Voice range profiles

The voice profiles for the speaking and the shouting voice can be recorded by equipment which picks up the faintest and loudest voice through all possible frequencies of the singing voice.

In a normal voice profile for the singing, speaking and shouting voice, the field for the shouting voice is always situated in the frequencies between chest and head registers. The voice range profile measurements are clinically useful in diagnosis and therapy.

Sonography

Sonography is a commonly used method for acoustic analysis of voice production. Figure 4.5 shows a sonographic analysis of a normal sustained vowel 'a'.

Speech colour transformation

The two-channel 'speech colour transformation' was developed by Esser for speech therapy of hearing-impaired children. By means of colour filters frequencies can be determined by the mixture of colours to be seen on a screen; high frequencies, for instance, appear as the colour blue. This method is very useful as an audiovisual feedback for speech therapy. The therapist may produce a correct 'sss' sound which

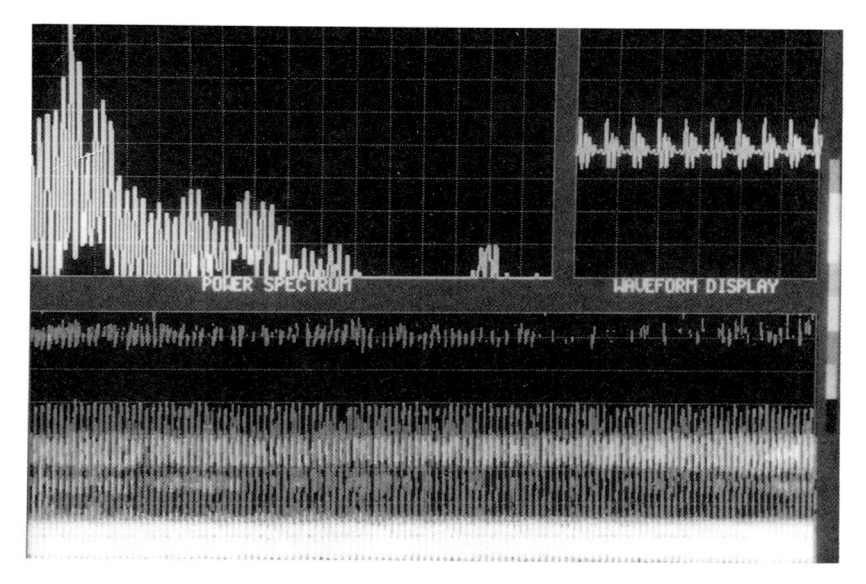

Figure 4.5 Normal sonogram

is represented by the blue colour in the upper channel. The patient may use the lower channel and try to find the correct colour imitation.

In our experience the speech colour transformation system is also suitable for the treatment of motoric articulation disorders.

Conclusion

The methods described in this chapter should be used before and after surgical procedures of the larynx, pharynx and the neck; and also before and after radiotherapy or voice therapy. The documentation is needed for clinical use and particularly for expert opinion.

Chapter 5

The role of computers

W. A. Ainsworth

There are three main areas where computers play a part in the investigation of voice problems. Firstly, they may be used to estimate the fundamental frequency of the voice and its variation; some pathological conditions may be predicted by the irregularity of the fundamental frequency. Secondly, computers may be used to analyse individual glottal pulses; asymmetric vibrations and imperfect closure may be detected in this way. Thirdly, computers may be employed in the administration of speech training exercises and in intelligibility testing, making the results of speech therapy more reliable and easier to assess.

Digitization

The electrical signal obtained when a sound impinges on a microphone is a continuous variable, whereas information is stored in a computer as a set of discrete numbers. In order to analyse a speech signal by computer the sound must first be converted into numbers: this process is known as digitization. It is achieved by sampling the amplitude of the microphone voltage at regular instants in time. The device for doing this is an analogue to digital converter (ADC). The resulting numbers are stored in the memory of the computer and then transferred to disk (Figure 5.1).

The signal is often first recorded on audiotape, but this introduces phase distortions which are deleterious for some voice analysis procedures. It is therefore best to digitize the signal directly if environmental conditions allow. The presence of the computer itself, however, may introduce extraneous noise which will distort the speech signal.

When digitizing a signal two parameters need to be considered: the sampling rate and the quantization level. In order to avoid aliasing (recording an ambiguous signal), the Nyquist theorem states that the sampling rate should be at least twice the highest frequency in the signal. This condition can be satisfied in one of two ways: either the signal can be passed through a low-pass filter with a cut-off frequency of less than half the sampling rate, or the signal can be sampled at more than twice the highest frequency in the unprocessed signal. The former technique is usually employed, but the antialiasing filter may introduce phase distortion. The latter technique may require a very high sampling rate and consequently use much storage for the digitized signal.

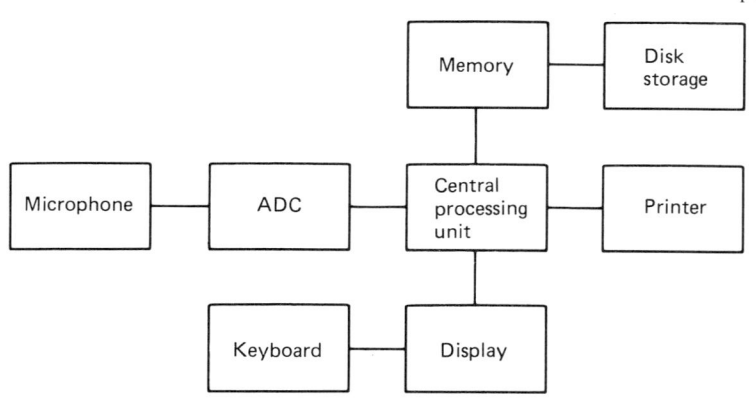

Figure 5.1 Block diagram of the computer system used for investigating voice problems

Voiced speech signals have most of their energy below 5 kHz, so an antialiasing filter with a cut-off of this frequency and a sampling rate of 10 kHz is appropriate. Some speech sounds, however, especially fricatives, have significant energy up to about 10 kHz, so a sampling rate of 20 kHz or greater is required if no filter is employed. These high rates are preferred for some signal processing techniques such as perturbation analysis.

The other parameter which must be considered is the number of quantization levels, or bits, with which to represent each sample of the waveform. If the number of bits is too small quantization noise will be introduced which will distort any further analysis. On the other hand, the larger the number of bits the more storage will be needed and the more processing will be required in any subsequent analysis. In practice it has been found that 8 bits is too small for many forms of speech analysis but that 16 bits is more than adequate. A compromise of 12 bits is usually adopted.

Waveform analysis

Voiced speech sounds are produced by pulses of air from the larynx exciting the resonances of the vocal tract and radiating from the lips (and the nasal tract and nostrils, in the case of nasalized sounds). The signal that is stored in the computer is the waveform of this radiated sound. A typical digitized waveform of a voiced speech sound is shown in the upper part of Figure 5.2. This is the vowel 'a', as in the word 'hard', spoken by a middle-aged male speaker. Note the periodic structure.

If the larynx needs to be removed, other means of voice excitation have to be employed. Figure 5.3 shows the waveform of an 'a' vowel spoken by a male oesophageal speaker of about the same age as the speaker of the vowel in Figure 5.2. The waveform is similar, but less regular.

In parsimonious laryngectomy (near-total laryngectomy with myomucosal valved neoglottis), speech is restored by fashioning a dynamic tracheopharyngeal shunt resulting in neoglottal speech (Singh, 1989). The vibrations of the new voice source are more regular and sustained longer compared with those in oesophageal speech,

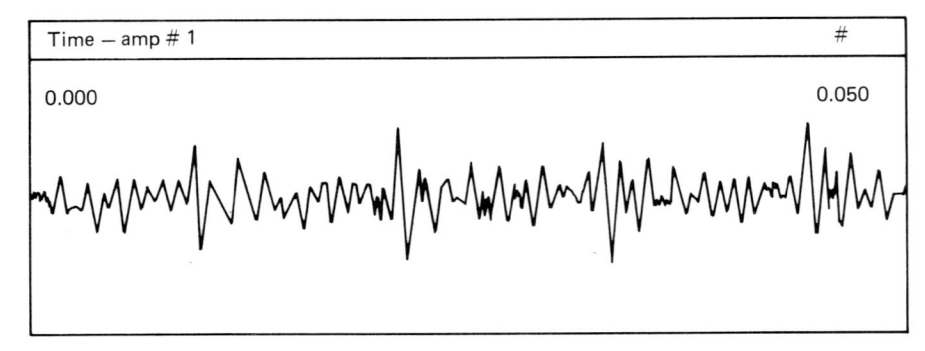

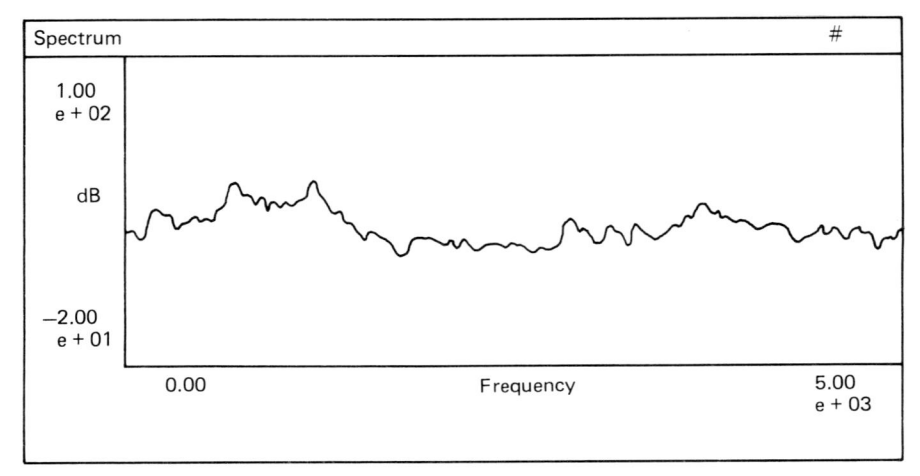

Figure 5.2 Waveform (upper) and spectrum (lower) of the vowel 'a' spoken by a normal male speaker

thus resulting in more intelligible speech (Ainsworth and Singh, 1990). A typical 'a' waveform produced by a male neoglottal speaker is shown in Figure 5.4.

Spectral analysis

Computer programs are made up of procedures consisting of lists of instructions which enable the output data to be calculated from the input data. These procedures are known as algorithms. One such algorithm is the fast Fourier transform (FFT) which produces a representation of the speech known as its spectrum.

The spectra of each vowel are shown in the lower halves of Figures 5.2–5.4. These show the distribution of energy as a function of frequency. The peaks in the spectrum are known as formants and reflect the resonances of the vocal tract. The two highest peaks, at about 700 Hz and 1200 Hz in Figure 5.2, are characteristic of a particular vowel. These are typical of the vowel 'a' in the word 'hard'. The small peak at a lower frequency, in this case at about 200 Hz, is sometimes known as the glottal formant and occurs at the frequency of vibration of the voice sourse. The spectra of oesophageal speech (Figure 5.3) and neoglottal speech (Figure 5.4) lack the glottal formant. Neoglottal speech does, however, show the two major formants which enable vowel sounds to be distinguished from one another.

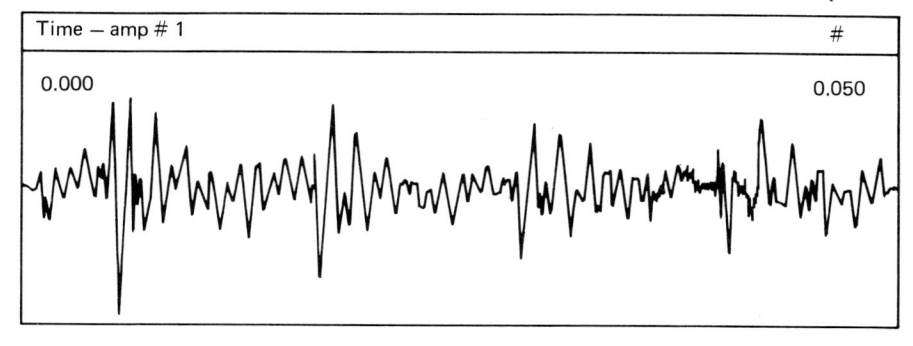

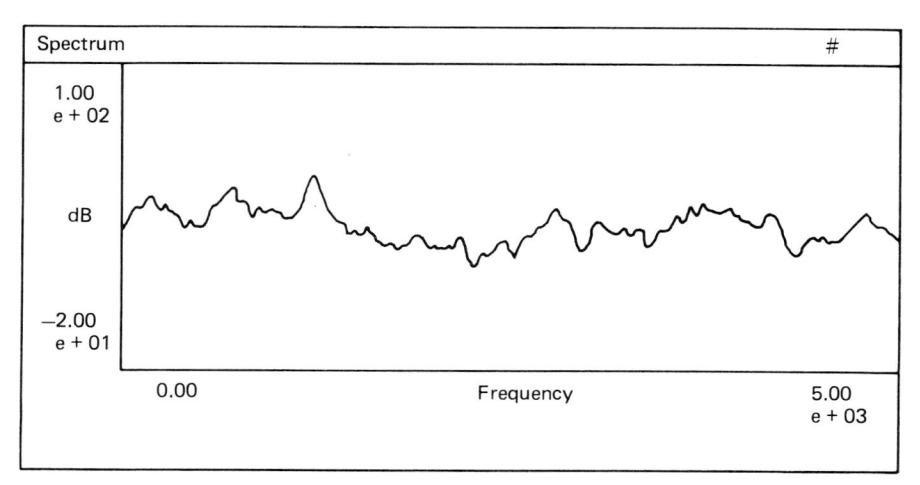

Figure 5.3 Waveform (upper) and spectrum (lower) of the vowel 'a' spoken by a oesophageal male speaker

Fundamental frequency estimation

The waveform shown in Figure 5.2 has a pseudoperiodic structure whose period is determined by the time intervals between the pulses produced by the opening and closing of the glottis. This is sometimes called the glottal period. The fundamental frequency of the voice is the reciprocal of this glottal period, and is the physical quantity corresponding to what is subjectively known as the pitch of the voice.

In normal speech the glottal period varies smoothly, but if there is some malfunctioning of the larynx successive glottal periods are often irregular in duration. It is of interest, therefore, to be able to estimate the fundamental frequency of the voice from the speech waveform.

There are two classes of techniques used for fundamental frequency estimation: frequency analysis and temporal analysis. A comprehensive survey of fundamental frequency estimation techniques is given by Hess (1983).

In frequency analysis the waveform is first transformed into its spectrum, then further processing, such as cepstral analysis (Noll, 1967), is performed to estimate the fundamental frequency. Frequency analysis techniques, however, are not usually appropriate for estimating fundamental frequency as a means of investigating voice problems. An FFT is applied to a section of the speech waveform a few glottal

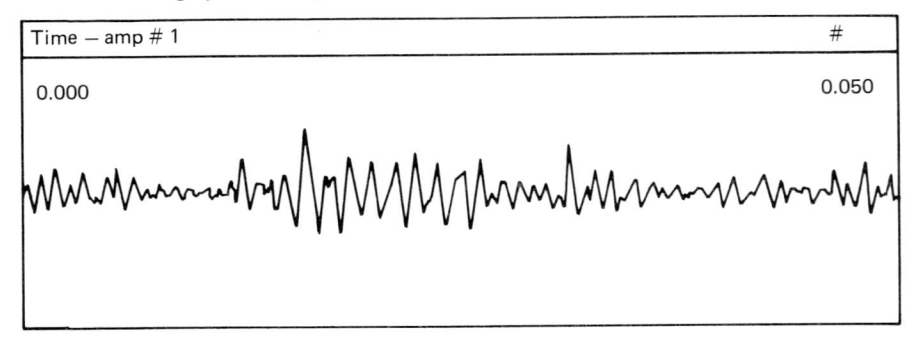

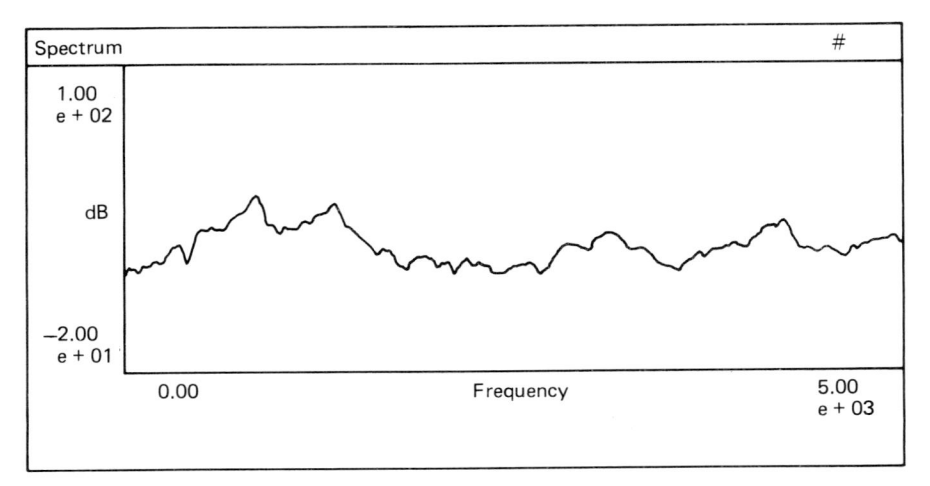

Figure 5.4 Waveform (upper) and spectrum (lower) of the vowel 'a' spoken by a neoglottal male speaker

periods long, and this leads to an estimate of fundamental frequency which is the average of several adjacent periods. For normal speech this increases the accuracy of the estimation, but for abnormal speech this obscures the irregular phonation.

Temporal analysis is therefore more appropriate for investigating voice problems. One of the first of these techniques was described by Gruenz and Schott (1949); this is sometimes known as a 'peak-picking' algorithm because it works by marking the peaks in the waveform. A more sophisticated algorithm based on a generalization of this technique was developed by Gold and Rabiner (1969). This employs six features of the waveform: the amplitudes of both the positive and negative peaks, the differences in amplitude between each peak and the previous one of the same polarity, and the differences in amplitude between each peak and the previous one of opposite polarity. The time intervals between each of these features and the previous occurrence of that feature are measured by an algorithm similar to the peak-picking algorithm outlined above, and the correlations between these time intervals and the previous time intervals are computed. The time interval that gives the highest correlation is then taken to be the duration of the current glottal period.

Many other algorithms have been developed for the estimation of fundamental frequency. These include the simple inverse filter tracking (SIFT) algorithm based on linear prediction analysis (Markel, 1972), and the average magnitude difference function (AMDF) algorithm based on the fact that the difference between a periodic waveform and a delayed version of itself exhibits minima in the difference function at delays equal to the periodicity (Ross et al., 1974). The survey by Hess (1983) describes these and other frequency estimation algorithms.

Perturbation analysis

One of the acoustic features that distinguishes pathological voices from normal is the amount of 'jitter' and 'shimmer' present. Jitter is the irregularity of the durations of successive glottal periods and may be defined as the standard deviation of the durations of successive glottal periods of a sustained vowel spoken on a monotone. Shimmer is the irregularity of the amplitude of the signal in successive glottal periods and may be defined similarly as the standard deviation of the amplitude of the signal from period to period.

For normal voices Horii (1979) found an overall mean jitter of only 36 microseconds. This was for six male voices. With a sampling rate of 40 kHz (i.e. a sampling interval of 25 μs) this kind of measurement becomes inaccurate. One possible technique is to employ an algorithm such as that of Gold and Rabiner (1969) to determine the approximate start of each glottal period, then to insert extra samples around this point by interpolation (such as a parabolic fit around three points) in order to determine the position of the peak more accurately. The alternative is to sample at a higher rate and to bear the consequent extra costs.

For pathological voices, however, the magnitude of the jitter is much greater. Van Michel (1966) reported a mean jitter of 70–570 μs for a sustained 'a' vowel judged perceptually to be pathological, and Smith (1977) found jitter ranging from 0.62 ms to 5.13 ms for sustained vowels produced by oesophageal speakers. Hence a sampling rate of 40 kHz (a sampling interval of 25 μs) should give sufficient temporal resolution for investigating pathological voices.

Glottal pulse shape estimation

In order to investigate some voice problems it is desirable to perform an analysis of the airflow characteristics during individual glottal periods. This can be achieved by a technique known as 'inverse filtering'. Speech production can be modelled by a system in which pulses of air from the larynx are modified by a complex filter representing the action of the vocal tract and the radiation of the sound from the lips. It is, of course, the signal radiating from the lips that is transduced by the microphone, sampled by the analogue to digital converter and stored in the computer. The process of inverse filtering consists of estimating the characteristics of the vocal tract filter, inverting it, then passing the speech signal through this inverted filter in order to obtain a signal from which the glottal airflow can be estimated.

Each glottal period consists of an open phase, during which air flows through the glottis, and a closed phase, during which the vocal folds are together. During this closed phase there is no input to the vocal tract so the column of air inside performs a free oscillation. By measuring the resonances of this oscillation the characteristics of the vocal tract filter can be estimated. This is normally done by linear prediction analysis (Markel and Gray, 1976).

Linear prediction is a technique for predicting the value of the next point in a sampled waveform given the values of the immediate past samples and a set of linear prediction coefficients (LPC). The coefficients are computed in such a way that the difference between the predicted waveform and the measured sample points is minimized. One form of linear prediction analysis, known as covariance method, can be applied to a small part of the waveform. In fact it requires just twice as many points as there are resonances in the waveform. As speech contains no more than five or six significant formants (Figure 5.2), the covariance method can be applied with 10 or 12 sample points. In male speech the average value of the fundamental frequency is about 120 Hz so the duration of a glottal period is some 8 ms. If the vocal folds are together for half of the glottal period the duration of the closed phase will be 4 ms. If the waveform is sampled at 10 kHz, 40 points are available for LPC calculations. In the case of female speech the fundamental frequency is at least an octave higher, so the number of closed-phase sample points available at any given frequency is halved. In addition the glottal waveform of female speech is more sinusoidal so the duration of the closed phase is further reduced (Lobo and Ainsworth, 1988). The number of points available for closed-phase analysis is scarcely sufficient at a sampling frequency of 10 kHz.

Once the linear prediction coefficients have been computed, the characteristics of the vocal tract filter can be estimated. The filter is then inverted with resonances (poles) changed to antiresonances (zeros) and vice versa. The original speech waveform is then passed through this inverted filter. This effectively cancels out the formants. The new signal is integrated to remove the effects of lip radiation, and the resulting waveform represents the air flow as a function of time through the vocal folds.

This technique only gives valid results if the position of the closed phase is correctly located. In practice it is necessary to choose the portion of the waveform for closed-phase analysis that gives the minimum ripple in the closed phase of the resulting glottal air flow waveform.

Aids to diagnosis

One of the potential advantages of using computers for investigating voice problems is that they present the possibility of aiding the diagnosis of various voice conditions. They can do this in two ways: data display and pattern recognition.

One way of characterizing the variation in a voice is by means of a time interval histogram. If a passage is read aloud and the duration of each glottal period of voiced speech is measured, the intervals can be sorted into bins and the number of intervals in each bin can be plotted. The resulting distribution shows the modal frequency of the voice and its range; the greater the range, the wider the distribution.

A similar display can be used to estimate the amount of jitter in a voice. A steady vowel spoken on a monotone is produced, then a time interval histogram is computed as above. The width of the distribution reflects the amount of jitter in the voice.

Another useful display is one that shows the digram statistics of the voice. The durations of every glottal period of a phrase are estimated as above, but instead of calculating a histogram from the intervals, the duration of the first period is plotted as the abscissa and the duration of the second period as the ordinate of an x–y display. The process is repeated, plotting the second period against the third, and so on. The result is a digram display. If the voice is regular a single diagonal line results, but if the voice is irregular a different pattern, symmetric about the diagonal, is obtained. If the glottal periods are random a scatter of points about the centre of the display is made, but if there is some structure more regular patterns are produced. For example, if the voice consists of alternating long and short glottal periods, two diverging lines are produced.

There appears to be some potential in using computers in dysphonic voice screening. The idea is that patients who are referred to hospital consultants for further investigation could be given immediately a simple test which involved speaking into a computer. The computer could analyse their voices and decide whether they required an urgent consultation. In this way patients with serious, progressive voice pathologies could be seen and treated quickly in preference to those requiring less urgent treatment.

The problem lies in deciding what measurements should be made during the screening process and what criteria should be used to decide that immediate treatment is necessary. Laver et al. (1984) investigated four measures of jitter and shimmer: (a) mean, (b) standard deviation, (c) rate (percentage of points in the sample where the magnitude of the excursion is equal to or greater than 3% of the trend value), and (d) directional perturbation factor (DPF), the percentage of changes in sign in the excursion values (Hecker and Kreul, 1971). The best single measure was found to be shimmer DPF. Using a criterion of 2 or more standard deviations from the mean value of a group of normal controls, about 60% of a mixed group of voice pathologies were detected using this measure with only about 3% false positives (normal voices wrongly detected as pathological).

Voice pathologies, however, manifest themselves in many different forms so it is unlikely that a single measure would be sufficient to separate all pathological from normal subjects. Laver et al. (1984) showed that better discrimination between pathological and normal voices maybe obtained from a two-dimensional plot of shimmer DPF versus mean fundamental frequency. Research is in progress to see if better discrimination can be obtained if more measures are employed and more complex pattern recognition algorithms are used.

Rehabilitation

After surgery or other treatment, speech therapy is often employed to try to restore the voice to a normal condition. There is a potential role for computers in automating this process. Instead of dealing with one patient at a time, the therapist could select a computer program and leave the patient with the computer while dealing with the next patient. The program could present on screen the words that the patient needs to practise. The words could be presented in different orders, or randomly, and could be interspersed with messages or graphics in order to motivate the patients and retain their attention. It might be useful to employ a speech synthesizer for this purpose.

In research it is often necessary to compare the effectiveness of one technique with another. Research is being carried out on various aspects of newer surgical voice restoration procedures at the voice research laboratory at St John's Hospital, Livingston, Scotland, in collaboration with the Department of Communication and Neuroscience of the University of Keele. One of the goals of laryngeal surgery is to restore or retain intelligible speech. The only objective way to ensure that this has been achieved is to ask the patient to record lists of words or phrases, which a panel of listeners then attempts to identify. Many word lists have been proposed for investigating hearing problems (Egan, 1948; House et al., 1965; Voiers, 1977; Foster and Haggard, 1979), and some of these are also useful for investigating voice problems. One such word list is the modified rhyme test (House et al., 1965). This test has the advantage that it can be administered by computer. It consists of ten lists of 20 groups of words. Each group contains six monosyllabic words which differ only in their first consonant (e.g. ten, pen, den, fen, when, wren). Lists are assembled by choosing a rhyming word at random from each group, and having the speaker read them out. This process can be controlled by a computer. The program chooses one of the words and displays it on the screen. The speaker articulates each word as it appears. The test is administered by playing a recording of the spoken words synchronized with a computer program which displays all six words on the screen just before the recording of one of them is played; the listener is required to decide which word has been spoken and to press the appropriate key.

This technique makes it easy to ascertain which consonants are being confused. This is done by means of a confusion matrix. The rows are labelled with the consonants spoken and the columns with the consonants heard. Each cell in the matrix contains the number of responses to a particular stimulus. Ideally there should be non-zero entries in the diagonal and zero everywhere else. Any deviations from this can be quickly spotted, and the effectiveness of different techniques can be compared. The construction of confusion matrices by hand is a time-consuming business, so the use of a computer is recommended.

Conclusion

Computers have a number of uses in the investigation of voice problems. The major use at present is in research into normal and abnormal functioning of the larynx. With increasing knowledge it is expected that the techniques currently being developed will be adapted to provide effective tools for the rapid diagnosis of voice problems.

References

Ainsworth W., Singh W. (1990). Analysis of fundamental frequency and temporal characteristics of neoglottal, esophageal and normal speech. *Proc. Inst. Acoust.*, **12**, 25–32.
Egan J.P. (1948). Articulation testing methods. *Laryngoscope*, **58**, 955–91.
Foster J.R., Haggard M.P. (1979). FAAF — an efficient analytical test of speech perception. *Inst. Acoust. Autumn Conf.*, 9–12.
Gold B., Rabiner L.R. (1969). Parallel processing techniques for estimating pitch periods of speech in the time domain. *J. Acoust. Soc. Am.*, **46**, 442–8.
Gruenz O.O., Schott L.O. (1949). Extraction and portrayal of pitch of speech sounds. *J. Acoust. Soc. Am.*, **21**, 487–95.
Hecker M., Kreul E. (1971). Descriptions of the speech of patients with cancer of the vocal folds. Part 1: Measures of fundamental frequency. *J. Acoust. Soc. Am.*, **49**, 1275–82.
Hess W. (1983). *Pitch Determination of Speech Signals.* Berlin: Springer.
Horii Y. (1979). Fundamental frequency perturbation observed in sustained phonation. *J. Acoust. Soc. Am.*, **66** (A), S65.
House A.S., Williams C.E., Hecker M.H.L., Kryter K.D. (1965). Articulation testing methods: consonantal discrimination with a closed-response set. *J. Acoust. Soc. Am.*, **29**, 487–95.

Laver J., Hiller S., Mackenzie J. (1984). Acoustic analysis of vocal fold pathology. *Proc. Inst. Acoust.*, **6**, 425–30.

Lobo A.P., Ainsworth W.A. (1988). Variation of glottal pulse shape with fundamental frequency. *Proceedings of the 7th FASE Symposium*, Edinburgh, **2**, pp. 217–24.

Markel J.D. (1972). The SIFT algorithm for fundamental frequency estimation. *IEEE Trans.*, **AU-20**, 154–60.

Markel J.D., Gray A.H. (1976). *Linear Prediction of Speech*. Berlin: Springer.

Noll A.M. (1967). Cepstrum pitch determination. *J. Acoust. Soc. Am.*, **41**, 293–309.

Ross M.J., Shaffer H.L., Cohen A. et al. (1974). Average magnitude difference function pitch extractor. *IEEE Trans.*, **ASSP-22**, 353–61.

Singh W. (1989). Near total laryngectomy. In *Proceedings of the International Voice Symposium*, Edinburgh (Singh W., ed.) pp. 53–58.

Smith S.L. (1977). Electroglottography. In *Proceedings of the XVIIth International Congress of the International Association of Logopedics and Phoniatrics*, Copenhagen.

Van Michel C. (1966). Mouvements glottiques phonatoires sans émission sonore. Etudes electroglottographique. *Folia Phoniatr.*, **18**, 1–8.

Voiers W.D. (1977). Diagnostic evaluation of speech intelligibility. In *Benchmark Papers in Acoustics*, vol. II: *Speech Intelligibility and Speaker Recognition* (Hawley M., ed.) Stroudsburg: Dowden, Hutchinson & Ross, pp. 374–87.

Chapter 6

The voice research laboratory in clinical practice

W. Singh and G. McKenna

Laboratory-based studies of speech can be divided into two separate (though related) types: the clinically oriented and the research oriented. These two undertakings have different goals and different time-scales. Research is fundamentally a long-term undertaking which in the case of the voice laboratory at St John's Hospital, Livingston, involves a series of experiments under controlled conditions, the aim of which is to provide a body of knowledge concerning a particular aspect of voice and speech, in this case alaryngeal speech. Such experimentation requires time to be assessed and evaluated in relation to previous research.

Clinically oriented investigations, on the other hand, require a much shorter time-scale, typically requiring on-the-spot analysis of some aspect of speech for diagnostic or assessment purposes. This can only be done reliably after a great deal of experience with a wide range of examples of the problems which are being investigated, as well as of previous findings in the field. Typically, such investigations should follow on from the more general type of research outlined above. It should then be possible to apply research findings to derive clinical procedures which can be carried out on a day-to-day basis. This must be done by a clinician and a researcher in cooperation, taking account both of clinical requirements and of the restrictions on the amount and type of information that can reasonably be provided in a clinical setting.

Diagnosis and assessment

The distinction between diagnosis and assessment is important. *Diagnosis* involves the use of instrumental techniques to ascertain the cause and nature of a speech pathology. *Assessment*, on the other hand, involves the measuring of various speech parameters in patients whose speech problem has already been diagnosed.

The following sections describe several instrumental techniques that are being used in our research studies on alaryngeal speech, and specifically on the characteristics of *neoglottal* speech (Singh, 1985, 1989, 1991, 1992). The assumption underlying this chapter is that instrumental studies of speech and voice production allow a more objective and more precise quantification of many features of the process than is possible through purely auditory analysis by the clinician. It is hoped that these analysis techniques will therefore be seen to be widely applicable in the field of speech pathology research.

Speech production and the limitations of instrumental investigation

Speech is produced by a complex interaction between three functionally separate components: *respiration* (which provides the air stream), *phonation* (by which the vocal folds make this air stream audible) and *articulation* (by which the basic tone produced by the vocal folds is modified by the tongue, lips and soft palate to form the vowel and consonant sounds which make up speech).

These various components of speech can be investigated using a number of laboratory-based experimental techniques, at a number of different stages in the process. Attention can be directed, for example, to the acoustic features of speech, as in *sound spectrography* or *phonetography*; to the movements of the vocal organs that give rise to these acoustic features, as in *electrolaryngography* or *stroboscopy*; or even to the neurophysiological stage of the process, as in *electromyography*.

Given the complexity of speech production, each particular method of analysis can only focus on a portion of the total process at a time; no single instrumental technique can provide a complete account of the production of even a single sound. These limitations must be borne in mind when the results of instrumental investigations are being interpreted. Electrolaryngography, for example, provides information *only* about the functioning of the vocal folds (or other voicing source), and nothing at all concerning the activities of the supralaryngeal vocal tract. Sound spectrography provides a wealth of acoustic information from which much can be inferred about the movements of the articulatory organs, though it gives no direct information about such movements. Phonetography, another acoustic technique, deals only with the fundamental frequency and intensity characteristics of speech, not with the supralaryngeal organs. Stroboscopy is another technique which focuses almost exclusively on vocal fold activity — both in the transverse and vertical axis.

Electrolaryngography

Four different types of glottography (electrolaryngography, photoglottography, glottography by inverse filtering and ultrasound glottography) are generally recognized. In the St John's Hospital voice research laboratory electrolaryngography (electroglottography) is used in clinical practice and for research.

Electrolaryngography (Abberton and Fourcin, 1984; Fourcin, 1986; Singh, 1987, 1988, 1989; Abberton at al., 1989; Hacki, 1989; Motta et al., 1990; Singh and Ainsworth, 1992) allows the investigation of voicing source activity by means of two electrodes which are placed superficially on the neck at the level of the voicing source; either the vocal folds for normal speakers, or the pharyngo-oesophageal segment or the neoglottis for alaryngeal speakers. A small current of 3–5 milliamperes is passed between these electrodes and the resistance offered by the soft tissue in the neck to this current is measured by the laryngograph. When the vocal folds are open, resistance is high; when they are closed, resistance is low (Figure 6.1). This time-varying resistance can then be displayed either on an oscilloscope or on the computer monitor (for those systems which include the appropriate software) and can be printed or stored on a disk (Figure 6.2). This trace is known as the L_x trace, and provides a non-invasive record of voicing source activity.

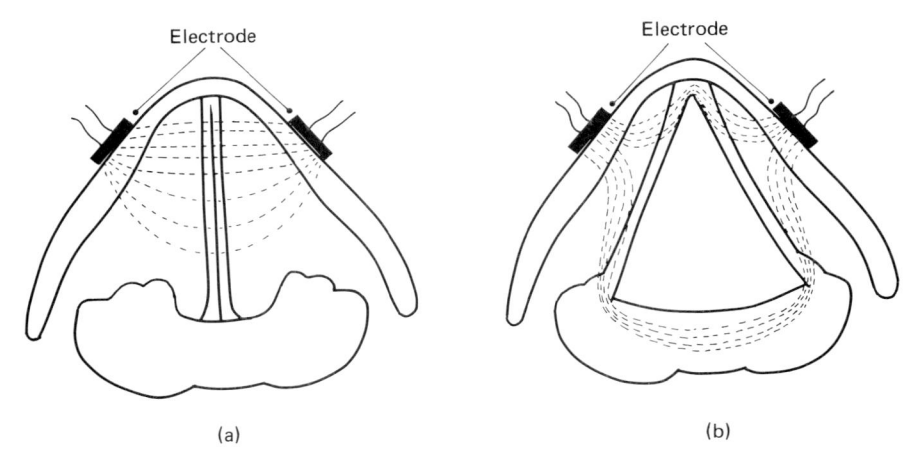

72 Functional Surgery of the Larynx and Pharynx

Figure 6.1 Passage of electric current through the glottis: (a) vocal folds in the closed position; (b) vocal folds fully apart. From Singh (1988), reproduced by kind permission of the editor of the *Journal of Laryngology and Otology*

L_x displays

Figure 6.3 shows an example of the kind of traces that are produced by the electrolaryngograph. These traces were produced by male subject, aged 57 years, while pronouncing the vowel 'ah'. The top trace shows the acoustic signal picked up by a microphone placed 30 cm from the speaker's mouth, while the bottom trace shows the L_x wave picked up by the electrodes at the speaker's larynx. Each peak in the L_x waveform corresponds to a complete closure of the vocal folds; each trough corresponds to the open phase. Each cycle of the wave corresponds to one complete opening and closing cycle of the vocal folds.

In Figure 6.3, the duration of the various phases of vocal fold vibration have been marked using five vertical line cursors. This clearly shows the difference in duration

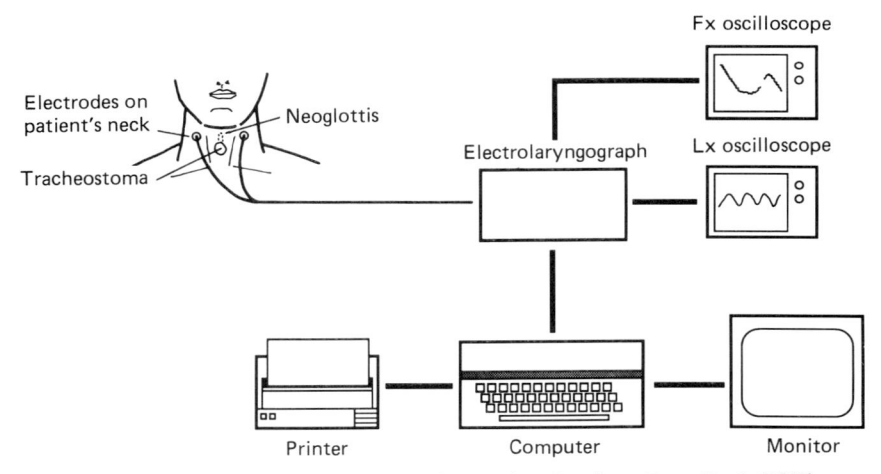

Figure 6.2 Recording the L_x and F_x waveforms of a neoglottal patient. From Singh (1988), reproduced by kind permission of the editor of the *Journal of Laryngology and Otology*

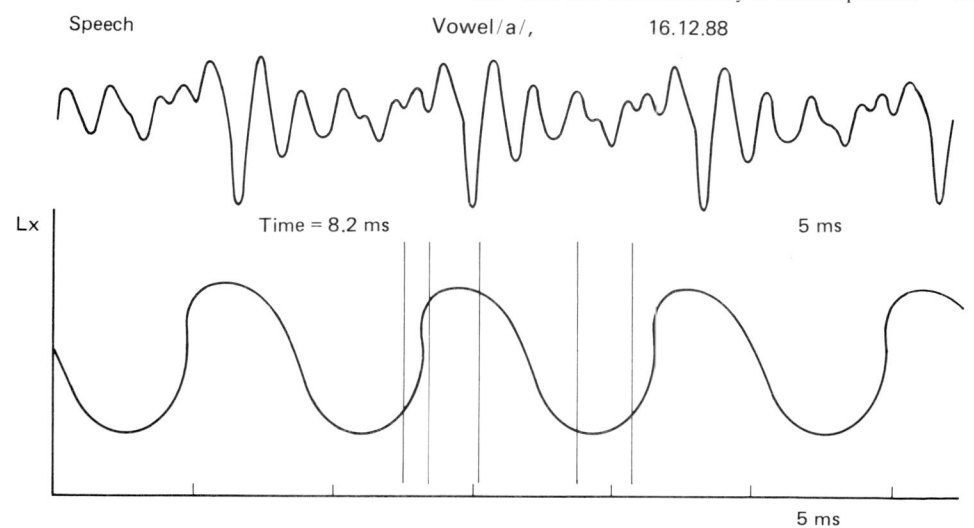

Figure 6.3 L_x and speech waveforms produced by a normal male speaker, aged 57 years, during a sustained vowel 'ah'. Note the correlation between the peaks in the L_x trace and those in the speech waveform

between the closing and opening phases. The normal waveform shows a relatively steep closing phase, when compared to the more gradual opening phase. This indicates that the vocal folds are coming together relatively quickly, but peeling apart more gradually, as predicted by the aerodynamic–myoelastic theory of vocal fold vibration. The number in the centre of the display is the duration of one complete cycle of vocal fold vibration, in this case 8.2 ms. It is clear that there is also a high correlation between the peak in the L_x waveform and the point of maximum acoustic excitation of the vocal tract on the speech waveform (shown by the point of maximum amplitude).

Figure 6.4 shows an example of the traces produced by 63-year-old female subject, again during production of the vowel 'ah'. Although the time-scale on Figures 6.3 and 6.4 is the same, there are far more cycles of vibration on the L_x trace produced by the female speaker, indicating that this speaker's vocal folds are vibrating at a faster rate than those of the male speaker above. For the female speaker, one complete cycle of vibration is completed in only 4.5 ms, just over half the time taken by the male speaker.

Figure 6.5 shows an example of the traces produced by a male neoglottal speaker, aged 61 years, this time during a sustained 'ee' vowel. While this speaker's L_x trace is quite clear, it is also more symmetrical than that produced by the normal male speaker in Figure 6.3, indicating that for the neoglottal speaker the closing and opening phases of the vibratory cycle of the neoglottis are more similar in duration, while the duration of one cycle of vibration is 5.7 ms, intermediate between the values shown by the normal male and female above. There is also a high degree of correlation between the L_x peaks and the peaks in the speech waveform.

D_x displays

The rate of vibration of the vocal folds is more usually known as the *fundamental frequency* (measured in cycles per second or hertz), and is the main physiological

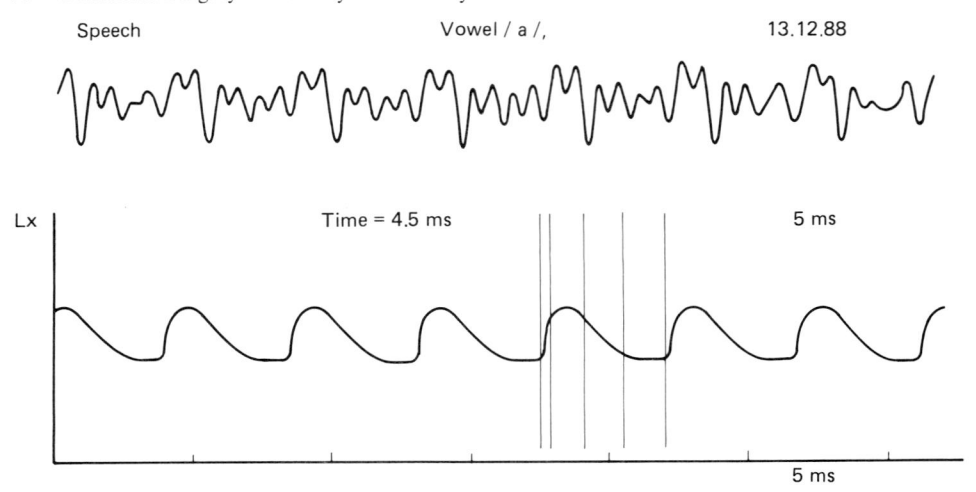

74 Functional Surgery of the Larynx and Pharynx

Figure 6.4 L_x and speech waveforms produced by a normal female speaker, aged 63 years, during a sustained vowel 'ah'

correlate of what the listener perceives as the speaker's pitch. The L_x wave can also be used to calculate the fundamental frequency (F_0) of the speaker's voice during the course of an utterance. While the fundamental frequency fluctuates continuously during speech, it does so within certain limits imposed by the speaker's vocal physiology, and also by his or her habitual preference (see below). Differences in mean F_0 during speech are a major factor distinguishing male and female speakers, for example.

The long-term average fundamental frequency, as well as the range of fundamental frequencies used by the speaker, can be plotted in a distribution histogram of the type shown in Figure 6.6. This shows a typical distribution produced by a

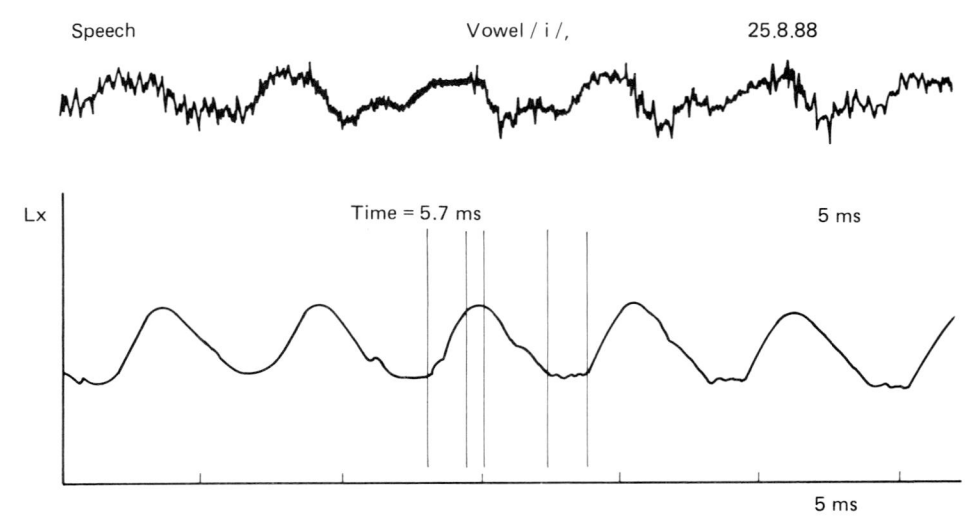

Figure 6.5 L_x and speech waveforms produced by a male neoglottal speaker, aged 61 years, during a sustained vowel 'ee'

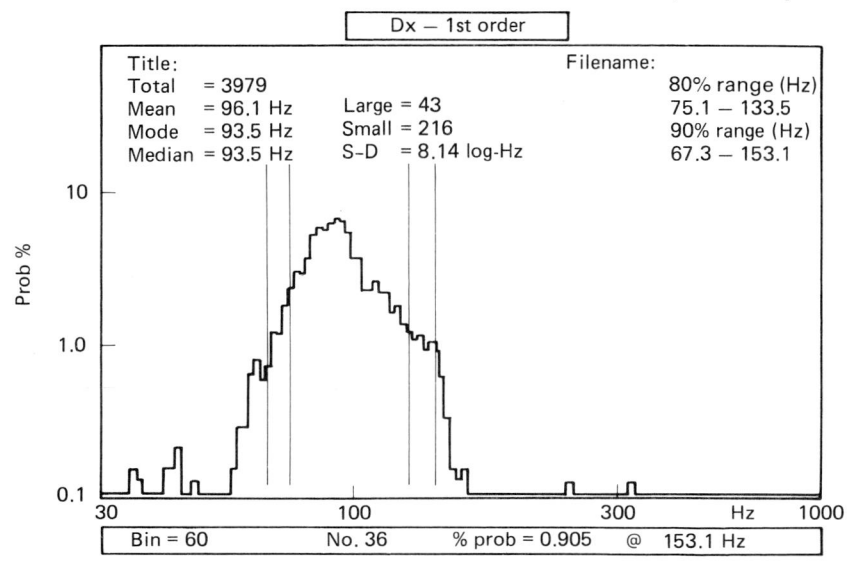

Figure 6.6 Fundamental frequency distribution histogram produced by a normal male speaker, aged 57 years; first order

57-year-old male speaker while reading the first paragraph of the Rainbow passage (Fairbanks, 1940). The central tendency of the distribution is shown by a very clear peak, with a modal frequency of 93.5 Hz, while the width of the main distribution shows the range of frequencies produced by the speaker during this task. The 80% and 90% ranges are also marked by four vertical line cursors.

The numbers at the top of the display provide more accurate quantification of these variables. Central tendency is shown by the mean, mode and median; while range is shown both by the standard deviation of F_0, and by the 80% and 90% ranges. So for this speaker the vocal folds vibrate at around 93 Hz (i.e. 93 times per second), although this can be as low as 67 Hz or as high as 153 Hz. The other figures show the total number of vocal fold cycles which were registered during this task, as well as the number which were calculated to fall outside the 30–1000 Hz limit of the laryngograph.

Figure 6.7 shows the second-order D_x distribution for the same speaker, which is calculated by using only those vocal fold cycles whose frequencies fall into the same histogram bin (i.e. only those whose frequency is relatively close). Periods of voicing where F_0 is not changing in a smooth fashion are therefore removed, as are artefacts caused by movement of the electrodes.

Figures 6.8 and 6.9 show the first and second order distributions produced by a male neoglottal speaker, again based on a reading of the Rainbow passage. This speaker clearly shows a modal F_0 of around 157 Hz, while F_0 ranges from around 75 Hz to 218 Hz. This speaker's F_0 is therefore somewhat higher than that of the normal male shown in Figures 6.6 and 6.7, and the range of F_0 movement is also wider, especially at the upper end.

The D_x distributions can be related to Figures 6.10 and 6.11, which show a plot of F_0 by time for these speakers, while producing the first and second sentences of the Rainbow passage. Clearly, while F_0 rises and falls continuously during these sentences, it does so within clearly defined limits (for the normal speaker, roughly

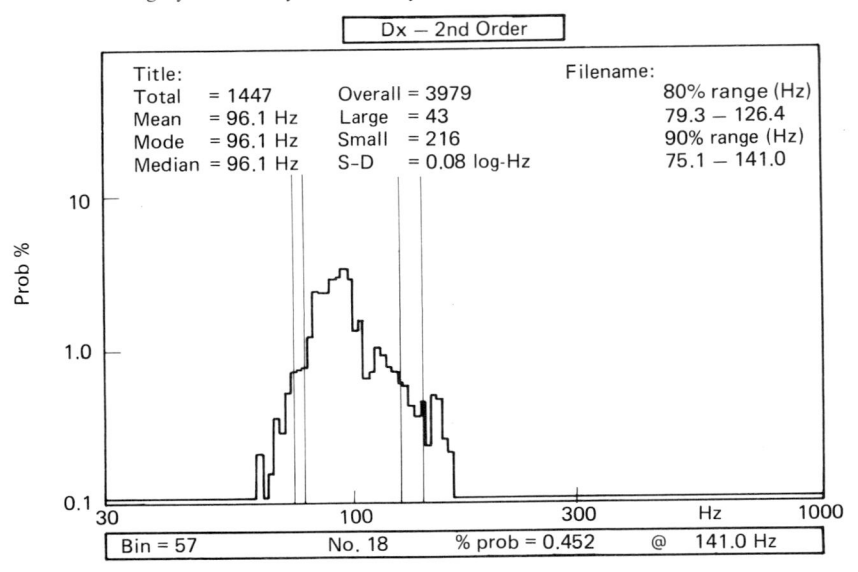

76 Functional Surgery of the Larynx and Pharynx

Figure 6.7 Fundamental frequency distribution histogram produced by a normal male speaker, aged 57 years; second order

60–160 Hz; for the neoglottal speaker, 90–190 Hz). Isolated cycles of vibration whose frequencies fall outside these limits are filtered out by second-order processing.

Figures 6.12 and 6.13 show another way of examining the data, this time with a view to determining the regularity of F_0 vibration. In this type of plot, the frequency of each cycle is plotted against that of the preceding cycle. In voices where F_0 is

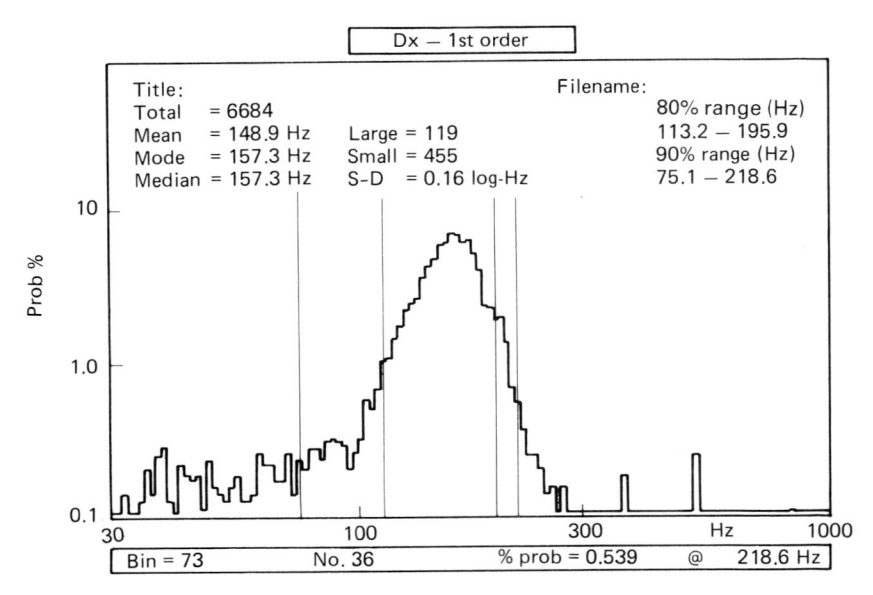

Figure 6.8 Fundamental frequency distribution histogram produced by a male neoglottal speaker, aged 59 years; first order

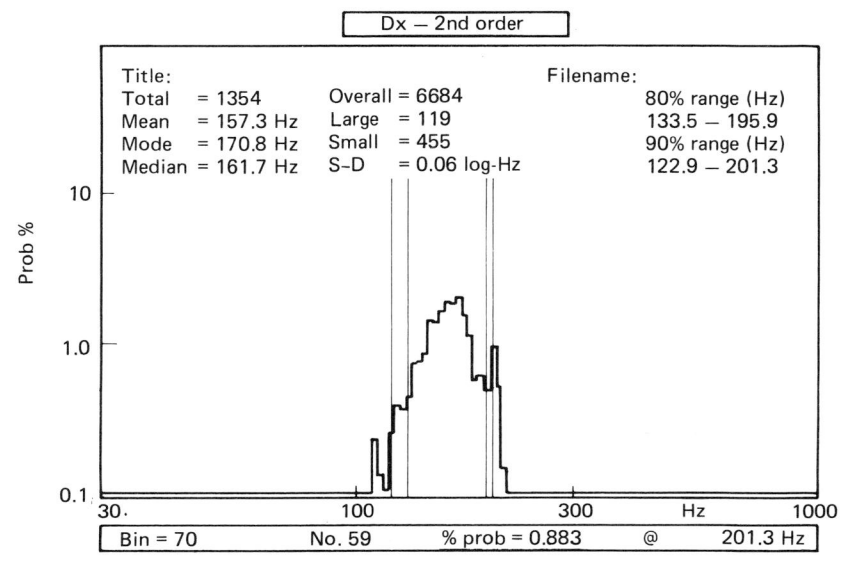

Figure 6.9 Fundamental frequency distribution histogram produced by a male neoglottal speaker, aged 59 years; second order

changing in a smooth fashion, there will be a concentration of points along the diagonal, with relatively little scatter around this group. The position of the main group along the diagonal is determined by the speaker's long-term average F_0. The

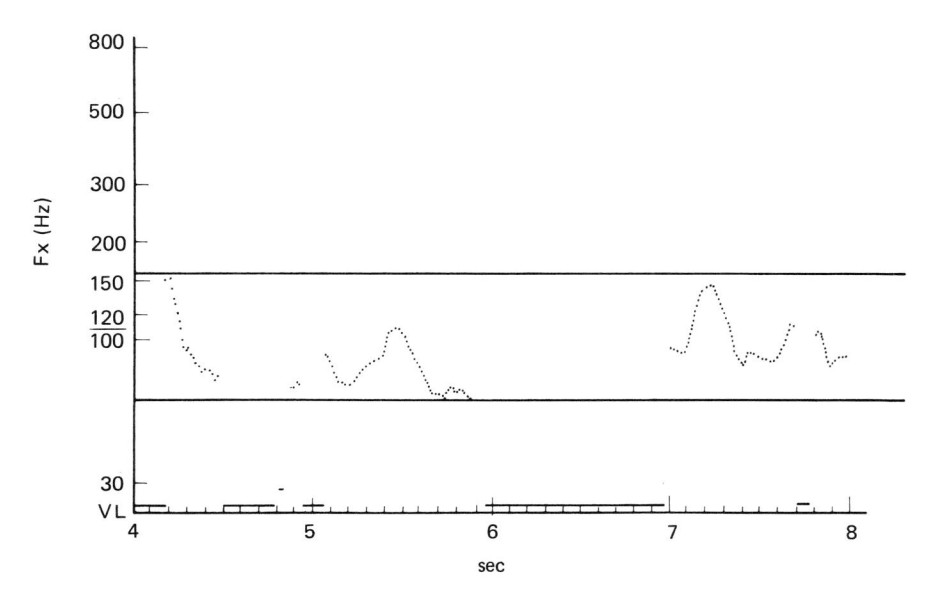

Figure 6.10 Fundamental frequency contour produced by a normal male speaker, aged 57 years, taken from the first paragraph of the Rainbow passage. The approximate upper and lower ranges of the speaker's fundamental frequency are marked by two horizontal lines. Note the isolated points which fall outside this limit and which will be filtered out by second-order processing

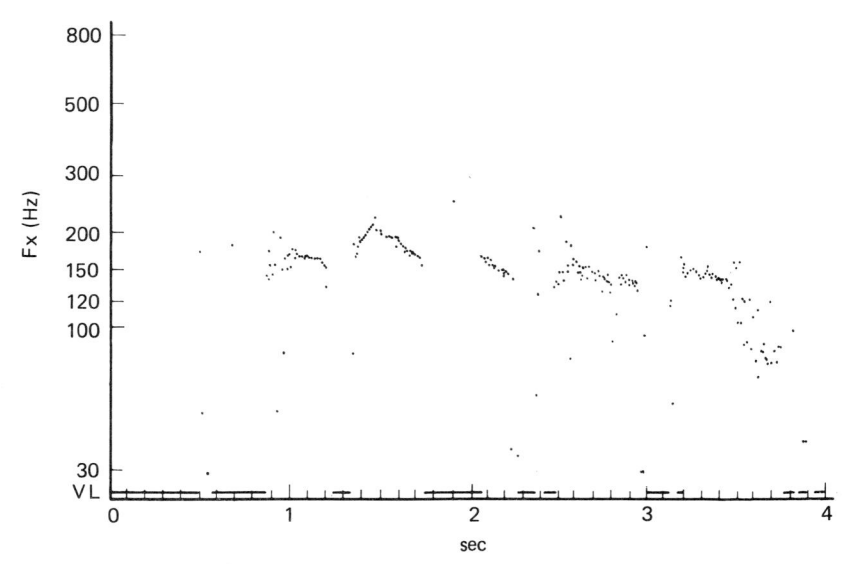

78   Functional Surgery of the Larynx and Pharynx

Figure 6.11 Fundamental frequency contour produced by a male neoglottal speaker, aged 59 years, taken from the first paragraph of the Rainbow passage

main group in the neoglottal speaker's plot is thus nearer the middle of the diagonal than that of the normal speaker, indicating the neoglottal speaker's high pitch. For the neoglottal speaker there is also a greater degree of scatter around the main

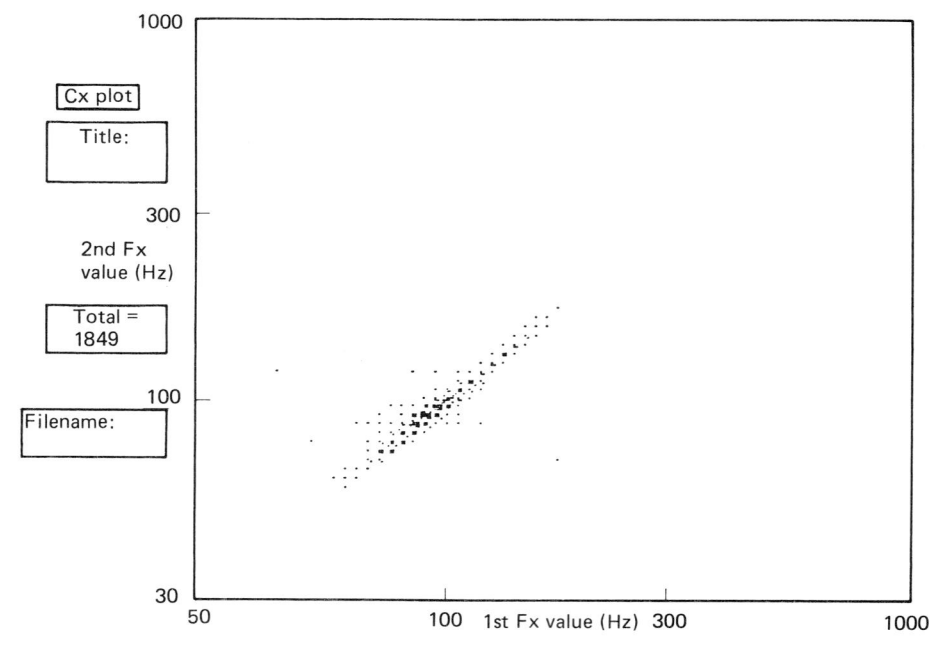

Figure 6.12 The frequency of each cycle of vibration plotted against that of the previous cycle for a normal male speaker, aged 57 years; note the concentration of points along the diagonal

group, indicating a less smooth transition from cycle to cycle than is the case for the normal speaker. This can also be seen by comparing the relative smoothness of the curves in Figures 6.10 and 6.11.

F_x displays

The F_x display provides a way of examining the *pattern* of F_0 movement during speech, in a similar fashion to Figure 6.11, but in this case over a much shorter period of time, with simultaneous display of the F_0 pattern on the screen (F_x is the term used for the pattern registered by the laryngograph, and can be considered to be equivalent to F_0). This facility can be used to assess the speaker's ability to control the direction of F_0 movement. In Figure 6.14, the speaker (a 57-year-old male) was asked to imitate four F_0 patterns, while pronouncing the vowel 'ah': a rise, a fall, a rise–fall, and a fall–rise. This allows us to assess not only whether the speaker can control the direction of F_0, but also whether he can change the direction of F_0.

Movements of F_0 of this kind are important in a number of ways in speech. A rising F_0 can be used to distinguish phrases intended as questions (e.g. 'John's coming tonight?') from phrases intended as statements of fact (e.g. 'John's coming tonight'), which are typically pronounced with a falling F_0. Also, F_0 movement is one of the factors that distinguish such phrases as '*black*board' (as found in the classroom) from 'black *board*' (a board that is black). The F_0 patterns produced during the reading of the Rainbow passage (see Figure 6.11) are due to a combination of these kind of movements.

Clearly, the ability of the alaryngeal speaker to produce such F_0 movements will

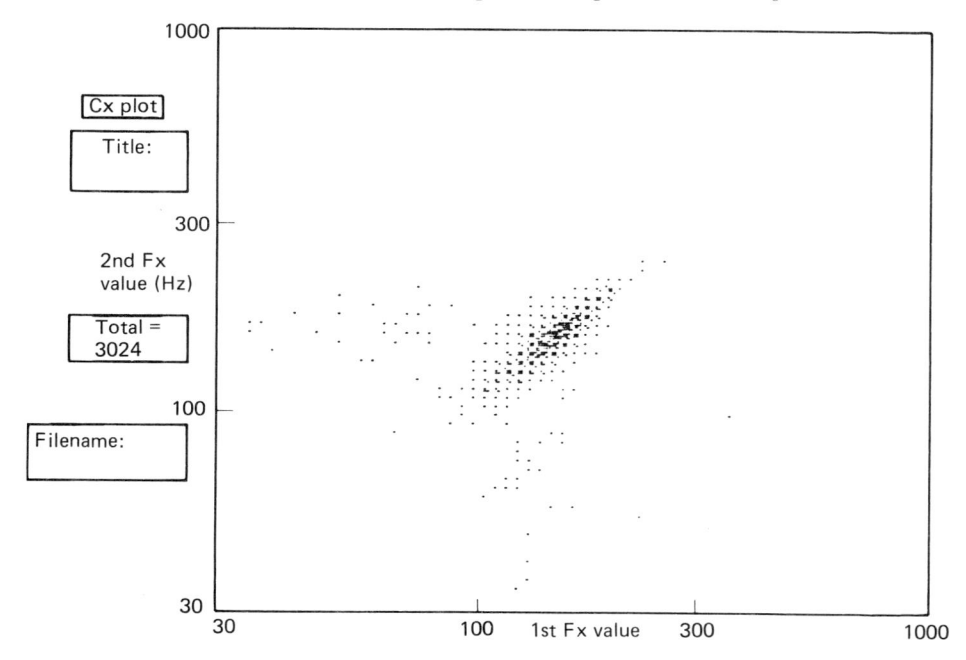

Figure 6.13 The frequency of each cycle of vibration plotted against that of the previous cycle for a male neoglottal speaker, aged 59 years

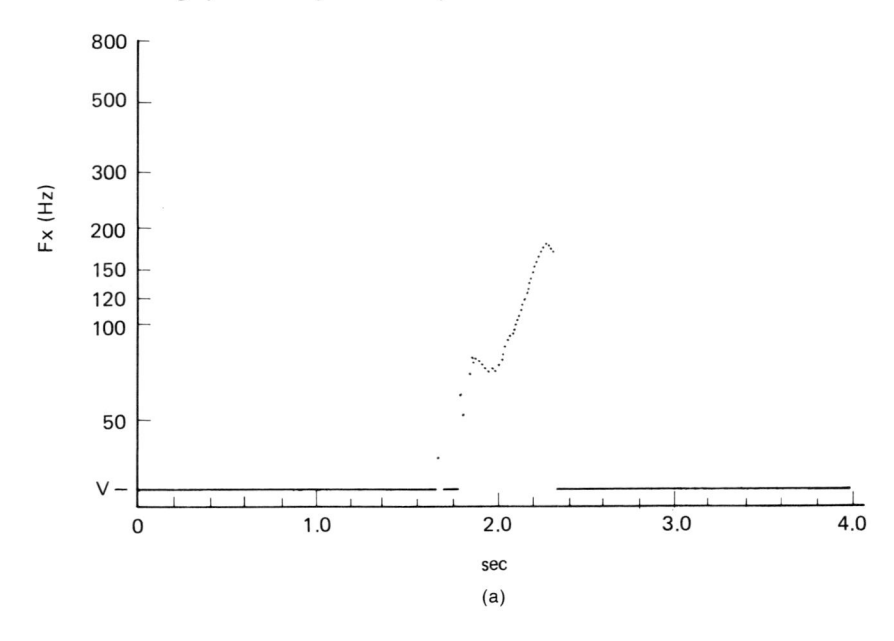

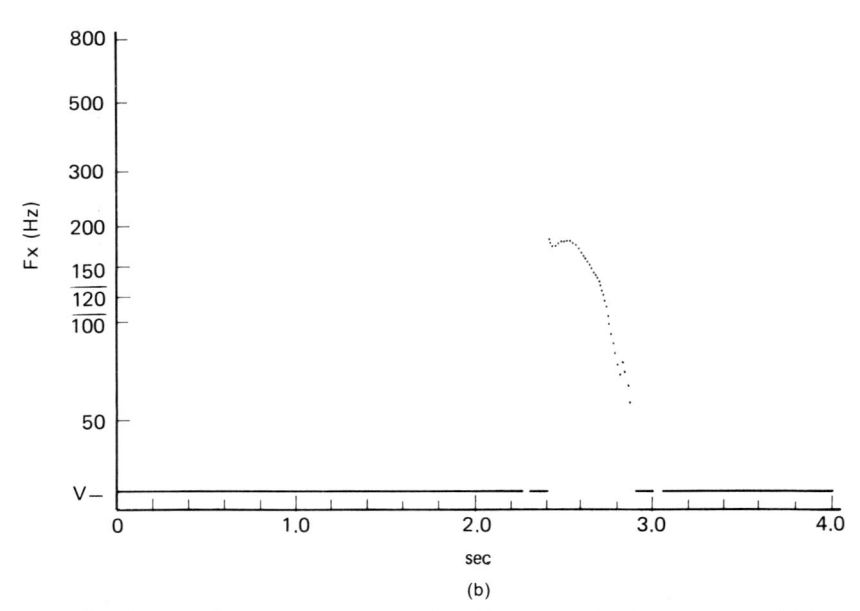

Figure 6.14 Fundamental frequency contours produced by a normal male speaker, aged 57 years: (a) a rise (/); (b) a fall (\); (c) a rise–fall (/\); (d) a fall–rise (\/)

(c)

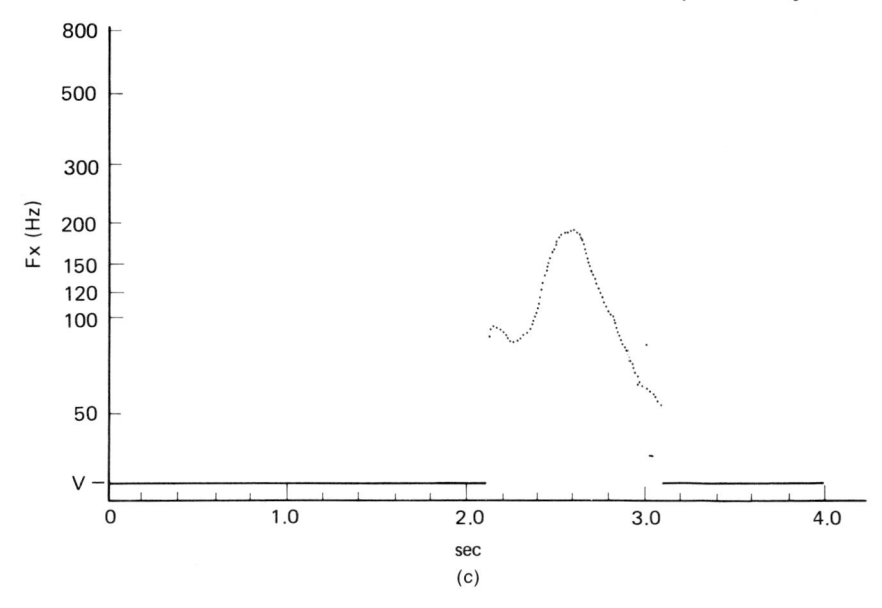

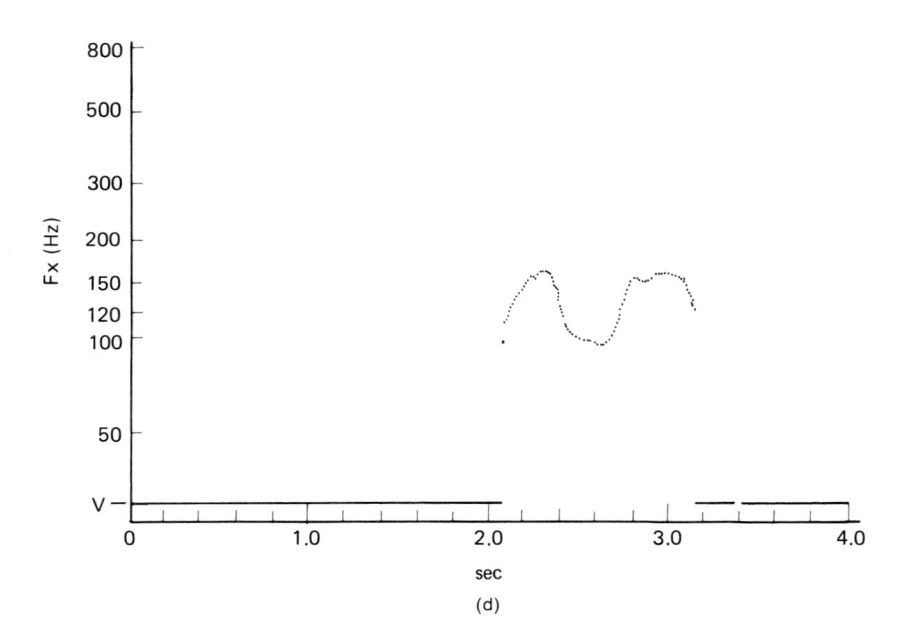

(d)

contribute a great deal to the naturalness and overall intelligibility of his or her speech. Figure 6.15 shows the same F_0 patterns as Figure 6.14, this time produced by a neoglottal speaker. These displays show that this speaker *is* capable of producing the desired F_0 movements, although the traces are not as smooth or regular as those produced by the normal speaker.

As the body of electrolaryngographic data accumulates and various waveform patterns are recognized and analysed by researchers (Singh, 1987, 1988, 1989; Hacki, 1989; Motta et al., 1990; Singh and Ainsworth, 1992), it may be possible to diagnose a variety of laryngeal pathologies in the near future. Clinically, electrolaryngography (electroglottography) is useful for differential diagnosis of early laryngeal cancer and recurrence after radiotherapy. It has proved a useful non-invasive technique to provide a visual feedback in pattern matching and thus improve the speech of the patients, both qualitatively and quantitatively (Singh, 1987). This justifies its use in clinical practice for rehabilitation of laryngectomy patients.

Phonetography or voice field measurement

The automatic phonetograph (Damsté, 1970; Schutte and Seidner, 1983; Komiyama et al., 1984; Gramming and Sundberg, 1988; Hacki, 1988; Frokjaer-Jensen, 1989; Loebell, 1989; Pabon, 1989; Singh, 1989; Titze, 1992) is a computer-based program that supplements information provided by the laryngograph, in that it automatically measures information not only about frequencies used by the speaker during ordinary speech, but also about the intensity (sound pressure level or loudness) of the voice at these frequencies, in ordinary speech, singing and shouting. A given speaker, for example, might be able to produce voicing at both 100 Hz and 150 Hz, but louder at 150 Hz than at 100 Hz. In the past a tone generator was used and the patient had to match the tone of the generator, which many patients found very difficult. This information was plotted manually by the operator and was a time-consuming process.

The phonetogram provides a two-dimensional graphical representation of frequency ranges and loudness in ordinary speech, singing and shouting. It works by producing a series of tones at various frequencies which the speaker is asked to imitate as loudly and as softly as possible, using an 'ah' vowel. The microphone is kept at a standard distance of 30 cm in front of the patient. This can be repeated at various points along the frequency scale until the speaker reaches the upper and lower limits of his or her range. The area enclosed within these limits is known as the speaker's *phonetogram* or *voice field* (Figure 6.16). This shows the potential intensity of the speaker's voice at a number of different frequencies.

In this way, the phonetograph tests the physiological limits of the speaker. This is perhaps the main difference between this technique and laryngography; the laryngograph is most useful for measuring the speaker's *habitual* frequency and range during ordinary speech, whereas the phonetograph tests the speaker's full *potential* frequency range. Preliminary results tend to suggest that the habitual range is smaller than the potential range; in other words, speakers seem not to use their entire vocal range during ordinary conversational speech. Wider ranges may be used when the speaker is shouting or singing.

Figure 6.17 shows the phonetogram produced by a male neoglottal speaker. This speaker was able to produce voicing at all frequencies. This can be compared to the range of F_0 shown by this speaker during the reading of the Rainbow passage (see

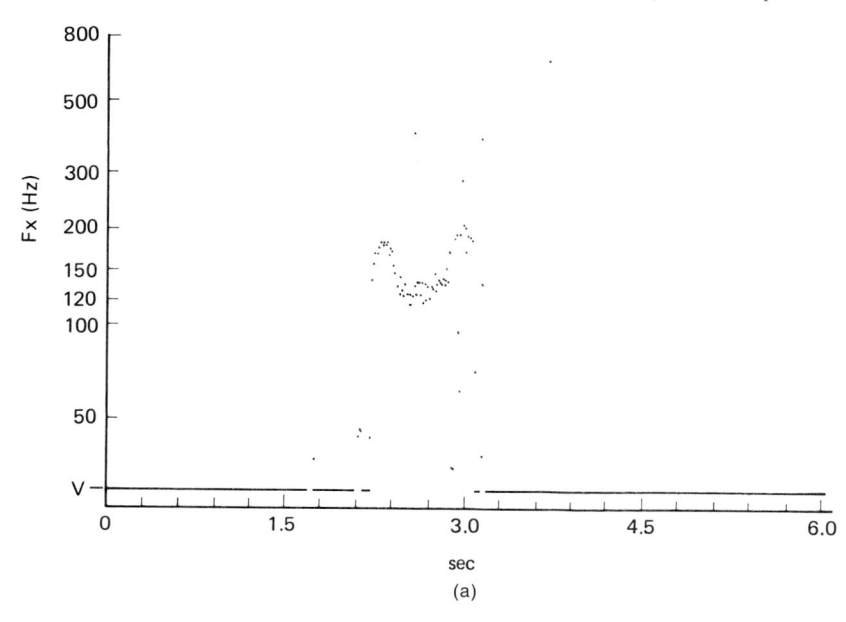

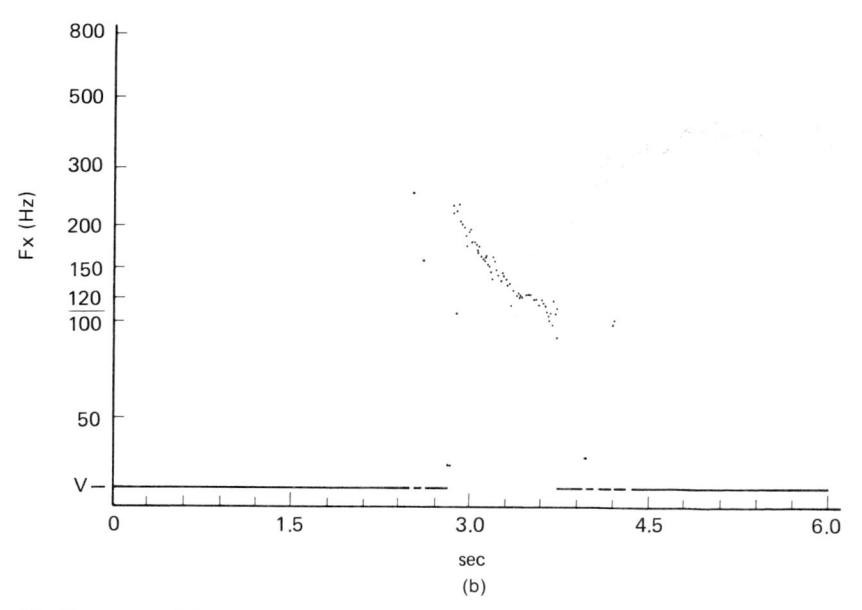

Figure 6.15 Fundamental frequency contours produced by a male neoglottal speaker, aged 59 years: (a) a rise (/); (b) a fall (\); (c) a rise–fall (/\); (d) a fall–rise (\/)

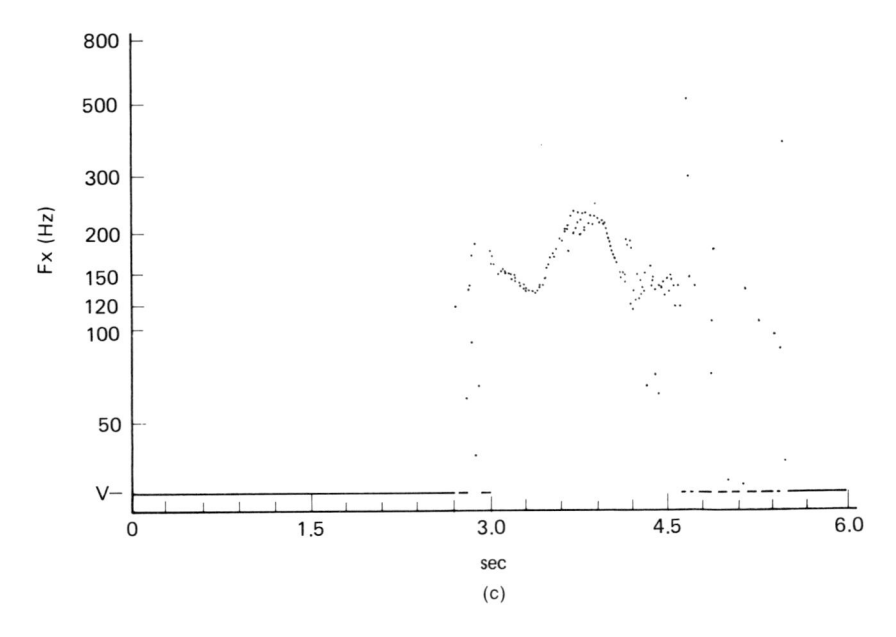

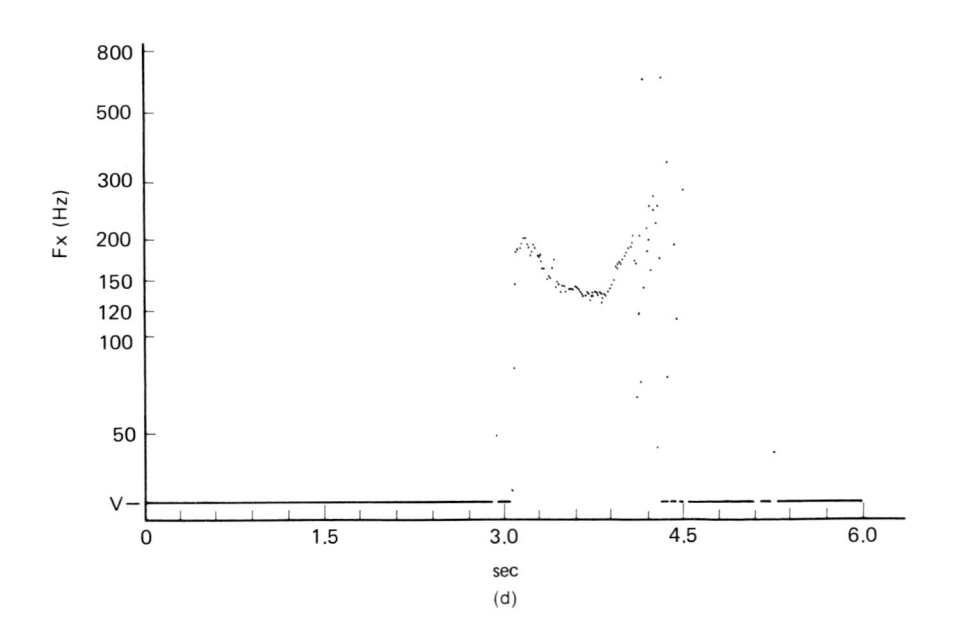

84 Functional Surgery of the Larynx and Pharynx

(c)

(d)

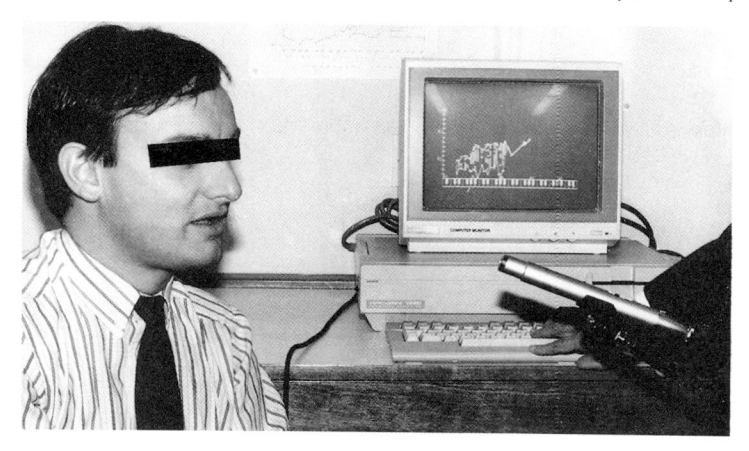

Figure 6.16 Phonetogram produced by a normal male speaker during repeated production of the vowel 'ah' at varying frequencies and loudness levels

Figure 6.11); clearly, he was able to produce higher frequencies than he actually did during normal speech.

Figure 6.18 shows the phonetogram produced by a speaker with cancer of the larynx. Clearly, this speaker's potential range of frequency has been much reduced. The maximum F_0 produced is only 103 Hz; the range only 73–103 Hz. In terms of intensity, there is again a very narrow range, only 62–75 dB. Comparing this with Figure 6.17 shows the greater frequency and intensity ranges (resulting in a much larger voice field) produced by the neoglottal speaker.

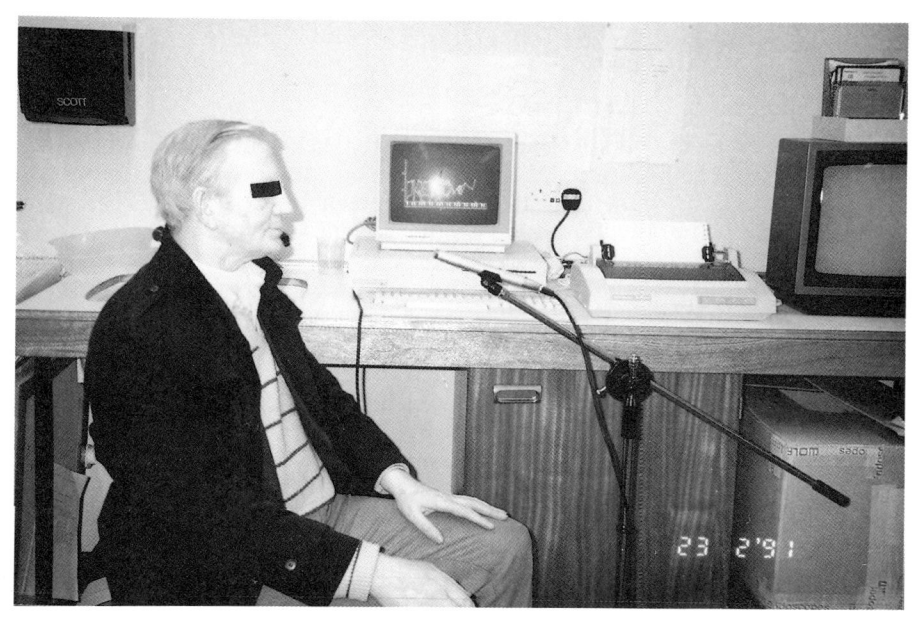

Figure 6.17 Phonetogram produced by a male neoglottal speaker during production of the vowel 'ah' at varying frequencies and loudness levels

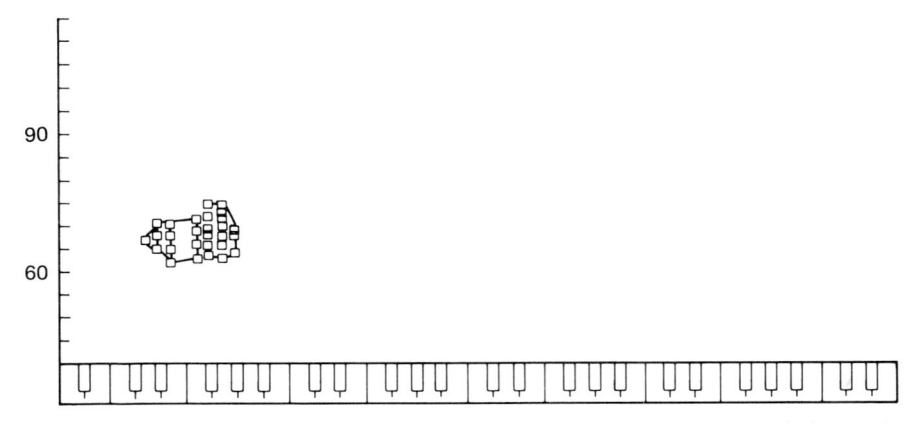

Figure 6.18 Phonetogram produced by a male suffering from cancer of the larynx, during production of the vowel 'ah' at varying frequencies and loudness levels

Clinically, the phonetogram can be used as part of an assessment of the potential of the voice, both conversational speech and singing voice, and can thus be used as a diagnostic aid in voice disorders. It is also used for assessment of results of voice therapy, especially in voice-dependent profesionals such as teachers and singers.

Sound spectrography

Sound spectrography is a very flexible technique for the acoustic analysis of speech, which provides a large amount of information on the frequency, duration and intensity characteristics of the acoustic signal produced by the speaker. The acoustic signal picked up from the microphone is analysed into its various frequency components, both the fundamental frequency produced by the vibration of the vocal folds, and the various resonant frequencies that are added to this by the movements of the tongue, the lips and the soft palate in the upper vocal tract. The spectrograph then displays these frequency components and their relative intensity, and also shows how these components change during the course of a short sentence.

Figure 6.19 shows a sample spectrogram of the word 'cease', which illustrates the various types of information that the spectrograph provides. This word consists of two high-frequency 's' sounds at the beginning and end of the word, and a short 'ee' sound in the middle. This spectrogram clearly shows that the final 's' is longer than the initial 's'. The dark low-frequency band present during the 'ee' sound is the voicing or fundamental frequency produced by the vocal folds (and which is absent during the 's' sounds, which are hence termed *voiceless*). The narrower higher-frequency bands represent the resonances produced by the particular vocal tract configuration associated with the 'ee' sound (and indeed contribute to our recognition of it). Intensity, finally, is shown by the relative darkness of the various

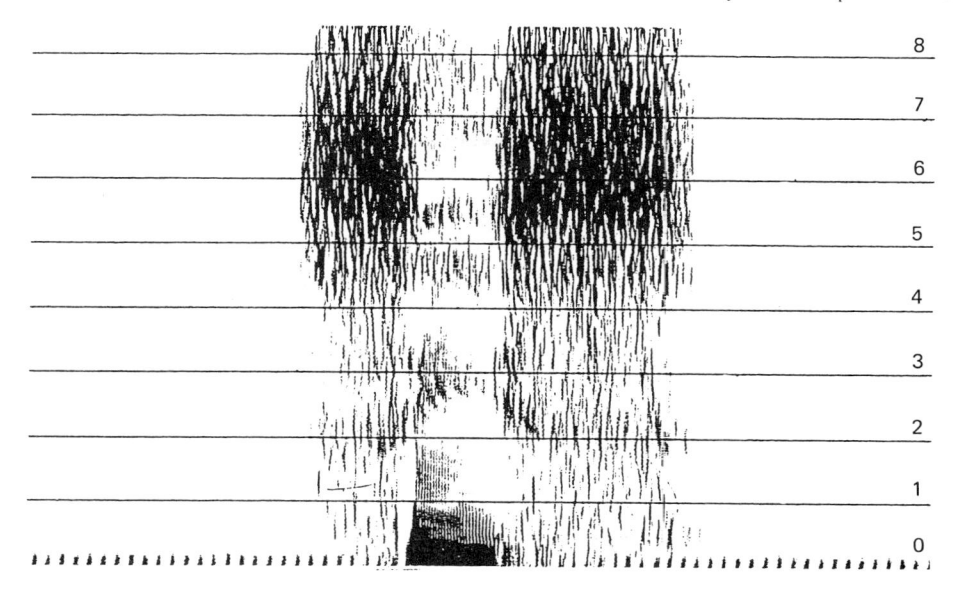

Figure 6.19 Sample spectrogram of the word 'cease'

frequency components. The two 's' sounds, for example, are both very dark (and therefore very intense). The lower frequencies of the 's' sounds are much less intense, and therefore much lighter on the spectrogram. The 'ee' vowel is also fairly dark, and in this case it is the lower frequencies that are more intense.

Sound spectrography can be used for a wide range of speech analyses, but in the St John's Hospital voice laboratory it is specifically used to assess the ability of alaryngeal speakers to produce the linguistic distinction known as *voicing contrast*.

Electrostroboscopy

The role of stroboscopy in research has been known for over a century. Oertel in 1878 was the first to apply this principle to the study of the larynx. Since the pioneering work of Schonharl (1960), laryngostroboscopy has become established as a diagnostic and research tool in phoniatrics. It works on the principle that if light is flashed at the same frequency (synchronization) as that of periodic vocal cord vibrations, the vocal cords appear to stand still. Similarly, a light source that flashed at a very slightly different frequency from the vibration of the vocal cords would make them appear to be moving in slow motion. This gives the clinician more information than could be obtained by conventional laryngoscopic examination of the fast-moving cords (Figure 6.20).

It is well recognized that vocal cords vibrate not only in the transverse axis but also in the vertical axis. There is a phase difference between the lower and upper part of the medial margins of the phonating vocal cords producing a fluid-like travelling mucosal wave (Berke et al., 1989). Traditional laryngoscopy has the disadvantage that the vocal cords cannot be observed with great precision by the naked human eye because of the high rate of vibrations (100 Hz or more). The detailed and precise assessment of the pathology of the vibrating vocal cords can be achieved by produc-

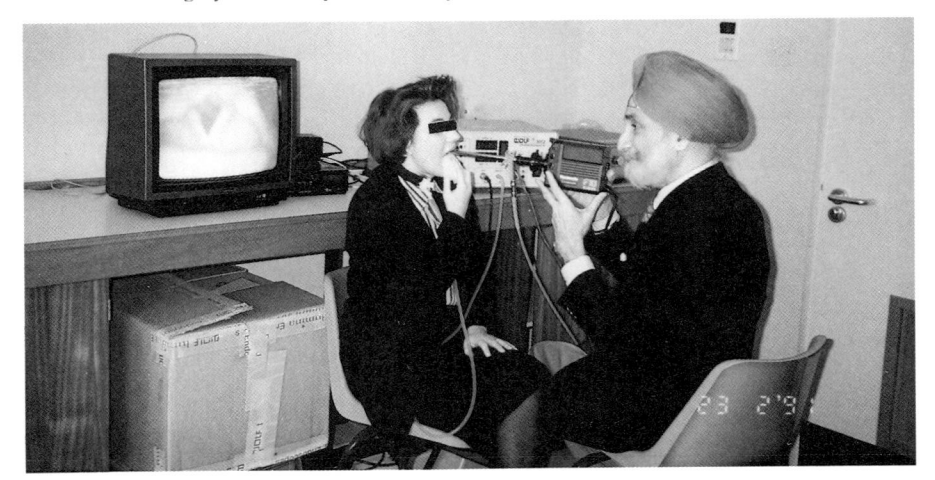

88   Functional Surgery of the Larynx and Pharynx

Figure 6.20   Technique of videolaryngostroboscopy. A member of staff (acting as the patient) holds her tongue while the examiner views the larynx, through a video camera, on monitor. A stethoscope attached to a microphone is held by the speaker against the neck at the level of the vocal cords and the patient is asked to say 'ah'. The fundamental frequency of the vibrating cords automatically synchronizes with the flashing frequency of the light source when the examiner presses the foot pedal of the stroboscope, thus making the cords appear stationary for detailed examination

ing illusory slow motion or stillness with the aid of a stroboscope. Secondly, conventional laryngoscopy only detects the lateromedial movements; it ignores the role of the vertical fluid-like travelling mucosal wave which can best be studied by laryngostroboscopy (Kitzing, 1985). Absence of the travelling mucosal wave may be pathognomonic of serious disease, e.g. glottic cancer.

Stroboscopic light can be used in conjunction with a laryngeal mirror, a rigid or flexible endoscope or an operating microscope. A video camera could be attached and the illuminated images of the vocal cords may be seen on the monitor and also recorded on videotape for a permanent record (videostroboscopy). A stethoscope attached to a microphone is held by the speaker against the side of the neck at the level of the vocal cords. The fundamental frequency of the vibrating vocal cords is detected by the microphone and is varied by 0–2 Hz to supply the flash frequency of the light source. The light source is usually supplied via a fibre-optic cable which can be attached to an endoscope or operating microscope, which in turn can be attached to a video camera and a video recording system.

Rigid endoscopy provides high-resolution images of the vocal cords, whereas the image quality and resolution attained by the small-diameter flexible endoscope is of comparatively inferior quality. However, the flexible endoscope allows examination of the larynx in a more natural posture during connected speech and while phonating sustained vowels. With improved imaging techniques the flexible (stereoscopic) endoscope may well be the instrument of choice in the near future. Microstroboscopy allows magnification and the use of both eyes for better optic resolution.

Videostroboscopy is a useful tool clinically and in research. It helps in the diagnosis of voice disorder, both organic and functional (Loebell, 1989). It is extremely useful for the detection of early cancer of the larynx (von Leden, 1961; Loebell, 1989). It is useful for the differential diagnosis of vocal fold paresis from cricoarytenoid joint ankylosis, and for monitoring the course of laryngeal paresis (Kitzing, 1985). It also provides a visual display for group discussion and teaching. The videostroboscopic images can be used as visual feedback in speech therapy for patients, especially for professional voice users such as teachers, actors and singers. In research, videostroboscopy has contributed much to our knowledge of the phonatory function of the larynx.

Stroboscopy has proved to be useful qualitatively but its quantitative role is not substantiated. Recently, attempts have been made to quantify stroboscopic data (Kitzing, 1985; Wendler et al., 1986), with limited success. With continued interest, this objective may be achieved in the near future.

Subglottal pressure in alaryngeal speakers

Subglottal pressure in speakers with an intact larynx can be measured in various ways: directly, by puncturing the subglottal space with a needle (Loebell, 1969; Schutte, 1980), by using a transglottal catheter (van den Berg, 1956) or by using an ultraminiature pressure transducer (Schutte and Miller, 1986, 1988); or indirectly by using an oesophageal balloon (van den Berg, 1956). Although subglottal pressure is of some clinical value in laryngeal speech, it is not routinely measured. In normal phonation the subglottal pressure varies from 6 cmH$_2$O to 10 cmH$_2$O (Beukelman et al., 1980). Isshiki (1959) reported subglottal pressure of 5–25 cmH$_2$O in normal subjects. Subglottal pressure is of great clinical significance in patients who have undergone near-total laryngectomy (parsimonious laryngectomy) or total laryngectomy with tracheo-oesophageal fistula operation (alaryngeal speakers). Subglottal pressure is here taken to mean the pressure below the voicing source used by the patients — below the neoglottis in near-total laryngectomy (parsimonious laryngectomy) patients (Singh, 1985, 1989, 1991), and below the pharyngo-oesophageal segment and prosthesis in patients who have undergone total laryngectomy with a tracheo-oesophageal fistula operation.

Subglottal pressure is routinely measured in the voice research laboratory at St John's Hospital in neoglottal speakers and tracheo-oesophageal speakers using the Singh fistula valve. It is well known that a certain amount of pressure must be exerted by the pulmonary expiratory air flow to set the voicing source in vibration and to maintain that vibration during the course of phonation. It is also clear that the greater the pressure required, the greater will be the strain on the cardiopulmonary system. This becomes of utmost importance in alaryngeal speech, where most of the speakers are between 50 and 70 years old. Fortunately, the types of alaryngeal speech that use pulmonary air to power a substitute voicing source (neoglottis in parsimonious laryngectomy or pharyngo-oesophageal segment in tracheo-oesophageal fistula speakers) offer us the opportunity to measure the subglottal pressure directly and non-invasively (Figures 6.21 and 6.22), because the pressure measuring device can be positioned in the tracheostoma (this technique is inapplicable in oesophageal speech since the lungs do not provide the air stream for speech). The Modified Singh tracheostoma valve fitted to the stoma is connected by tubing to a Mercury electromanometer which in turn is connected to a microcomputer (Figures 6.21 and 6.22). The speaker is asked to produce a prolonged 'ah' vowel, and the subglottal pressure can be shown as a time-varying trace on the computer monitor (the trace can also be printed or stored on disk for future reference). A typical trace produced by a neoglottal speaker, aged 76 years, is shown in Figure 6.21. After the initial rise in pressure which is required to set the neoglottis in motion, the trace stabilizes at around 15 cmH$_2$O, where it remains until the end of the utterance; while for the

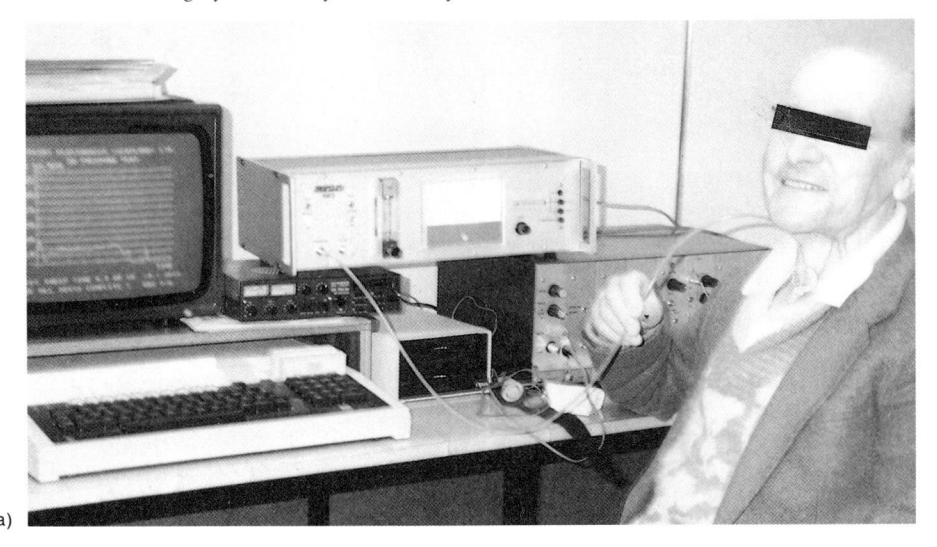

Figure 6.21 Measurement of subglottal pressure in a neoglottal speaker: (a) patient connected to measuring apparatus (b); (c) a typical subglottal pressure trace produced by a male neoglottal speaker during a sustained vowel 'ah'

tracheo-oesophageal speaker aged 70 years, the trace stabilizes at around 30 cmH$_2$O (Figure 6.22).

Subglottal pressure is also routinely measured in all the follow-up cases who have undergone near-total laryngectomy (parsimonious laryngectomy). Establishing the subglottal pressure that allows easiest phonation will help to determine the optimum diameter for the neoglottis in parsimonious laryngectomy. The majority of these patients use a pressure of around 15 cmH$_2$O for phonation (approximate diameter of the neoglottal tube 5–6 mm). The patients are advised to report immediately if they require more effort than usual to phonate. The increase in pressure may herald early local recurrence, the presence of a second primary tumour in the same region, or secondaries in the neck pressing on the neoglottis. The sinister pathology would probably be missed by visual examination or by palpation in the early stage. It is strongly recommended that every voice clinic or laboratory should have this facility.

Conclusion

The analysis techniques discussed in this chapter can provide a large amount of objective, quantitative information on several aspects of the speech production process. This can be used to provide both normative data and data on the characteristics of various types of speech pathology, in this case specifically on the various types of alaryngeal speech. This allows for more precise quantification of speech characteristics than would be the case with a purely auditory analysis.

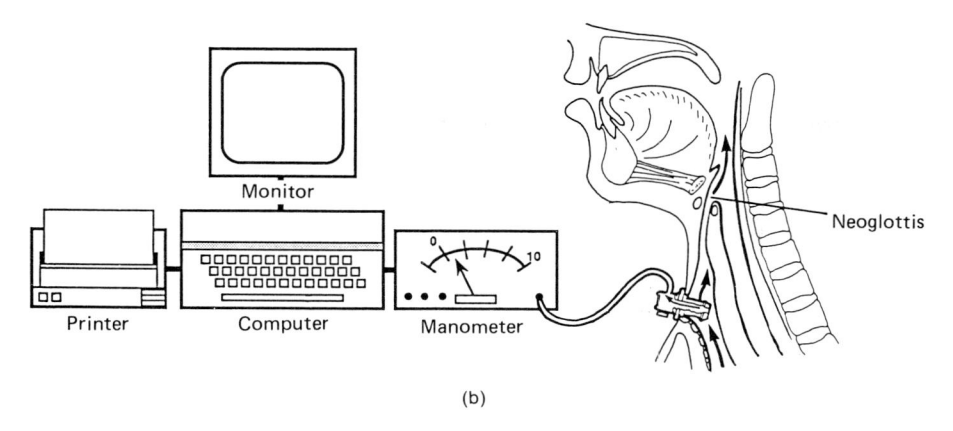

Monitor — Computer — Printer — Manometer — Neoglottis

(b)

SG pressure test

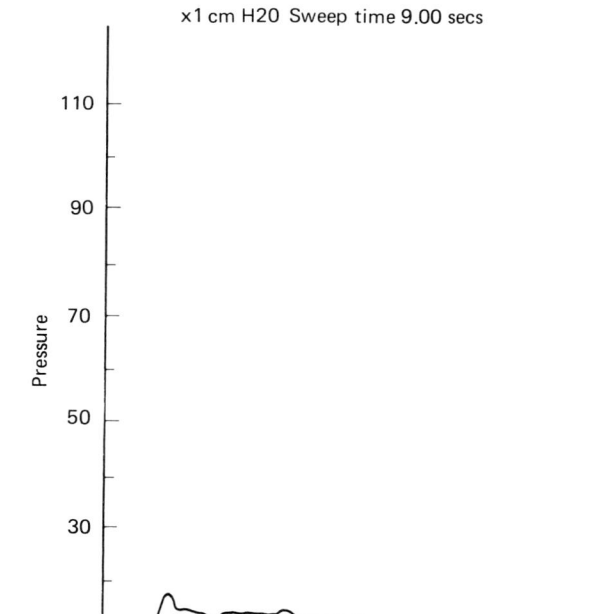

x1 cm H20 Sweep time 9.00 secs

Pressure (110, 90, 70, 50, 30, 10) vs Time

(c)

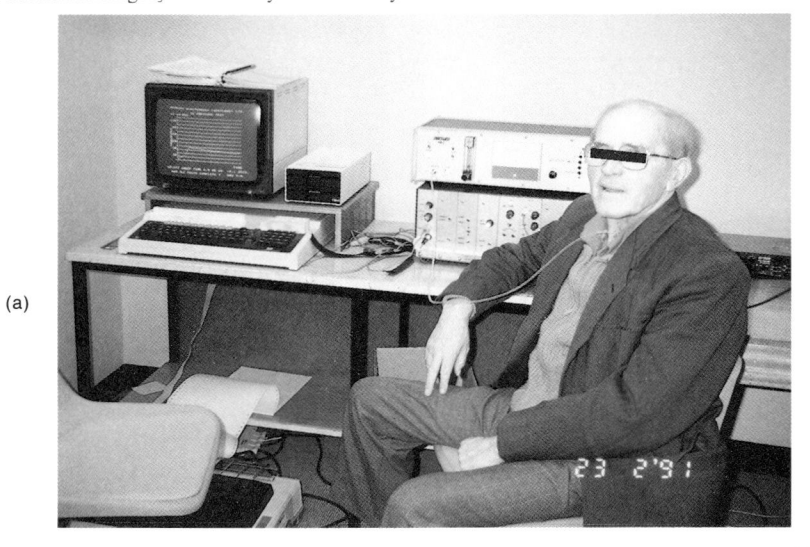

92   Functional Surgery of the Larynx and Pharynx

(a)

Figure 6.22 Measurement of subglottal pressure in a tracheo-oesophageal fistula speaker: (a) patient connected to measuring apparatus (b); (c) a typical pressure trace produced by a male tracheo-oesophageal fistula speaker during a sustained vowel 'ah'

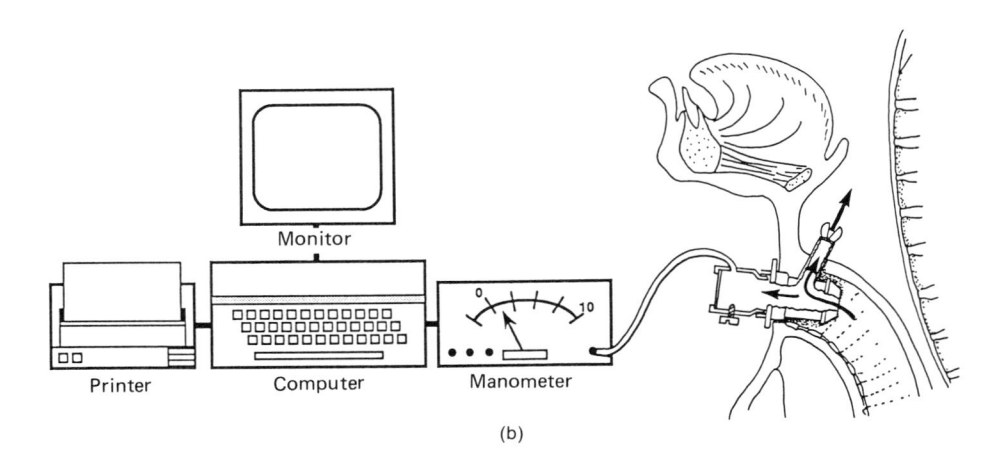

(b)

SG pressure test

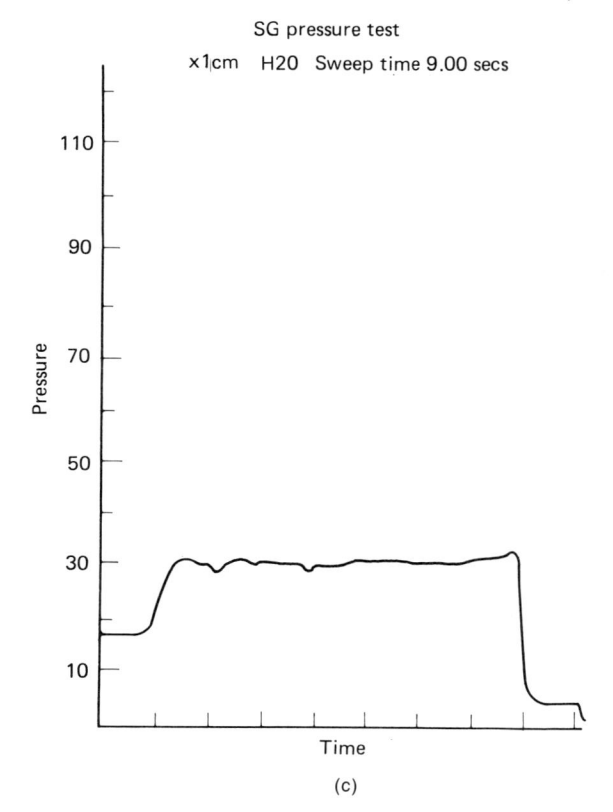

x1 cm H20   Sweep time 9.00 secs

Pressure (y-axis: 10, 30, 50, 70, 90, 110)

Time

(c)

References

Abberton E., Fourcin A. (1984). Electrolaryngography. In *Experimental Clinical Phonetics* (Code C., Ball M., eds) Beckenham: Croom Helm, pp. 62–78.

Abberton E., Howard D., Fourcin A. (1989). Laryngographic assessment of normal voice: a tutorial. *Clin. Ling. Phon.*, **3**, 281–96.

Berke G.S., Hanson D.G., Trapp T.K. et al. (1989). Office based system for voice analysis. *Arch. Otolaryngol.*, **115**, 74–7.

Beukelman P.R., Cummings C.W., Dobie R.A., Weymuller E.A. (1980). Objective assessment of laryngectomised patients with surgical reconstruction. *Arch. Otolaryngol.*, **106**, 715–18.

Damsté P.H. (1970). The phonetogram. *Pract. Otorhinolaryngol.*, **32**, 185–7.

Fairbanks G. (1940). *Voice and Articulation Drillbook*. New York: Harpers, p. 168.

Fourcin A. (1986). Electrolaryngographic assessment of vocal fold function. *J. Phon.*, **14**, 435–42.

Frokjaer-Jensen B. (1989). PC-based instrumentation for speech analysis. In *Proceedings of the International Voice Symposium*, Edinburgh (Singh W., ed.) pp. 30–3

Gramming P., Sundberg J. (1988). Spectrum factors relevant to phonetogram measurement. *J. Acoust. Soc. Am.*, **83**, 2352–60.

Hacki T. (1988). Die Beurteilung der quantitativen Sprechstimmleistungen. Das Sprechstimmfeld im Singstimmfeld. *Folia Phoniatr.*, **40**, 190–6.

Hacki T. (1989). Klassifizierung von Glottisdysfunktionen mit Hilfe der Electroglottographie. *Folia Phoniatr.*, **41**, 43–8.

Isshiki N. (1959). Quoted by Hirano M. (1981). Aerodynamic tests. In *Clinical Examination of Voice*. New York: Springer.

Kitzing P. (1985). Stroboscopy — a pertinent laryngological examination. *J. Otolaryngol.*, **14**, 151–7.

Komiyama S., Watanabe H., Ryu S. (1984). Phonographic relationship between pitch and intensity of the human voice. *Folia Phoniatr.*, **36**, 1–7.

Loebell E. (1969). Direct measurement of subglottal pressure. *Arch. Otorhinolaryngol. Belg.*, **194**, 316–20.

Loebell E. (1989). Aids to diagnosis. In *Proceedings of the International Voice Symposium*, Edinburgh (Singh W., ed.) p. 25.

Motta G., Cesari U., Iengo M., Motta G. Jr (1990). Clinical application of electroglottography. *Folia Phoniatr.*, **42**, 111–17.

Pabon J.P.H. (1989). Acoustic phonetogram recording supplemented with acoustical voice quality parameters. In *Proceedings of the International Voice Symposium*, Edinburgh (Singh W., ed.) p. 42.

Schonharl E. (1960). *Die Stroboskopie in der Praktischen Laryngologie*. Stuttgart: Thieme.

Schutte H.K. (1980). Examination of voice qualities by phonetography. *HNO – PRAXIS* 5/2, 132–9.

Schutte H.K., Miller D.G. (1986). Transglottal pressures in professional singing. *Acta Otorhinolaryngol. Belg.*, **40**, 395–404.

Schutte H.K., Miller D.G. (1988). Resonanzspiele der Gesangsstimme in ihren Beziehungen zu supra- und subglottalen Druckverlaufen: Konsequenzen fur die Stimmbildungstheorie. *Folia Phoniatr.*, **40**, 65–73.

Schutte H.K., Seidner W. (1983). Recommendation by the Union of European Phoniatricians (UEP): standardising voice area measurement/phonetography. *Folia Phoniatr.*, **35**, 286–8.

Singh W. (1987). Electrolaryngography in near-total laryngectomy with myo-mucosal valved neoglottis. *J. Laryngol. Otol.*, **101**, 815–18.

Singh W. (1988a). A simple surgical technique and a new prosthesis for voice rehabilitation after laryngectomy. *J. Laryngol. Otol.*, **102**, 332–4.

Singh W. (1988b). Clinical application of electrolaryngograph for speech rehabilitation in near-total laryngectomy with myo-mucosal valved neoglottis. *J. Laryngol. Otol.*, **102**, 335–6.

Singh W. (1989). Near-total laryngectomy. In *Proceedings of the International Voice Symposium*, Edinburgh (Singh W., ed.) pp. 53–8.

Singh, W. (1991). Preservation of voice in laryngectomy. *Acta Phoniatrica Latina*, **13**, 302–4.

Singh W., Hardcastle P. (1985). Near-total laryngectomy with myo-mucosal valved neoglottis. *J. Laryngol. Otol.*, **99**, 581–8.

Singh, W., Ainsworth, W. (1992). Computerised measurement of fundamental frequency in Scottish neoglottal patients. *Folia Phoniatr.*, **44**, 231–7.

Titze, I.R. (1992). Acoustic interpretation of the Voice Range Profile (Phonetogram). *J. Speech Hear. Res.*, **35**, 21–34.

van den Berg J.W. (1956). Direct and indirect determination of the mean subglottic pressure. *Folia Phoniatr.*, **8**, 1–24.

von Leden H. (1961). The electric synchron-stroboscope: its value for the practising laryngologist. *Ann. Otorhinolaryngol.*, **70**, 881–93.

Wendler J., Koppen K., Fischer S. (1986). The validity of stroboscopic data in terms of quantiative measures. In *Proceedings of the International Conference on Voice*. Kurume (Hirano M., ed.) pp. 36–42.

Part Three

Surgery of the Larynx and Pharynx

Chapter 7

Laryngeal and pharyngeal surgery: past, present and future

D.A. Shumrick and L.W. Savoury

Diseases of the larynx and pharynx have fascinated inquisitive minds for centuries. In few other regions of the body are the symptoms of pathology so evident. Obstruction of either the alimentary or respiratory tract produces intolerable distress in the patient.

The region from the oropharynx to the cricopharyngeus is one of the most highly innervated and coordinated regions of the body. This fact alone destines major surgical resections to produce frequently suboptimal results. Knowledge of the historical progression of surgical events in this region is not only interesting, but also important in providing a perspective of modern-day therapy.

History

Knowledge of laryngeal and pharyngeal disorders dates back to the ancient Greeks in 400 BC. Hippocrates spent much of his time attending oropharyngeal inflammatory disorders and makes clear reference to the larynx and pharynx in his work. It appears, however, that the ancient Greeks did not appreciate the difference between the larynx and pharynx (Jones and Withington, 1923); these two terms were used interchangeably, and no obvious knowledge of function is discernible in writings from that time. Hippocrates did, however, perform oropharyngeal intubation for obstructive inflammatory disease. The hollow tubes used did not extend far beyond the obstructing site, and probably acted as nothing more than oropharyngeal airways.

One of the first major advances in medicine came with the work of Galen in AD 150. His writings so influenced medicine that many teachings remained unchanged for over a thousand years. It is astounding to realize that the work of Galen dominated medical thinking until the Renaissance in the sixteenth century. He displayed an astute knowledge of the larynx and pharynx and clearly separates the two structures. Much to the surprise of his contemporaries, he proposed the larynx as the organ of voice. He went further to prove that the recurrent laryngeal nerves were essential in the production of voice, and proposed that they worked on a mechanical pulley system (May, 1968). Galen also makes reference to malignant ulcerations of the throat but provides no insight into surgical treatment.

The first suggestion of surgical intervention in laryngeal and pharyngeal disease appears in the Babylonian Talmud at about AD 360 (Stevenson and Guthrie, 1949). Reference is made to an incision of the trachea, or *arteria aspira* as it was called, for the relief of airway obstruction. It was noted that a transverse incision of the trachea invariably proved fatal, but longitudinal ones relieved the obstruction and allowed survival of the patient. Paul or Aegina in AD 560 also made reference to surgical intervention (laryngotomy) for airway obstruction (Stevenson and Guthrie, 1949).

Although knowledge of tracheostomies is clearly recorded prior to the Renaissance, it appears that very few people performed this operation.

It is Antonio Musa Brasavola who is credited with performing the first tracheotomy in 1546 (Wright, 1914). Boerhaave, in the latter part of the seventeenth century, makes clear reference to carcinoma of the larynx but provides no insight into surgical treatment of that disease. In the latter part of the eighteenth century, a surgical opening of the larynx was performed; subsequently, Desault was credited with performing one of the first laryngectomies for the removal of a laryngeal growth.

One of the major advances in laryngology came in 1855 when a singing teacher named Manoel Garcia became the first to visualize the larynx in a live patient (himself) using indirect laryngoscopy. Although there are claims prior to this of physicians using a similar instrument, these claims largely went unnoticed. Shortly after this, in 1866, Patrick Watson was credited with having performed the first total laryngectomy for syphilis of the larynx. Subsequently, in 1873, Theodore Billroth performed the first laryngectomy for carcinoma (Wright, 1914). Subsequent examination of this laryngectomy specimen, however, revealed that the pathology might have been tuberculosis. Billroth also performed the first resection of the oesophagus and thus did much to herald an era of surgery which exploded in the early twentieth century.

Multiple reports of total laryngectomies and pharyngectomies appeared at the turn of the century and were met with mixed reviews. Most surgeons of this time recognized the grave prognosis of patients with malignant growths in this region. Multiple reports of partial laryngectomies also appeared and were met favourably by most surgeons, as this procedure represented a somewhat conservative approach to a devastating disease. Reports also began to surface on the transoral removal of laryngeal growths by indirect means and the use of laryngotomy for the removal of laryngeal polypi and other growths.

Present techniques

A discussion on current techniques in pharyngeal and laryngeal surgery has to include the philosophies introduced at the turn of the century, since many of these procedures are applicable today. Laryngology has developed rapidly following the advent of indirect laryngoscopy and open procedures on the larynx. At the turn of the century, endoscopic techniques were becoming popular for diagnostic and therapeutic purposes. Knowledge increased and probably culminated with the formation of the Chevalier Jackson Clinic in Philadelphia in the early 1900s. (Stevenson and Guthrie, 1949). The prevalence of tuberculosis and polio at that time helped broncho-oesophagology to reach its height.

It soon became obvious to surgeons at the turn of the century that extirpation of extensive laryngeal and pharyngeal lesions was not a problem. The real problem came with reconstruction of the alimentary tract. Since that time, a multitude of techniques have been developed. The poor prognosis of patients with hypopharyngeal malignancy led to the challenge being directed at techniques providing the best function, least morbidity and least complications. With current survival rates ranging from 10% to 30%, these criteria still apply (Silver, 1981). Most techniques provide a conduit from oropharynx to oesophagus, although full replacement of the coordinated pharynx is an unrealistic goal.

At the turn of the century, the first tissue to be used for reconstruction was local skin. Since that time, the use of skin has been modified in many ways, recent applications being the tubed deltopectoral flap, tubed myocutaneous flaps and, most recently, free transfer of skin by microvascular anastomosis.

Besides full-thickness skin, split-thickness skin grafts have been used over a stent. Reconstruction by these techniques has notoriously been associated with a high fistula rate and stenosis. An added disadvantage is that it often requires multiple procedures and many patients develop recurrence before completion of the reconstruction.

In the 1920s viscera were first used for reconstruction following total removal of the larynx and pharynx. These were all pedicled reconstructions and usually involved a subcutaneous route. Although stomach was initially used, colon and small bowel were also experimented with early on (Surkin and Lawson, 1984). In 1960 Ong and Lee, and later LeQuesne and Ranger, revitalized the use of stomach by performing a total laryngopharyngo-oesophagectomy, passing the mobilized stomach through the posterior mediastinum and anastomosing it to the pharynx (Ong and Lee, 1960; LeQuesne and Ranger, 1966). This technique has received minor modification since that time and remains one of the viable alternatives in laryngopharyngeal reconstruction.

One of the major advances in this field of reconstruction was the introduction of free tissue transfer by microvascular anastomosis. The first successful report was by Seidenberg in 1959 when he performed a reconstruction in a dog using jejunum (Seidenberg and Rosenak, 1959). Since that time, small bowel, gastric antrum and sigmoid colon have been used, but free jejunal transfer remains the tissue of choice with this technique.

The availability of these varied surgical techniques has brought about useful introspection as to when and why these procedures should be done. Several authors have shown that large hypopharyngeal tumours are often much more aggressive and extensive histologically than is appreciated clinically (Harrison, 1969, 1970; Kirchner, 1975; Gluckman and Weissler, 1987).

Most surgeons consequently feel that a wide surgical margin is necessary if the aim is cure. Those utilizing gastric pull-up procedures argue that the total oesophagectomy not only provides a wide surgical margin but removes potential for the development of a second primary tumour (Harrison, 1979). Surgeons utilizing free visceral transfer for reconstruction insist on a margin of at least 5 cm from the tumour, and argue that survival rates are not significantly different for both procedures (Gluckman and McDonough, 1985). More than 60 free jejunal transfers have been performed at the University of Cincinnati Medical Center with a mortality rate of only 2% and an overall success rate of 90%. This one-stage procedure allows early rehabilitation of the patient and remains the authors' technique of choice.

Today the laryngologist enjoys a high degree of sophistication with the use of fibre-optic and video techniques in laryngoscopy and improvements in radiological examination. These allow a thorough assessment of any pharyngeal or laryngeal disorder. The head and neck surgeon can perform excision of minor abnormalities with minimal sequelae through various endoscopic or external approaches to the larynx or pharynx. The introduction of lasers has allowed the removal of benign laryngeal lesions with minimal damage to a finely tuned organ. Partial excision of larger lesions through any number of external approaches can now be performed. Finally, total excision of the larynx, pharynx and oesophagus for extensive lesions with immediate reconstruction is now possible. However, surgeons are limited in what they can do for the survival of patients with extensive malignancies.

Future techniques

The future in laryngeal and pharyngeal surgery no doubt lies in a refinement of current methods. Improved radiographic techniques will hopefully lead to better assessment of these tumours preoperatively and help to define more clearly the role of conservative surgery. The application of such techniques as photodynamic therapy may prove very useful in the early detection and treatment of these disorders.

Spurred on by the ingenuity of the surgical giants at the turn of the century we are quickly approaching the limit of our surgical capabilities. The future in that regard can only be expected to refine our current technical ability. Despite major technological advancements, we are still faced with similar problems to our predecessors. Improvements in the prognosis for hypopharyngeal malignancy will come with a clearer understanding of the biology of cancer, improved preventive techniques and the introduction of new chemotherapeutic agents.

References

Gluckman J.L., McDonough J.J. (1985). Complications associated with free jejunal graft reconstruction of the pharyngoesophagus — a multi-institutional experience with 52 cases. *Head Neck Surg.*, **7**, 200–5.
Gluckman J.L. Weissler M.C. (1987). Partial vs total oesophagectomy for advanced carcinoma of the hypopharynx. *Arch. Otolaryngol. Head Neck Surg.*, **113**, 69–72.
Harrison D.F.N. (1969). Surgical management of cancer of the hypopharynx and cervical oesophagus. *Brit. J. Surg.*, **56**, 95–103.
Harrison D.F.N. (1970). Pathology of hypopharyngeal cancer in relation to surgical management. *J. Laryngol. Otol.*, **84**, 349–67.
Harrison D.F.N. (1979). Surgical management of hypopharyngeal cancer. *Arch. Otolaryngol.*, **105**, 149–52.
Jones W.H., Withington E.T. (1923). *The Works of Hippocrates*. London: Loeb Classical Library.
Kirchner J.A. (1975). Pyriform sinus cancer: a clinical and laboratory study. *Ann. Otol. Rhinol. Laryngol.*, **84**, 793–803.
LeQuesne L.P., Ranger D. (1966). Pharyngolaryngectomy, with immediate pharyngogastric anastomosis. *Brit. J. Surg.*, **53**, 105–9.
May M.T. (1968). *Galen — On the Usefulness of the Parts of the Body*. New York: Cornell University Press.
Ong G.B., Lee T.C. (1960). Pharyngogastric anastomosis after oesophagopharyngectomy for carcinoma of the hypopharynx and cervical oesophagus. *Brit. J. Surg.*, **48**, 193–200.
Seidenberg B., Rosenak S.S. (1959). Immediate reconstruction of the cervical oesophagus by a revascularised isolated jejunal segment. *Ann. Surg.*, **149**, 162–71.
Silver C.E. (1981). Surgical treatment of hypopharyngeal and cervical oesophageal cancer. *World J. Surg.*, **5**, 499–507.
Stevenson R.S., Guthrie D. (1949). *A history of Otolaryngology*. Edinburgh: Livingstone.
Surkin M.I., Lawson W. (1984). Analysis of the methods of pharyngooesophageal reconstruction. *Head Neck Surg.*, **6**, 953–70.
Wright J. (1914). *A History of Laryngology and Rhinology*. New York: Lea & Febiger.

Chapter 8

Pharyngo-oesophageal reconstruction and rehabilitation

D.S. Soutar

The overriding principles of pharyngo-oesophageal reconstruction are to provide a suitable conduit for the passage of foodstuffs from the oral cavity to the oesophagus and at the same time protect the airway from aspiration of foodstuffs into the lungs. Cases requiring pharyngo-oesophageal reconstruction most commonly encountered by the author are shown in Table 8.1. The complexity of the reconstruction is greatly variable depending on the extent of the defect and this, in part, explains the wide variety of methods that have been described in the past, many of which remain useful today.

In the most complete form of reconstruction, the aerodigestive tract is completely separated into a respiratory tract with a permanent tracheostomy and a separate digestive tract. In the most incomplete form, a portion of pharyngeal wall can be reconstructed using a skin graft or skin flap while the integrity of the larynx and respiratory tract is maintained. Between these extremes, there is a wide variety of variations that require the attention of the surgeon.

It should be borne in mind that malignant tumours requiring this extensive reconstruction carry a poor prognosis, with survival rates embarrassingly low at between 10% and 30% (Vandenbrouck et al., 1977; Silver, 1981; Van den Bogaert et al., 1983). This has led to the debate centring on the mortality and morbidity of the various methods of reconstruction. As surgical techniques and anaesthesia have improved, the perioperative mortality has fallen, even in very complex reconstructions. The emphasis is now slowly shifting towards rehabilitation and the patient's ability to swallow and speak.

Functional rehabilitation is not solely dependent on the method of reconstruction used but also reflects the extent of the defect. There is a significant difference between partial and total pharyngo-oesophageal reconstruction (Soutar, 1985) and the extent of the surgery involved is therefore of vital importance in assessing what type of reconstruction will be required, the associated mortality and morbidity, and the likely functional outcome.

Preoperative assessment

The likely cases requiring pharyngo-oesophageal reconstruction have already been shown in Table 8.1. Unfortunately, it is notoriously difficult to investigate this area of the body and to determine the extent of tumours or fistulae, or even the exact defect in secondary surgery following pharyngotomy. The author relies on two main areas

102   Functional Surgery of the Larynx and Pharynx

Table 8.1   Indications for pharyngo-oesophageal reconstruction

1. Cancer of the hypopharynx
2. Advanced carcinomas of the larynx involving the pharynx
3. Salvage surgery for radiotherapy recurrent tumours
4. Secondary surgery for fistula or wound breakdown
5. Secondary surgery for established pharyngostome and oesophagostome
6. Ingestion of corrosive substances

of investigation, namely an examination under anaesthesia which includes endoscopic examination, and radiological investigations.

Examination under anaesthesia

Anaesthesia provides the best conditions for a full and detailed examination of any tumour or fistula. Endoscopic examination is part of this procedure, together with direct laryngoscopy and palpation of the tumour and the neck. The aim is to identify the areas of tumour involvement and to assess whether a complete or partial laryngopharyngo-oesophagectomy will be required.

Radiological investigations

The author favours videofluoroscopy which allows a dynamic contrast examination to be performed. Areas of incoordination can be identified, together with irregularities resulting from tumour involvement. Radiological examination can also be used to determine the extent of any sinus or fistula where secondary reconstruction is required. Occasionally computed tomography (CT) has proved a useful additional examination, but is not used routinely.

There is a third criterion which the author has found most useful in preoperative assessment and that is a high index of suspicion. For example, in tumours recurring after radiotherapy, although the recurrence may appear small, the surgery required to eradicate the disease will be much more extensive. This is because the pattern of invasion, particularly of radiorecurrent squamous cell carcinoma, is different from that of the primary tumour. Furthermore, irradiated tissues will not heal satisfactorily and require a wider excision prior to any reconstruction.

Postcricoid carcinomas and cancers of the hypopharynx should be regarded with suspicion since the histological spread of the tumour is often much greater than would be expected from gross examination (Harrison, 1970; Gluckman et al., 1987). Similarly, an apparently small fistula may require a fairly radical operation, particularly if associated with previous radiotherapy or failure of a previous method of reconstruction.

Once the extent of the expected defect has been mapped out then the appropriate method of reconstruction can be planned.

Reconstruction

A wide variety of reconstructive techniques have been used (see Chapter 7). Many of these techniques proved unreliable and have been replaced with techniques which have a proven record and are associated with a low mortality and morbidity. The modern techniques in common usage are outlined in Table 8.2.

Table 8.2 Pharyngo-oesophageal reconstruction

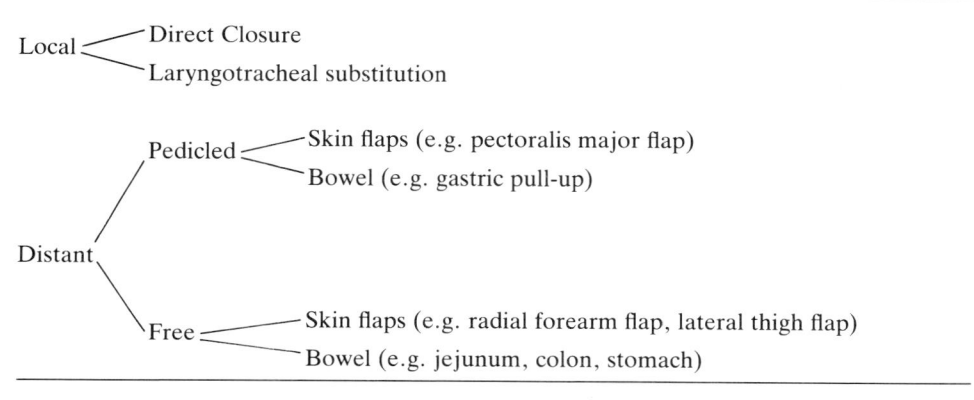

```
Local ─┬─ Direct Closure
       └─ Laryngotracheal substitution

Distant ─┬─ Pedicled ─┬─ Skin flaps (e.g. pectoralis major flap)
         │            └─ Bowel (e.g. gastric pull-up)
         │
         └─ Free ─┬─ Skin flaps (e.g. radial forearm flap, lateral thigh flap)
                  └─ Bowel (e.g. jejunum, colon, stomach)
```

Local reconstruction

Direct closure of the pharynx is only possible where there has been little tissue loss. Fortunately, the great majority of standard laryngectomies only require pharyngeal repair by direct wound closure. In more extensive lesions when the tumour extends into the pharynx or originates in the hypopharynx, tissues have to be imported from other sites.

One other means of local reconstruction is to utilize the anterior portion of the larynx and trachea as a laryngotracheal substitution to replace the resected portion of hypopharynx. This operation was described by Arsherson for the treatment of a postcricoid carcinoma (Arsherson, 1954).

For such tumours, this author prefers a circumferential excision with a total pharyngolaryngectomy because of the difficulty in obtaining local and regional control.

Distant reconstruction

Because of the lack of available tissue locally, the great majority of cases of pharyngo-oesophageal reconstruction require the import of tissue from a distance. This can be achieved using a pedicled technique, where the vascular pedicle remains intact, or by free techniques, where the vascular anatomy is reconstructed by microsurgery.

Pedicled skin flaps

The early pedicled flaps using cervical flaps and tubed pedicles have been largely superseded. The deltopectoral flap (Bakamjian, 1965) remains useful and provides an adequate tube comprised of relatively thin, pliable skin. It does, however, require a two-stage procedure.

This technique has been largely superseded by the pectoralis major myocutaneous flap method (Ariyan, 1979a; Ariyan and Cuono, 1980), which has now become one of the workhorses for head and neck reconstruction (Figure 8.1). It provides abundant tissue but often the skin is difficult to tube. The muscle can be used to advantage to protect the carotid vessels and to provide an extra layer of cover to minimize fistulae. In postirradiated cases particularly, this can assume great importance, especially if there are problems with the overlying skin. The affected skin can be

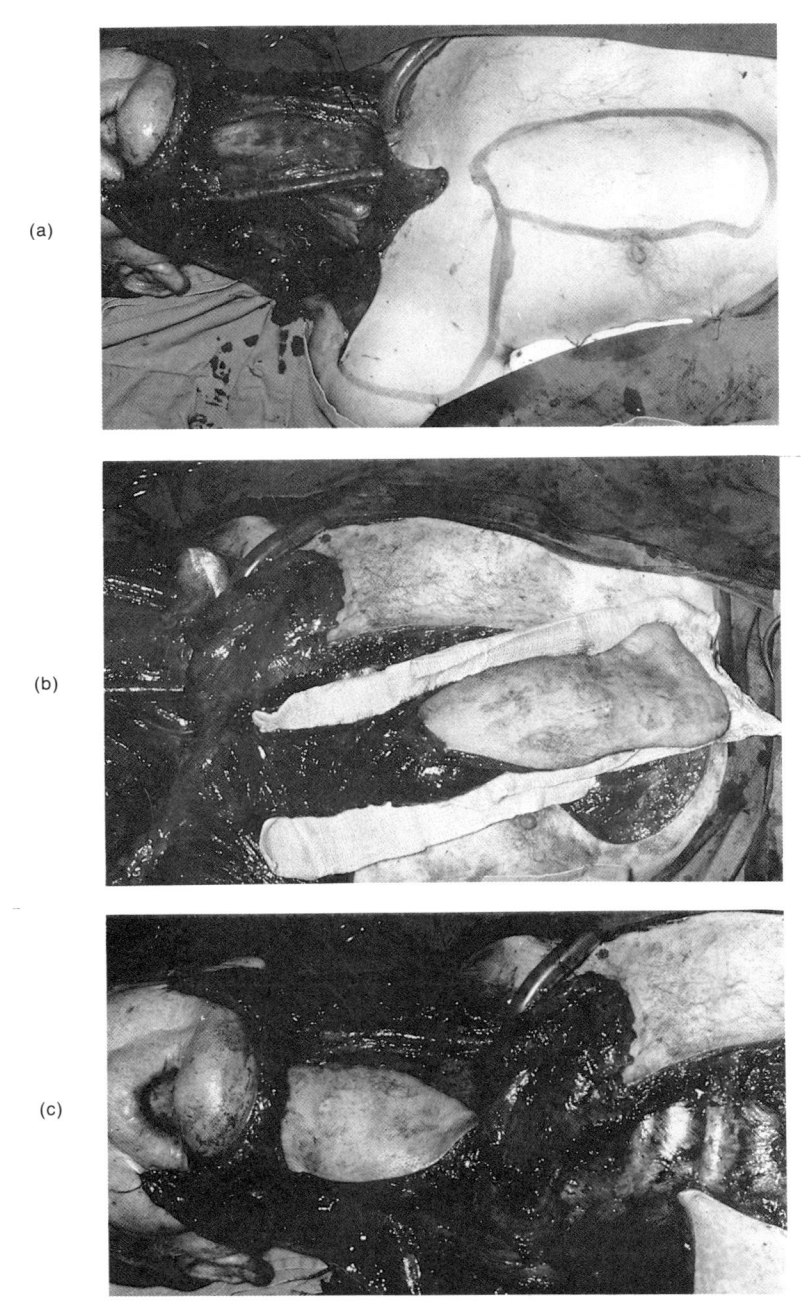

Figure 8.1 A total laryngopharyngo-oesophagectomy has been performed; (a) reconstruction is planned using a pectoralis major flap via a defensive approach which preserves the deltopectoral flap. (b) The pectoralis major myocutaneous flap is raised as a skin island flap. (c) The flap is tubed and inset into the neck. (d) A wide skin flap is required to accommodate the upper oropharyngeal diameter. (e) Appearance at 18 months following surgery

(d)

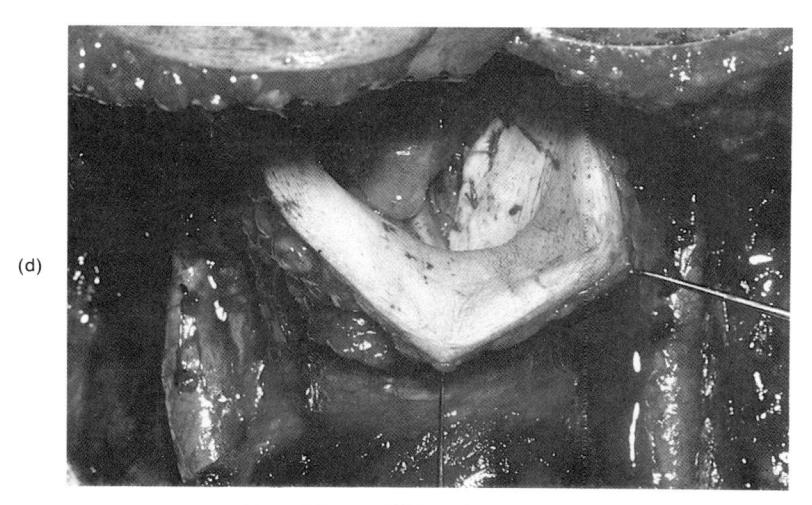

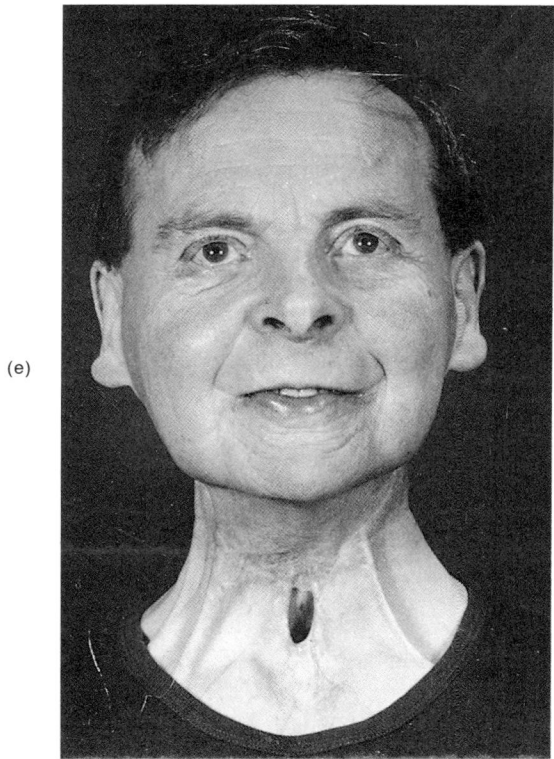

(e)

excised and the muscle exposed and subsequently skin-grafted with a good cosmetic result. Other myocutaneous flaps such as the sternocleidomastoid flap (Ariyan, 1979b), latissimus dorsi myocutaneous flap (Watson et al., 1982) and the trapezius myocutaneous flap (Demergasso and Piazza, 1979) have similar uses.

The author finds the sternocleidomastoid flap the least reliable of the pedicled myocutaneous flaps and in cancer surgery its use is extremely limited, since it often comes into the zone requiring surgical or radiotherapy treatment.

Of the remaining three pedicled myocutaneous flaps, the pectoralis major remains by far the most useful as it is readily accessible; but all three flaps tend to be bulky. Although the muscle can be used to advantage as mentioned previously, it is often very difficult to form an adequate tube. These pedicled flaps therefore are less useful in circumferential defects of the pharynx and oesophagus. They are most useful in partial reconstructions, particularly in cases where a strip of posterior pharyngeal wall mucosa has been maintained intact. They are also very useful in the closure of any fistula that requires the local excision of one wall of the pharynx, and also in some cases of pharyngeal reconstruction following injection of corrosive substances.

Pedicled bowel transfers
Pedicled bowel transfers such as reversed gastric tubes and pedicled colonic transfers have in the past been associated with a high morbidity and mortality and are no longer in common practice. The pedicled bowel transfer that is still commonly used is the gastric pull-up (Ong and Lee, 1960). Proponents of this technique point out the radical nature of the surgery, particularly excision of the oesophagus and the control of submucosal spread distally. They also point out the fact that only one anastomosis is required and this is safely sited in the neck.

Others less enthusiastic about this technique point out its high mortality and morbidity, the mortality varying widely between 0% and 31% (Stell, 1970; Lam et al., 1981). Gastric pull-up is a major operative procedure and requires significant surgical expertise and experience. The results from Queen Mary Hospital, Hong Kong, of a very large series show a marked reduction in hospital deaths from 31% to 4.5% and an overall morbidity reducing from 53% to 32% (Lam, 1987).

The gastric pull-up is at its best when there is a long segment defect requiring reconstruction. On oncological grounds, it allows radical excision of the oesophagus where this is deemed advisable.

Unfortunately, the majority of recurrences in hypopharyngeal cancer occur at the upper margin; but in expert hands, the fundus of the stomach can be mobilized well into the oropharynx, and its size allows for an end-to-end single bowel anastomosis.

Free tissue transfer
The difficulties in reconstructing circumferential defects of the pharynx and upper oesophagus proved to be an essential stimulus for the development of microvascular surgery. It was Seidenberg in 1959 who first transplanted a loop of jejunum and revascularized it by anastomosing the artery and vein to vessels in the neck (Seidenberg et al., 1959). Over the years, free jejunal transfer has become an established method of reconstructing total pharyngo-oesophageal defects (Flynn and Acland, 1979; Gluckman et al., 1982). Free colonic transfer has also been employed (Nakayama et al., 1964), and recent work suggests that colon offers several advantages over jejunum when it is transplanted into the neck (Smith et al., 1987a, b). One further free bowel transfer utilizes a portion of stomach formed into a tube (Hiebert and Cummings, 1961; Papachristou et al., 1979; Baudet, 1979).

Free bowel transfers

The advantage of using the jejunum and colon is that they provide ready-made conduits for pharyngeal reconstruction, whereas the stomach mucosal flap has first to be formed into a tube. On the other hand, free gastric transfer allows the incorporation of omentum which can be fully utilized in reconstructing defects of the neck, at the same time as pharyngo-oesophageal reconstruction.

Free bowel transfers are most useful in dealing with circumferential pharyngo-oesophageal defects, particularly those involving a short segment, and they are best suited for reconstruction in the cervical region. In cases where there is some continuity of the pharynx and oesophagus and a patch is required, a laparotomy appears to be unwarranted when compared with pedicled skin flaps or free skin flap reconstruction. There are occasions, however, when a free jejunal mucosal patch may offer some advantages (Sasaki et al., 1982), but this is a rare requirement in pharyngo-oesophageal reconstruction.

Proponents of free bowel transfer point to the low mortality and morbidity associated with this technique, particularly with small bowel surgery involving the jejunum. It allows ready access proximally well into the oropharynx without any tension or difficulties. Distally, however, the resection is limited to the cervical region. Monitoring of such free bowel transfers can prove difficult unless special measures are taken, such as exteriorizing a portion of bowel as described by Katsaros et al. (1985).

Free skin flaps

A wide variety of free skin flaps can be used as a patch on any surface of the pharynx for pharyngo-oesophageal reconstruction. The most useful, however, incorporate thin, pliable skin. Where a tube is required for circumferential defects, then the two most popular flaps are the radial forearm flap (Harii et al., 1985) and the lateral thigh flap (Hayden, 1989). These flaps tend, on the whole, to be hairless, which is an important consideration, particularly if radiotherapy is not to be given postoperatively. The thin, pliable nature of the skin in both these regions allows it to be easily tubed to form a conduit for circumferential reconstruction (Figure 8.2). Both these donor sites offer large-sized vessels and a good vascular pedicle suitable for simple microvascular anastomosis. Proponents of skin flap techniques point out the benefits of the absence of a laparotomy wound with all that it entails, and the easier postoperative recovery in patients who are already severely debilitated. On the other hand, such skin tubes are adynamic and act purely as functionless conduits for the passage of food. As with all skin flaps there is a risk of contracture at the anastomosis between the skin and mucosa, and when this is circumferential, a stenosis can result.

The wide variety of methods of reconstructing pharyngo-oesophageal defects still persists. For defects that do not involve the whole circumference of the pharynx or oesophagus, the author favours applying a patch in the form of either a pectoralis major myocutaneous flap or a free flap, most commonly the radial forearm flap. When dealing with isolated losses of the posterior pharyngeal wall, for example, a free radial forearm flap can prove a most useful method of reconstruction. It maintains adequate diameter of the pharynx and oesophagus while preserving the larynx and respiratory tract intact. The most common patches, however, are to the lateral or anterior wall, and here the pedicled pectoralis major myocutaneous flap is often the first option.

For circumferential defects, the author's preference is for a bowel transfer offering a ready-made hollow conduit. For short segments confined in the cervical region, the

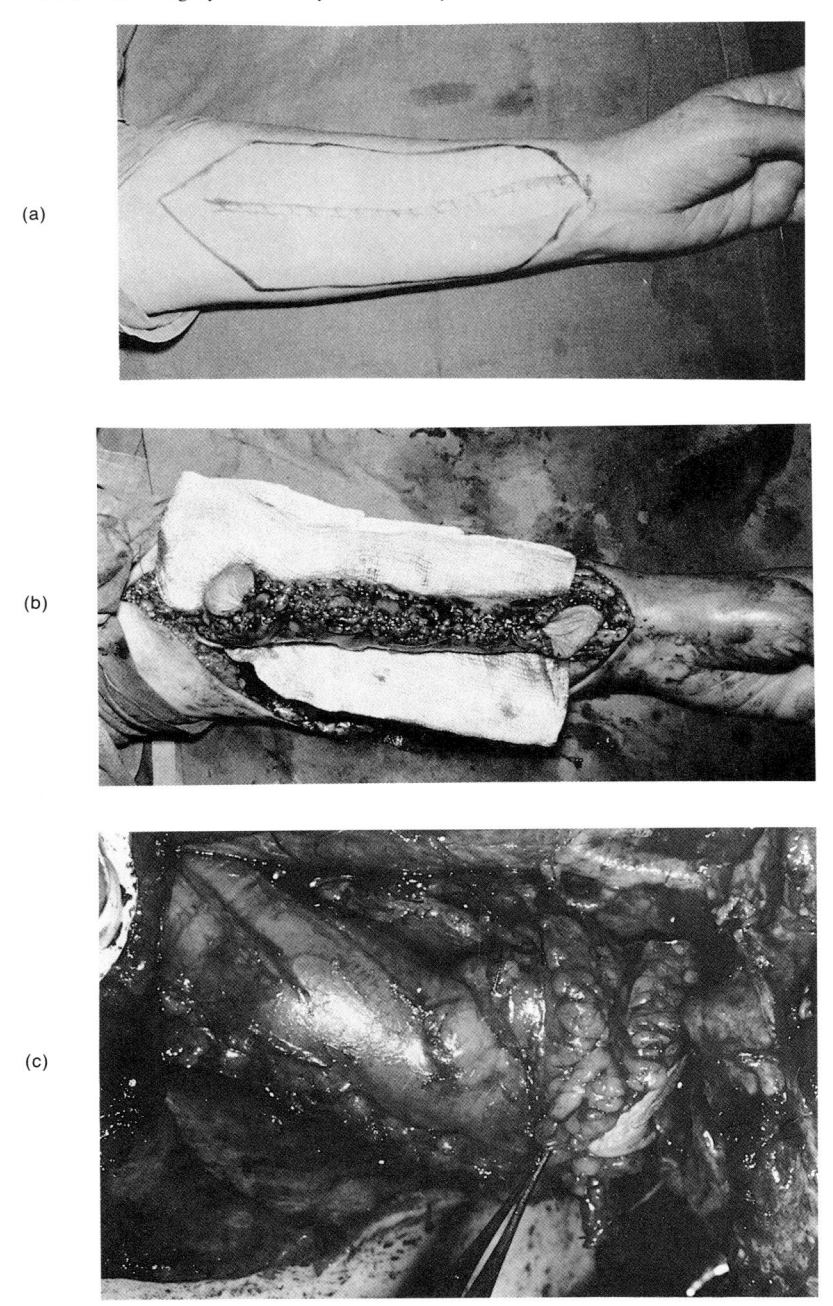

Figure 8.2 Reconstruction using a left radial forearm flap. (a) The flap is designed. (b) The flap is tubed in situ on the arm. The design at both ends increases the diameter of the tube. (c) The radial forearm skin tube is sutured into the defect in the neck. (d) Appearance 1 year following surgery

(d)

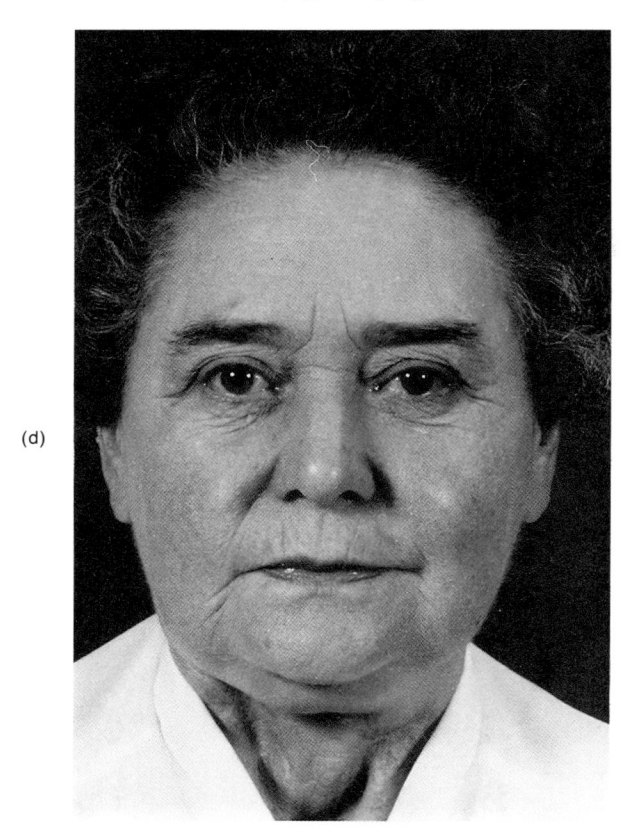

author favours free jejunal transfer. For more extensive lesions in which resection of a segment of oesophagus is deemed desirable, then the gastric pull-up is the author's first choice. In debilitated patients or in exceptional circumstances, a skin tube reconstruction may be required, accepting the likelihood of stenosis (particularly at the distal skin mucosal anastomosis). Where appropriate, the first choice is a free radial forearm flap; failing this, a tubed pectoralis major flap is a second option.

Rehabilitation

The main aim of pharyngo-oesophageal reconstruction, is to provide an adequate reconstruction for swallowing while safeguarding adequate respiration and ventilation. Swallowing, therefore, is an important measure of rehabilitation, as is the absence of developing pneumonia or any features associated with aspiration. One further consideration of rehabilitation in pharyngo-oesophageal reconstruction is the ability to speak and the production of voice.

In considering which method of reconstruction is most appropriate it is necessary to consider the type of defect, and whether it is circumferential or partial; as previously stated, different techniques appear to be more suited to coping with different defects. In addition, the extent of resection or the extent of the defect is important, whether this is a short segment defect, a long segment defect, a partial defect or a circumferential defect.

Swallowing

Swallowing is usually satisfactory when there is an intact strip of pharyngeal mucosa. This allows for a certain degree of distension and probably helps in the coordinated reflex which appears to control much of the swallowing mechanism. Patches, particularly incorporating skin flaps, can prove very useful in partial pharyngolaryngectomies, and although there is a risk of stenosis at the skin mucosal junctions these can often be dilated.

The same cannot be said for circumferential defects where the skin mucosal junctions are prone to fairly severe stenosis which does not readily lend itself to dilatation. By shaping the skin flaps an attempt can be made to widen the skin mucosal anastomosis to limit the incidence of stenosis (Figure 8.2). Ready-made conduits such as jejunum and colon appear to be better options here (Figure 8.3). Stenosis again can occur at the superior or inferior anastomosis but usually responds to dilatation. Superior anastomotic stenosis can be limited by widening the upper bowel anastomosis. This is most readily available in gastric pull-ups and colonic transfer, but can be achieved with the jejunum by performing a 'fish mouth' tech-

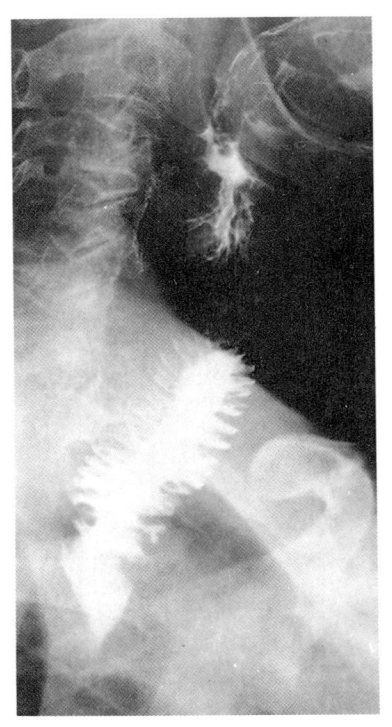

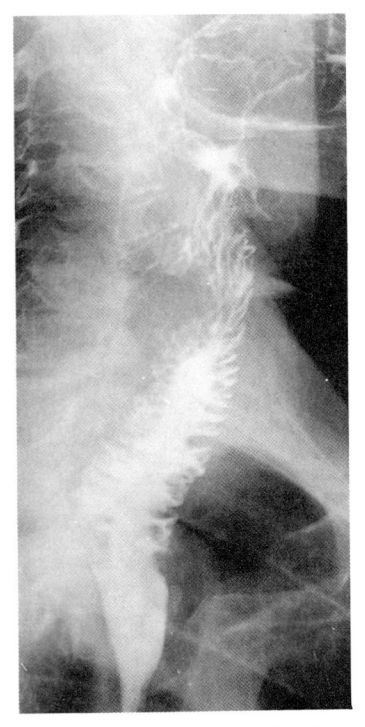

Figure 8.3 Barium swallow showing position of free jejunum reconstructing the pharyngo-oesophageal defect. The characteristic mucosal pattern of jejunum is still identifiable.

nique or, in severe cases, carrying out an end-to-side anastomosis between the jejunum and upper oropharynx (Nozaki et al., 1985). It is important not to put in too large a free jejunal graft, since the redundant bowel can result in slowing of deglutition and increasing difficulty in swallowing.

Even with a patent anastomosis, jejunal transfers do appear to be susceptible to a physiological dysphagia. This is thought to be due to the continued uncoordinated peristaltic movement of the jejunum, which persists following its transfer to the neck. The lack of coordination between the pharynx and the oesophagus and the uncoordinated peristalsis of the jejunal graft result in a functional dysphagia, despite the jejunal graft being inserted in a isoperistaltic fashion (Myers et al., 1980). Free colon transfer, on the other hand, does not appear to suffer from this intrinsic peristaltic activity (Smith et al., 1987b).

In gastric pull-ups, delay of food is seldom a problem as gastric emptying is much more rapid with the stomach in the pulled-up position. Regurgitation, however, is a significant problem which is present in at least a quarter of the patients (Wei et al., 1984).

Speech rehabilitation

There has been very little work on speech rehabilitation relating to the extent of excisional surgery, surgical defects in the pharynx and oesophagus and the various methods of reconstruction. Certainly, there has been less effort in this major type of surgery when compared with laryngectomy patients. This perhaps reflects the poor general prognosis and complications in patients undergoing total laryngopharyngectomy and reconstruction (Surkin et al., 1984). Gluckman has reported poor results with speech rehabilitation, following free jejunal transfers, when using the Singer and Blom duckbill prosthesis. His impression is that the failure may be related to the nature of the jejunal segment, or to the uncoordinated and unpredictable peristaltic activity of the jejunum (Gluckman and McDonough, 1989). Similarly poor results have been achieved with gastric pull-ups, with only a limited ability to communicate. A whisper often amplified by means of an electrolarynx was possible in only 11% of patients (Wei et al., 1984.)

The functional results of oropharyngeal surgery are currently under investigation in the West of Scotland Regional Plastic and Oral Surgery Unit at Canniesburn Hospital. A five-point scale has been designed to assess chewing, swallowing and speech (Table 8.3). This scale has proved to have statistically significant inter-rater reliability and therefore can be used as a means of self-assessment as well as assessment at routine clinic appointments (Nandagopal et al., 1990). It is hoped that this scale will provide the basis for further research and development into rehabilitation, and relate this both to excisional defects and to methods of reconstruction.

After successful laryngopharyngeal reconstruction there are three main avenues available for speech production:

(a) artificial larynx;
(b) speech by injection of air;
(c) fistula speech (Singh, 1988a, b, 1989a).

The conspicuous artificial sound produced by the artificial laryngeal devices limits their acceptance by patients. The speech produced by swallowing air to the reconstructed pharyngo-oesophagus and expelling it in small volumes is low-pitched and has a reduced intensity and rate of speech which results in poor intelligibility and acceptability.

Table 8.3 Functional intraoral Glasgow scale (FIGS)

Chewing	
Any food, no difficulty	5
Solid food, with difficulty	4
Semisolid food, no difficulty	3
Semisolid with difficulty	2
Cannot chew at all	1
Swallowing	
Any food, no difficulty	5
Solid food, with difficulty	4
Semisolid food only	3
Liquids only	2
Cannot swallow at all	1
Speech	
Clearly understood always	5
Requires repetition sometimes	4
Requires repetition many times	3
Understood by relatives only	2
Unintelligible	1

The introduction of fistula speech in combination with a voice prosthesis results in a more fluent and intelligible speech. The fistula between trachea and reconstructed pharyngo-oesophagus can be created primarily at the time of the original operation or as a secondary procedure (see Chapter 13). Finger occlusion of the tracheostoma allows the patient to use a greater volume of pulmonary air redirected into the pharyngo-oessophagus, rather than be restricted to the much smaller capacity of swallowed air. With the advent of tracheostoma valves, these patients can enjoy 'hands free' speech (Singh, 1985, 1987, 1989, 1990).

In fistula speech it is important to minimize the likelihood of aspiration of saliva or liquids as a result of the communication between respiratory and digestive tracts. In major pharyngo-oesophageal reconstruction it has been the author's practice to delay consideration of fistula speech until the patient has fully recovered from the extensive primary operation. This ensures that the patient has no difficulties in swallowing prior to any consideration of further surgery.

There is collaboration on fistula voice research between the West of Scotland Regional Plastic and Oral Maxillofacial Surgery Unit at Canniesburn Hospital in Glasgow and the Department of Otolaryngology Head and Neck Surgery Unit St John's Hospital, Livingston, which houses a well-equipped voice research laboratory (see Chapter 6).

Patients who have fully recovered from pharyngo-oesophageal reconstruction and who have no problems or difficulties in swallowing are referred to the voice research laboratory for detailed investigations. Amongst the various tests performed in the voice laboratory, subglottal pressure measurement is probably the most useful as it relates to back pressure on the cardiopulmonary system. Furthermore, it may herald the existence of local recurrence in the reconstructed pharyngo-oesophagus, especially when clinical examination is negative (see Chapter 9).

In suitable patients a fistula is created between the trachea and the reconstructed pharynx or residual oesophagus and an appropriate speaking valve inserted. The postoperative rehabilitation programme is carefully planned to return the patient successfully back to the community.

Conclusion

The type of pharyngo-oesophageal reconstruction advocated depends entirely on the defect to be reconstructed. Partial defects are suitable for skin flap reconstruction, either using pedicled myocutaneous flaps or free flaps using microvascular anastomosis. Complete circumferential defects can be divided into short segment or long segment defects. The short segment defects are suitable for reconstruction using free skin flaps or free bowel flaps revascularized by microvascular techniques. Longer segments are suited to free bowel transfers, particularly using the jejunum and colon, or in more extensive defects gastric pull-up procedures.

In experienced hands all of these techniques can be safe and reliable. In certain patients, however, a laparotomy may have to be avoided, particularly in severely debilitated or ill patients. In such cases skin flaps assume greater importance. In cases where there is extensive soft tissue damage, particularly affecting the neck skin or where the vessels in the neck are exposed, then additional protection to these vessels has to be provided over and above the pharyngo-oesophageal reconstruction. Myocutaneous flaps are most useful in this regard, as is the gastric mucosal flap incorporating omentum.

There are problems in swallowing with all these techniques: the skin flaps are prone to stenosis at the sites of anastomosis; the jejunum causes physiological dysphagia; and the stomach has a high incidence of regurgitation. Little is yet known about which method is best for producing speech in patients who have undergone a total pharyngolaryngectomy.

With operative mortality and morbidity rates decreasing with experience, attention should now be focused on the functional rehabilitation of these patients to improve the results of swallowing and speaking.

References

Ariyan S. (1979a). One stage repair of a cervical oesophagostome with two myocutaneous flaps from the neck and shoulder. *Plast. Reconst. Surg.*, **63**, 426–9.

Ariyan S. (1979b). One stage reconstruction for defects of the mouth using a sternomastoid myocutaneous flap. *Plast. Reconst. Surg.*, **63**, 618–25.

Ariyan S., Cuono C.B. (1980). Myocutaneous flaps for head and neck reconstruction. *Head and Neck Surg.*, **2**, 321–44.

Arsherson N. (1954). Pharyngectomy for post-cricoid carcinoma: one stage reconstruction of the pharynx using the larynx as an autograft. *J. Larygol. Otol.*, **68**, 550–9.

Bakamjian V.Y. (1965). A two stage method for pharyngoesophageal reconstruction with a primary pectoral skin flap. *Plast. Reconst. Surg.*, **36**, 173–84.

Baudet J. (1979). Reconstruction of the pharyngeal wall by free transfer of the greater omentum and stomach, *Int. J. Microsurg.*, **1**, 53–9.

Demergasso F., Piazza M.V. (1979). Trapezius myocutaneous flap in reconstructive surgery for head and neck tumour: an original technique. *Am. J. Surg.*, **138**, 533–6.

Flynn M.C., Acland R.D. (1979). Free intestinal autografts for reconstruction following pharyngolaryngo-oesophagectomy. *Surg. Gynaecol. Obstet.*, **149**, 858–62.

Gluckman J.L., McDonough J.J., Donegan J.O. (1982). The role of the free jejunal graft in reconstruction of the pharynx and cervical oesophagus. *Head Neck Surg.*, **4**, 360–9.

Gluckman J.L., Weissler M.C., McCafferty G. (1987). Partial versus total oesophagectomy for advanced carcinoma of the hypopharynx. *Arch. Otolaryngol. Head Neck Surg.*, **113**, 69–72.

Gluckman J.L., McDonough J.J. (1989). Free jejunal grafts. In *Microsurgical Reconstructions of the Head and Neck* (Baker S.R., ed.) New York: Churchill Livingstone, pp. 229–54.

Harii, K., Ebihara, S., Ono, I., et al. (1985). Pharyngoesophageal reconstruction using a fabricated forearm free flap. *Plast. Reconst. Surg.*, **75**, 463–74.

Harrison D.F.N. (1970). Pathology of hypopharyngeal cancer in relation to surgical management. *J. Laryngol. Otol.*, **84**, 349–57.

Hayden R.E. (1989). Lateral cutaneous thigh flap. In *Microsurgical Reconstruction of the Head and Neck* (Baker S.R., ed.) New York: Churchill Livingstone, pp. 211–28.

Hiebert C.A., Cummings G.O. (1961). Successful replacement of the cervical oesophagus by transplantation and revascularisation of a free graft of gastric antrum. *Ann. Surg.*, **154**, 103–6.

Katsaros J., Banis J.C., Acland R.D., Tan E. (1985). Monitoring free vascularised jejunum grafts. *Br. J. Plast. Surg.*, **38**, 220–2.

Lam K.H., Wong J., Lim S.T.K., Ong G.B. (1981). Pharyngogastric anastomosis following pharyngolaryngo-oesophagectomy: analysis of 157 cases. *World J. Surg.*, **5**, 509–16.

Lam K.H. (1987). Reconstruction of the cervical oesophagus with a gastric pull-up procedure. In, *Cancer of The Head and Neck* (Ariyan S. ed.) St Louis: CV Mosby Co., pp. 490–501.

Myers W.C., Seigler H.F., Hanks J.P., et al. (1985). Post-operative function of 'free' jejunal transplants for replacement of the cervical oesophagus. *Ann. Surg.*, **192**, 439–48.

Nakayama K., Yamamoto K., Makino H., et al. (1964). Experience with free autografts of the bowel with a new venous anastomosis apparatus. *Surgery*, **55**, 796–802.

Nandagopal N., Batchelor A.G., Soutar D.S. (July 1990). Functional assessment of the oral cavity following reconstructive surgery. *British Association of Plastic Surgeons Meeting*, Belfast.

Nozaki M., Huang T., Hayashi M. (1985). Reconstruction of the pharyngoesophagus following a laryngo-oesophagectomy and irradiation therapy. *Plast. Reconst. Surg.*, **76**, 386–92.

Ong G.B., Lee T.C. (1960). Pharyngogastric anastomosis after oesophagopharyngectomy for carcinoma of the hypopharynx and cervical oesophagus. *Br. J. Surg.*, **48**, 193–200.

Papachristou D.M., Trichilis E., Fortner J.G. (1979). Experimental use of free gastric flaps for the repair of pharyngoesophageal defects. *Plast. Reconst. Surg.*, **64**, 336–9.

Sasaki T.M., Baker H.W., McConnell D.B., Vetto M. (1982). Free jejunal mucosal patch graft reconstruction of the oropharynx. *Arch. Surg.*, **117**, 459–62.

Seidenberg B., Rosenek S.S., Hurwitt E.S., Som M.L. (1959). Immediate reconstruction of the cervical oesophagus by a revascularized isolated jejunal segment. *Ann. Surg.*, **149**, 162–71.

Silver C.E. (1981). Surgical treatment of hypopharyngeal and cervical oesophageal cancer. *World J. Surg.*, **5**, 499.

Singh W. (1985). New tracheostoma flap valve for surgical speech reconstruction. In *New Dimensions in Otorhinolaryngology, Head and Neck Surgery*, vol. II (Myers E., ed.) Amsterdam: Elsevier, pp. 480–1.

Singh W. (1987). Tracheostoma valve for speech rehabilitation in laryngectomees. *J. Laryngol. Otol.*, **101**, 809–14.

Singh W. (1988a). A simple surgical technique and a new prosthesis for voice rehabilitation after laryngectomy. *J. Laryngol. Otol.*, **102**, 332–4.

Singh W. (1988b). Valvula fonatoria de Singh. In *Recuperacion De La Voz En Los laryngectomizados* (Algaba J., ed.) Madrid: Garsi, pp. 331–3.

Singh W. (1989a). Near-total laryngectomy. In *Proceedings of International Voice Symposium*, Edinburgh. (Singh W., ed.) W. Singh, pp. 53–8.

Singh W. (1989b). Singh Tracheostoma Valve. In *Proceedings of the International Voice Symposium, Edinburgh*. (Singh W., ed.) Edinburgh: W. Singh, pp. 81–2.

Singh, W. (1990). Singh Tracheostoma Valve. In *Proceedings of XXIst International Congress of the International Association of Logopedics and Phoniatarics*. Prague, Czechoslovakia, pp. 435–7.

Smith R.W., Garvey C.J., Taylor P.C., Davies D. (1987a). Experimental assessment of free jejunal and colonic grafts of the oesophagus. *Arch. Otolaryngol. Head Neck Surg.*, **113**, 187–92.

Smith R.W., Garvey C.J., Dawson P.M., Davies D.M. (1987b). Jejunum versus colon for free oesophageal reconstruction: an experimental radiological assessment. *Br. J. Plast. Surg.*, **40**, 181–7.

Soutar D.S. (1985). Pharyngoesophageal reconstruction using a fabricated forearm flap. Discussion. *Plast. Reconst. Surg.*, **75**, 475.

Stell P.M. (1970). Esophageal replacement by transposed stomach following pharygno-laryngo-oesophagectomy for carcinoma of the cervical oesophagus. *Arch. Otolaryngol.*, **91**, 166–70.

Surkin M.I., Lawson W., Biller F. (1984). Analysis of the methods of pharyngoesophageal reconstruction. *Head Neck Surg.*, **6**, 953–70.

Van den Bogaert W., Ostyne F., Van den Schueren E. (1983). The primary treatment of advanced vocal cord cancer: laryngectomy or radiotherapy? *Int. J. Radiat. Oncol. Biol. Phys.*, **9**, 329–34.

Vandenbrouck C., Sancho H., Lefur R., et al. (1977). Results of a randomized clinical trial of pre-operative irradiation versus post-operative in treatment of tumours of the hypopharynx. *Cancer*, **39**, 1445–53.

Watson J.S., Robertson J., Lendrum M. (1982). Pharyngeal reconstruction using the latissimus dorsi myocutaneous flap. *Br. J. Plast. Surg.*, **35**, 401–12.

Wei W.I., Lam K.H., Choi S., Wong J. (1984). Late problems after pharyngolaryngo-oesophagectomy and pharyngogastric anastomosis for cancer of the larynx and hypopharynx. *Am. J. Surg.*, **148**, 509–12.

Chapter 9

Near-total or parsimonious laryngectomy

W. Singh

Speech is a basic human instinct and a psychosocial necessity. Loss of speech may not only disrupt an individual's livelihood, but also produce serious psychological stress and behaviour changes. In the UK, approximately 2000 cases of cancer of the larynx occur every year, and about 300 laryngectomies are performed. The majority of these patients are 50–70 years old, and are potentially able to return to work, provided they can communicate. The condition rarely occurs in children (Singh and Kaur 1987).

The management of carcinoma of the larynx is complicated by the numerous treatment options available to the head and neck surgeon. There is no universal consensus as to which of the available treatments is best for cancer clearance with minimum associated morbidity. The ultimate aim of any treatment is eradication of cancer and preservation of maximum possible function. The minimum target of a conservative laryngeal procedure should be to preserve voice and also to achieve cure rates comparable to total laryngectomy in properly selected cases. The scientific basis of the near-total laryngectomy (parsimonious laryngectomy) procedure is well established (Singh, 1989b, 1991; Singh and Hardcastle 1985).

This chapter describes the procedure of near-total laryngectomy (parsimonious laryngectomy), omitting other currently available conservative surgical procedures which are described in detail elsewhere.

History

The mention of conservation surgery of the larynx dates from much earlier than the first total laryngectomy. In 1851, Gordon Buck performed the first laryngofissure for cancer of the larynx (Buck, 1853). Billroth performed the first hemilaryngectomy in 1878. All these partial procedures fell into disrepute, mainly because of aspiration and infection, not because of insufficient clearance of cancer. Though these procedures were superior to total laryngectomy, in that they allowed preservation of voice, nasal respiration and clearance of tumour, there was no experimental evidence to prove their logic.

Over the years it has been observed that glottic cancer grows slowly and remains localized to the larynx for a long time. Hajek (1932) was the first to demonstrate that dye injected into the submucosa of the larynx spreads in a specific manner. It was the work of Pressman in 1956 that established the basis of various conservative procedures; he and his colleagues published their observations on the injection of dyes and radioisotopes into the larynx (Pressman, 1956; Pressman et al., 1961). Dye or isotopes injected submucosally remained localized to certain specific regions or compartments, and were never observed to cross the midline from one side to the other. 'Cancer of the larynx does, for a long time at least, remain localised to specific areas of isolation that can be demonstrated by dyes to exist as isolated compartments within the larynx. These observations may have an important bearing upon our thinking relative to surgery in the laryngeal region, particularly in so far as technique of, and indications for, subtotal laryngectomies are concerned' (Pressman et al., 1961).

In detailed whole-organ serial section studies of 200 laryngeal cancers by Kirchner (1977), the specimens yielded information regarding site, unilateral patterns of growth and spread of the lesion submucosally and via lymphatics, thus determining the grounds for suitability of a laryngeal cancer for conservative surgery.

A further study based on whole-organ serial section technique by Robbins and Michaels (1985) supports the belief that a large number of patients who underwent total laryngectomy could have been treated successfully by subtotal laryngectomy with preservation of voice.

Principle

Near-total laryngectomy (parsimonious laryngectomy) is appropriate for extirpation of advanced cancer of the larynx (e.g. in T3 glottal carcinoma, supraglottic carcinoma, transglottal carcinoma and piriform sinus cancer with cord fixation). It will preserve a good voice and avoid aspiration. The underlying principle is to resect the tumour-bearing part of the larynx, as against removal of the whole larynx in total laryngectomy, using the tumour-free laryngeal remnant to fashion a sphincteric speaking tube which permits lung-powered phonation. The principles of safe conservative surgery in parsimonious laryngectomy are based on a study of the development of the larynx, its submucosal compartmentation, and observations based on experimental and clinical patterns of laryngeal cancer.

Terminology

Any cancer extirpation procedure, preserving lung-powered voice by creating a dynamic, innervated myomucosal tracheopharyngeal shunt, employed as an alternative to total laryngectomy, might best be termed a parsimonious laryngectomy. The reason for introducing this new terminology arises from the fact that there is a considerable variation in the widely used description of a subtotal laryngectomy (or near-total laryngectomy) in the literature. The author has described a procedure of near-total laryngectomy (Singh, 1985, 1989b); other authors include Hofmann Saguez (1951), Pressman (1956), Majer and Reider (1958), Ogura and Dedo (1965), Czigner (1972), Iwai and Koike (1973), Mozolewski et al. (1975) and Pearson (1981). However, different procedures under the same name are being compared, with erroneous conclusions. With hindsight, the procedure of near-total laryngectomy described previously (Singh, 1985, 1989b, 1991) might better have been termed 'parsimonious laryngectomy'. Parsimonious laryngectomy serves the same safe oncological concept as total laryngectomy, with the advantage that it retains healthy laryngeal and tracheal tissue and uses it for voice reconstruction, in the form of a dynamic sphincteric laryngotracheal speaking tube.

Basic concept and comments

The resection of the tumour-bearing portion of the larynx, with clear margins and conserving as much as possible of the tumour-free remnant larynx, is based on oncological principles and is a safe and sound concept. The route of spread and extent of the tumour within the larynx is determined by the site of its origin. Cancer of the larynx does remain localized for a long time to specific anatomic areas of origin. These specific submucosal anatomic compartments within the larynx have been demonstrated by injecting dyes and radioisotopes submucosally (Pressman, 1961) and by whole-organ serial section studies (Olofsson and van Nostrand, 1973; Kirchner, 1975a, b, 1977, 1984a, b).

The breakthrough from one compartment to the other occurs in a limited number of cases, in later stages. Of greater significance is the fact that submucosal laryngeal compartments of one side do not communicate with those of the other side. The two halves of the larynx are separated from each other and there is no submucosal spread either by direct extension or lymphatics. In each hemilarynx, the connective tissue barriers (conus elasticus and quadrangular membrane) and the cartilaginous framework determine the spread of cancer.

The surface extension of laryngeal tumours, in many cases, represents only the tip of the iceberg. The bulk of the growth lies in occult submucosal compartments and later in two well-defined and relatively discrete spaces, pre-epiglottic and paraglottic, depending on the site of the origin of the tumour.

Logical excision of cancer in parsimonious laryngectomy requires a clear understanding of the submucosal laryngeal compartments, connective tissue barriers, surrounding cartilaginous framework, anterior commissure and pre-epiglottic and paraglottic spaces.

Submucosal compartments

There is a very definite correlation between the arrangements of submucosal laryngeal compartments and the pattern of site of origin and route of spread of cancer within the larynx. The knowledge of this anatomical arrangement can enable us to predict the probable route and extent of the pathology, depending on the site of origin of the growth within the larynx. This concept of compartmentalization and the slow growth of tumours in known patterns helps in forming a clinical judgment of how much of the tumour-bearing larynx is to be removed with clear margins (in millimetres), and how much in millimetres of the remainder can be safely used to achieve the function of voice production and avoid aspiration in parsimonious laryngectomy.

The traditional division of the larynx into three levels (supraglottis, glottis and subglottis) is not justifiable, either on embryologic, anatomic, functional or oncologic grounds (Kleinsasser, 1988). Division of the larynx based on submucosal compartmentalization seems to be the most rational from the oncologic point of view. On oncological grounds, the following unilateral compartments of the larynx are identifiable:

(a) supraglottis;
(b) ventricle of larynx;
(c) free margin of true vocal cords and underlying Reinke's space;

(d) infraglottis — mobile subglottis (from below true vocal cord to upper border of cricoid) and fixed subglottis (bounded by cricoid cartilage).

Supraglottis

The supraglottis is bounded by the epiglottis (both suprahyoid and infrahyoid portions) in the midline, above and laterally by the aryepiglottic folds, below by the false cords and posteriorly by the arytenoid cartilages. It is separated below from the glottis by the ventricle which forms its inferior boundary on either side. Anteriorly it is related to the pre-epiglottic space and laterally to the paraglottic spaces on either side. The *pre-epiglottic space* (Figure 9.1) is bounded superiorly by the hyoid bone and by the hypoepiglottic ligament lying underneath the mucous membrane of the vallecula, anteriorly by the thyrohyoid membrane and upper part of thyroid cartilage, posteriorly by the epiglottis, and inferiorly by the thyroepiglottic ligament. The thyroepiglottic and hypoepiglottic ligaments merge with the perichondrium of the thyroid cartilage and periosteum of the hyoid bone respectively. Thus a compartment lined with fibrous tissue is formed; it is filled with loose connective tissue and fat, and is rich in lymphatics, but contains no lymph nodes. The tumours of the epiglottis have easy access to the pre-epiglottic space. The lympatics from the supraglottic region accompany the superior neurovascular bundle and penetrate the thyrohyoid membrane to reach the upper deep cervical lymph nodes.

The *paraglottic space* (Figure 9.2) is a paired laryngeal space which clinically is of

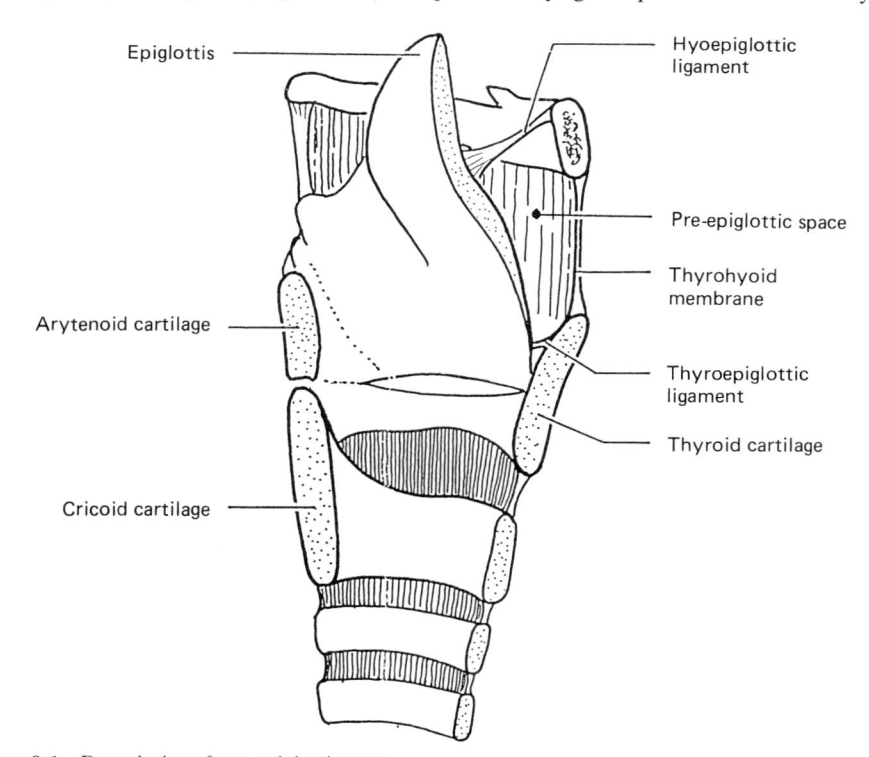

Figure 9.1 Boundaries of pre-epiglottic space

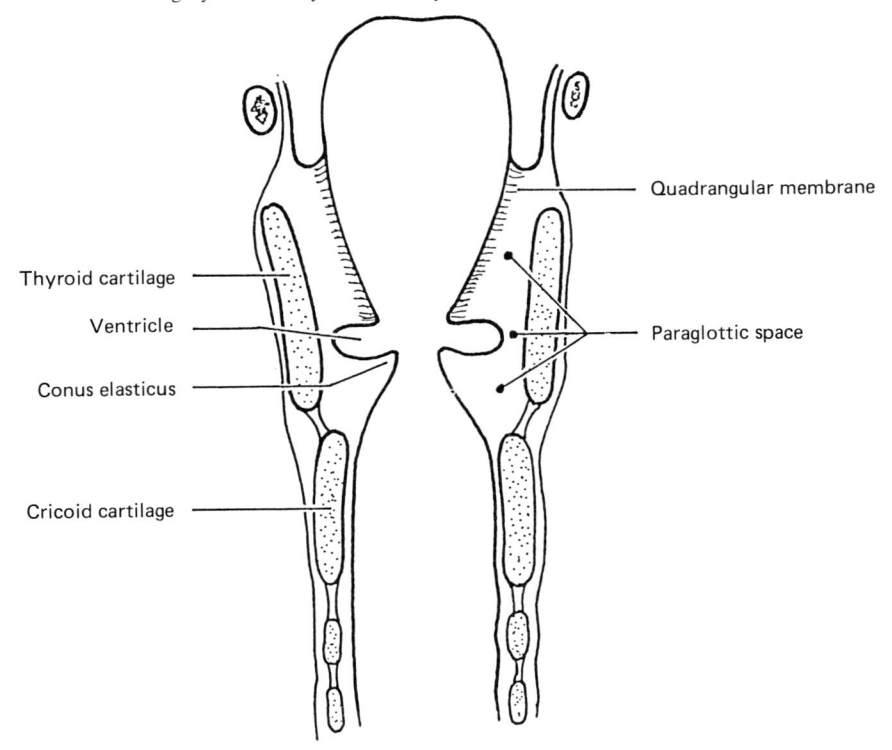

Figure 9.2 Boundaries of paraglottic space

paramount importance in the spread of cancer of the larynx. It lies lateral to supraglottis, infraglottis and ventricle. It is limited above and medially by the quadrangular membrane and ventricle, below and medially by the conus elasticus, anterolaterally by the thyroid cartilage, and posteriorly by the mucosa of the piriform sinus. Superiorly each paraglottic space is continuous with the pre-epiglottic space through an ill-defined corridor, but this is not the usual pathway of tumour spread. More commonly the cancer in the supraglottis region spreads to the paraglottic space through the ventricle which it surrounds and with which it is in close touch. Spread of the tumour into the paraglottic space is of great oncological significance in parsimonious laryngectomy and other conservative surgical procedures.

Comment
Based on the compartmentalization concept, supraglottic tumours can be removed safely with preservation of voice by supraglottic laryngectomy. In supraglottic laryngectomy, the whole of the pre-epiglottic space is removed. If the cancer has spread to the ventricle below and fixed the vocal cord (transglottic carcinoma T3) there is a serious risk that it has spread into the paraglottic space. Once the tumour is in the paraglottic space it cannot be extirpated by supraglottic laryngectomy. The option then is parsimonious laryngectomy with voice preservation as a standardized procedure; the alternative is total laryngectomy. Obviously the former is preferable, provided it is oncologically safe. Similarly, if the ipsilateral vocal cord is fixed in a glottic tumour, the paraglottic space is usually involved. The preferable surgical treatment is clearly parsimonious laryngectomy.

The precise involvement of the paraglottic space, thyroid cartilage infiltration and destruction can be detected by CT or magnetic resonance imaging (MRI) in many cases, though there are always some false positives and negatives.

In small numbers of cases of supraglottic cancer the tumour is reported to have approached the hyoid bone closely enough to require its removal. The author suggests that the hyoid bone be removed *in toto* in order to avoid any risk of leaving residual cancer behind. In parsimonious laryngectomy, removal of the hyoid bone *in toto* is the standard procedure, and is recommended as the most oncologically safe procedure.

Ventricle

The ventricle is the watershed between the supraglottis and glottis regions. In normal circumstances, and in the early stages of cancer in these regions, the ventricle forms a barrier between the two regions, both by direct continuity and by lymphatics. Cancer involving the ventricle either takes its origin in the ventricle itself and then grows upwards and downwards (Le Roux-Roberts, 1936; Baclesse, 1949) or, as most authors believe, it extends to the ventricle from the supraglottis or glottis regions. Involvement of the ventricle usually signifies spread to the paraglottal space (Figure 9.3). Whatever the initial starting point of the growth, a tumour crossing the ventricle in a vertical plane is a transglottic tumour. This term was first used by McGavran et al. (1961). Since then, many writers have reported that transglottal cancer invades

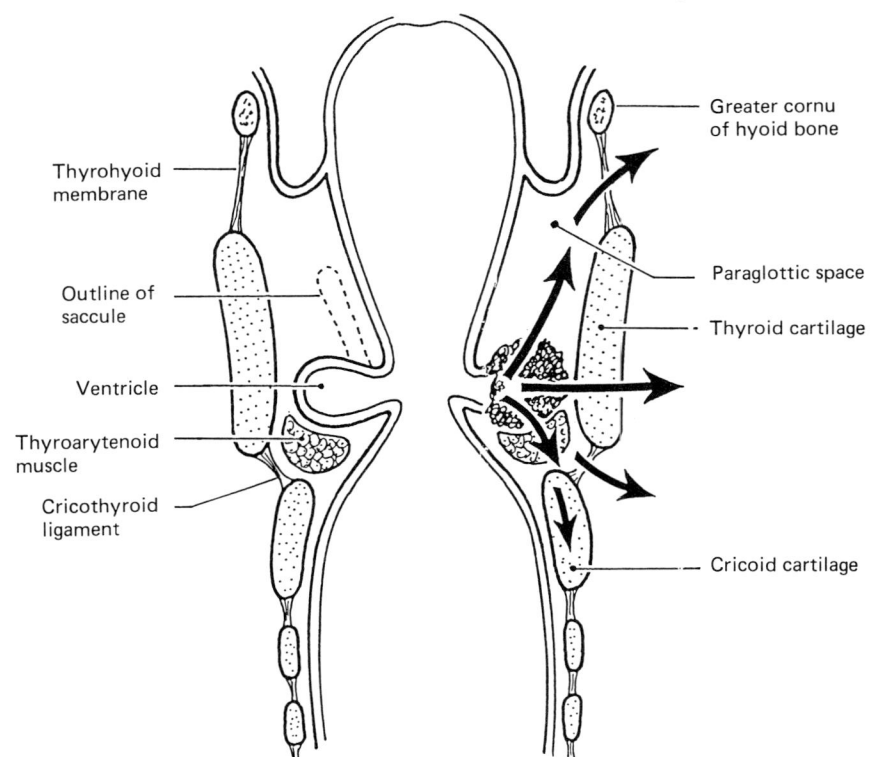

Figure 9.3 Direction of spread of left transglottic tumour

the laryngeal tissues deeply and shows a propensity towards regional metastases. The term 'ventricular (or ventriculosaccular) carcinoma' is used for tumours arising deep in the ventricle (Michaels and Hassmann, 1982). Whole-organ serial section studies by Kirchner et al. (1974) demonstrated that the laryngeal framework was involved in 76% of cases of transglottal cancer. The majority showed extensive involvement of the paraglottic space (and possibly the pre-epiglottic space), spread to the piriform sinus posteriorly and showed great propensity for spreading extralaryngeally through the cricothyroid membrane. Cervical node metastases were noted in 30% of cases. It has been observed by Pressman et al. (1961) and others that dye injected into a ventricle can spread to the ventricle of the other side as a very narrow dye-stained band. Cancer cells might also spread between right and left ventricles.

To sum up, cancer arising in a ventricle or invading it in the vertical plane from the supraglottis or glottis (transglottic cancer) has in the majority of cases the following features and patterns of growth.

(1) Most transglottic carcinomas are T3 or T4 neoplasms. They form a substantial percentage of the tumours that can be excised by parsimonious laryngectomy as a standard procedure, and which alternatively would require total laryngectomy with loss of voice.
(2) Relative to the small size of the clinically visible tumour, the extent of its spread deep into surrounding paralaryngeal space is much more extensive.
(3) In the majority of transglottic carcinomas, the laryngeal framework, especially the thyroid cartilage, is involved (Pittam and Carter, 1982). Destruction of the thyroid lamina is patchy, depending on scattered areas of ossification. The cricoid and arytenoid cartilages are infiltrated less frequently. The normal-looking thyroid lamina on the apparently uninvolved side can be affected by cancer, i.e. the laryngeal framework is invaded under the intact mucous membrane of the side opposite to the visible lesion (Kirchner, 1984b). This involvement of thyroid cartilage may represent bilateralization of the tumour, without the invasion of soft tissues (Micheau et al., 1976). Scanning by CT and MRI can identify invasion of cartilage, but neither is an entirely reliable indicator (Kirchner, 1984b).
(4) Seventy-five per cent of cases of transglottic carcinoma spread to the paraglottic and pre-epiglottic space (Pittam and Carter, 1982; Kirchner et al., 1974). When treating these patients, the potential involvement of these spaces must always be assumed unless proved otherwise.
(5) The tumour has a great predilection to spread outside the larynx, even at an early stage, by passing through the median cricothyroid ligament, involving the lymphatic network and possible Broyle's node lying on it. This region is drained by lymphatics to the lower cervical nodes of both sides. When a thyrocricotracheal (TCT) incision is planned, the cricoid cut on the unaffected side should be sited off-centre in order to avoid cutting through the potentially cancer-bearing lymphatics in the central cricothyroid ligament.
(6) Myers and Ogura (1979) wrote that the transglottic tumours, especially those with subglottic extensions, are associated with stomal recurrence. To avoid such a calamity, the tracheal part of the TCT incision should extend to or below the lower border of the first tracheal ring, in order to avoid cutting through potentially involved subglottic lymphatics (lymphatics of the infraglottis stop at the lower border of the cricoid cartilage).
(7) There is probable transventricular spread of carcinoma by lymphatics from one

ventricle to another. The saccule arising in the anterior part of the ventricle can harbour cancer which may not be visible. In ventricular tumours, bilateralization occurs across the anterior commissure (Micheau et al., 1976). Incision of paraglottic tissue and true and false cords on the uninvolved side should be at the posterior end of the ventricle, to avoid leaving any occult cancer in the anterior ventriculosaccular part.
(8) Neck node metastases are proportionately more common in transglottic carcinoma than in supraglottic or infraglottic tumours. Mittal et al. (1984) reported neck metastases in 45% of their cases with transglottal carcinomas. In the operating theatre it is important to palpate for neck nodes again when the neck muscles are relaxed under general anaesthesia. If neck nodes are clinically palpable, radical neck dissection can be done in conjunction with parsimonious laryngectomy.
(9) Twenty-five per cent of multiregional tumours (transglottal tumours) present with stridor (Stell and Bowdler, 1988). There is controversy regarding the best form of treatment for this. It has been suggested that transglottic tumours with cord fixation respond poorly to radiotherapy alone and would be better treated by surgery (Vermund, 1970).

Radiotherapy is advised as the primary mode of treatment only for patients who refuse surgery or whose general condition is too poor for surgery. In our experience, parsimonious laryngectomy is the standard surgical procedure in transglottic T3 and T4 cases where a small, oncologically safe laryngeal leftover can be used for production of voice. In irradiated cases of transglottic carcinoma where the tumour margins are well defined, the tumour can be safely excised with clear margins and the voice preserved. As reported earlier, inspection with a magnifying loupe is very helpful (Singh, 1989b), and great caution is needed. Whenever there is doubt, total laryngectomy or more radical procedures are necessary.

In the author's experience, parsimonious laryngectomy has been the standard operation in more than two-thirds of cases of transglottic carcinoma, including irradiated cases. Total laryngectomy is kept as an alternative in cases where, at operation, parsimonious laryngectomy seems to be contraindicated. In all cases preoperative permission for total laryngectomy, as an alternative, must be obtained routinely.

Glottis

The glottis includes the free margin of the true vocal cord and the underlying Reinke's space. Fortunately, this part of the larynx differs in the behaviour of cancer from the rest of the larynx. Study with dye injection and radioisotopes by Pressman et al. (1961) showed that this compartment is isolated from structures above and below, both for direct spread and lymphatic spread. It has sparse lymphatics.

Glottal carcinoma arises from the anterior part of the vocal cord and extends anteriorly to the anterior commissure. It spreads along the fibres of Broyle's tendon into the thyroid cartilage. It may cross over to the anterior part of the opposite vocal cord, inferiorly to the subglottis and superiorly to the ventricle and supraglottis. Very rarely it arises from the posterior part of the membrane covering the arytenoid or posterior commissure (Shaheen, 1959).

The conus elasticus and vocal ligament temporarily restrict deep infiltration to the subglottic space. Large tumours of the vocal cord infiltrate vocal muscles directly.

Before the conus elasticus is involved and destroyed it directs the tumour laterally into the paraglottic space. Most of these tumours find their way out of the larynx through the cricothyroid membrane and may invade the thyroid gland.

Glottal cancer is the most common and the most frequently curable form of laryngeal cancer. The earlier cordal cancer remains limited to its region and is treated by radiotherapy with good results.

In T3 glottal cancer, the ipsilateral vocal cord is fixed, usually with involvement of the paraglottal space. The involvement of thyroid or cricoid cartilage usually does not extend beyond the clinically obvious tumour. There is no consensus of opinion as to whether radiotherapy or radical surgery is the best method of treatment.

Based on the author's experience, parsimonious laryngectomy should be the standard surgical treatment for glottal T3 tumours. In cases of recurrence of the earlier cases of glottic cancer which have been treated by radiotherapy and recurrence of irradiated T3 tumours where the tumour margins are well-defined (as inspected with magnifying loupe), the tumour can be safely excised with clear margins and the voice preserved.

Where there is persistent post-irradiation oedema or a persistently fixed hemilarynx, a deep biopsy is mandatory to diagnose recurrence histologically. Imaging by CT or MRI may help in defining tumour extent, unfortunately rarely in cases that are otherwise difficult to assess. In these cases of post-irradiation recurrence there may be numerous false positive and false negative results.

The anterior commissure is inserted directly into the thyroid cartilage by Broyle's tendon and hence the tumour involving it may well have invaded the cartilage. This factor has to be kept in mind when considering conservative surgical procedures.

Subglottis

The subglottis or infraglottis extends from below the true vocal cords up to the inferior border of the cricoid cartilage. Primary subglottic carcinoma is rare. The lower border of the cricoid cartilage forms the watershed between larynx and trachea, both anatomically and in terms of lymphatic drainage. Spread of subglottal growth below this level contraindicates parsimonious laryngectomy.

Most of these tumours extend extralaryngeally either by lymphatics or directly by penetrating the cricothyroid membrane and invading the thyroid gland. Laterally they tend to invade laryngeal muscle and cartilage directly, while medially the growth encroaches upon the lumen.

The lymphatics from the subglottal region, above the upper border of cricoid, drain through the cricothyroid membrane to the ipsilateral lower cervical lymph nodes, while lymphatics from the subglottal region surrounded by the cricoid ring penetrate the cricothyroid membrane and enter the cricothyroid plexus, often spreading to cervical lymph nodes on both sides. This fact must be kept in mind while looking for cervical lymph nodes.

Piriform sinus

The piriform sinus is an inverted three-sided pyramid, bounded laterally by mucosa covering the posterior part of the thyroid lamina, medially by the aryepiglottic fold, arytenoid and cricoid cartilage, and above by the pharyngoepiglottic fold. Inferiorly its ill-defined apex lies just above and lateral to the cricopharyngeal muscle, leading to the oesophagus; anteriorly it lies in close proximity to the ipsilateral paraglottal space.

Piriform sinus tumours comprise the majority of all the hypopharyngeal tumours. Since most carcinomas of the piriform sinus are well advanced when first seen, the exact site of their origin can rarely be demonstrated precisely by whole-organ serial section studies. Piriform sinus carcinomas often grow medially into the ipsilateral larynx, fixing it, extending further through the paraglottal space and then penetrating the cricothyroid membrane to spread extralaryngeally, often involving the ipsilateral thyroid lobe. The ipsilateral vocal cord is already fixed in most cases by the time the diagnosis of piriform sinus cancer is made. Local infiltration occurs aggressively and rapidly because of lack of natural anatomic barriers. Cervical node metastases occur early because the piriform sinus is rich in lymphatics. Lateral extensions through the thyroid cartilage can be seen in a number of cases. Tumours with ipsilateral fixed vocal cord, thyroid cartilage involvement and involvement of the sinus apex are amenable to safe surgical resection and cure by parsimonious laryngectomy, but the involvement of postcricoid, interarytenoid area, fixation of the opposite vocal cord or involvement of the opposite piriform sinus are contraindications to parsimonious laryngectomy.

Previous radiotherapy in an otherwise resectable piriform sinus tumour with vocal cord fixation is no contraindication to parsimonious laryngectomy.

Because hypopharyngeal cancer is notorious for 'skip lesions', panendoscopy during parsimonious laryngectomy is essential to rule out any other lesion. The tumour clearance margin should be as wide as possible — the cancer in this region spreads submucosally for about 1 cm without surface involvement. The margins of clearance in a pharyngeal resection should be in centimetres, in contrast to T3 glottal cancer, where margin clearance in millimetres is safe oncologically.

Indications

Parsimonious laryngectomy is indicated in the following selected cases.

Non-irradiated patients

Larynx
Parsimonious laryngectomy is indicated in cases of T3 and T4 glottal carcinoma, supraglottal carcinoma and transglottal carcinoma with ipsilateral cord fixation.

Hypopharynx
Piriform sinus carcinoma with ipsilateral cord fixation is also an indication for parsimonious laryngectomy.

Recurrence after irradiation

Parsimonious laryngectomy is indicated for tumour recurrence in a patient after radiation for early glottal cancer and in selected cases of T3 glottal carcinoma where the margins are well defined for excision of tumour.

In cases of irradiated transglottal cancer and piriform fossa tumours one should be very wary. Unless the margins of clearance can be wide and are well defined, the alternative procedure of total laryngectomy or pharyngolaryngectomy is preferable.

Contraindications

Parsimonious laryngectomy (near-total laryngectomy) is contraindicated in the following situations:

(1) fixation of both vocal cords;
(2) interarytenoid area (posterior commissure) involvement;
(3) posterior (midline) subglottis extension;
(4) postcricoid involvement;
(5) radiation failures where margins of the tumour (under magnification) are indistinct;
(6) involvement of the opposite ventricle or paraglottal space (but involvement of the anterior end of the opposite vocal cord is not a contraindication so long as the opposite vocal cord is mobile);
(7) involvement of the posterior part of opposite thyroid lamina in the region of the cricothyroid joint (but involvement of the anterior part of the contralateral thyroid lamina is no contraindication as it can safely be removed in parsimonious laryngectomy).

Old age is not a contraindication for parsimonious laryngectomy, although the author is usually disinclined to attempt this procedure in patients over 80 years old.

Cervical node metastases are not a contraindication for parsimonious laryngectomy; the nodes can be removed by radical neck dissection in association with parsimonious laryngectomy.

Complications and solutions

Nerve injury

Injury to the recurrent laryngeal nerve on the normal side is extremely rare in experienced hands. The uninitiated are advised to use a magnifying loupe to recognize the position of this nerve, and to keep away from the cricothyroid joint. If an injured nerve does not recover and leads to aspiration, a Singh fistula valve (large size) can be used to prevent aspiration.

Stenosis

Stenosis of the speaking tube is rare and can be avoided by gentle handling of the mucosa and by taking care not to leave any raw area to heal and fibrose. A small (8 FG) ureteric catheter helps in the orientation and correct positioning of mucosa during suturing and minimal haematoma formation in the postoperative period. Use of a catheter larger than 8 FG is discouraged as it may cause stretching and injury to the mucosal surface resulting later in stenosis.

If stenosis occurs, it should be dilated with ureteric catheters in increasing diameters, from the stoma upwards; this procedure can be done in the outpatient department.

Dysphagia

Dysphagia is not a common problem after parsimonious laryngectomy. If the pharyngeal remnant is too narrow, a myocutaneous flap should be used to augment it.

In dysphagia caused by a slightly narrow pharyngo-oesophageal segment, bougie dilatation is advisable.

Infection

Preoperative antibiotics are recommended as a prophylaxis against infection. The author's practice is to give antibiotics in all cases undergoing parsimonious laryngectomy or total laryngectomy.

Mucocutaneous fistula

Mucocutaneous fistula formation is encountered rarely in patients who have been irradiated. In these cases a nasogastric tube should be kept *in situ* for feeding until the fistula has healed. We have not so far encountered a fistula in any of our irradiated or non-irradiated cases.

Aspiration

Aspiration is a rare complication of parsimonious laryngectomy in a non-irradiated patient. The following factors may contribute to the occurrence of aspiration:

(1) injury to the normal side recurrent laryngeal nerve;
(2) an unduly wide pharyngeal end of the speaking tube constructed by using a pharyngeal flap;
(3) a hypertonic cricopharyngeal sphincter;
(4) suturing of the remnant infrahyoid muscles to the suprahyoid musculature in the vertical plane with consequent elevation of the normal piriform fossa during swallowing;
(5) undesirable myotomy of constrictor muscle fibres above the cricopharyngeal muscle;
(6) stenosis of the pharyngo-oesophageal segment.

During normal swallowing there is coordination between pharyngeal peristalsis and relaxation of the cricopharyngeal muscle (Negus, 1949; Ardran and Kemp, 1951). The precise mechanism of this coordination is not well understood. The pharyngeal peristalsis and the upward and forward pull of the larynx mechanically stretching the cricopharyngeal muscle are regarded as some of the known coordinating factors in relaxation of the cricopharyngeal muscle. In parsimonious laryngectomy the lack of laryngeal pull can be a contributory factor. To rectify this anomalous factor we suggest cricopharyngeal myotomy.

It is easier to avoid aspiration than to rectify it surgically. If it does occur and causes symptoms, use of the Singh fistula valve (large size) may avoid aspiration while allowing the patient to retain phonation.

Procedure

The success of any surgical speech reconstruction procedure depends on the following requirements: the procedure should be simple and oncologically safe; it should be

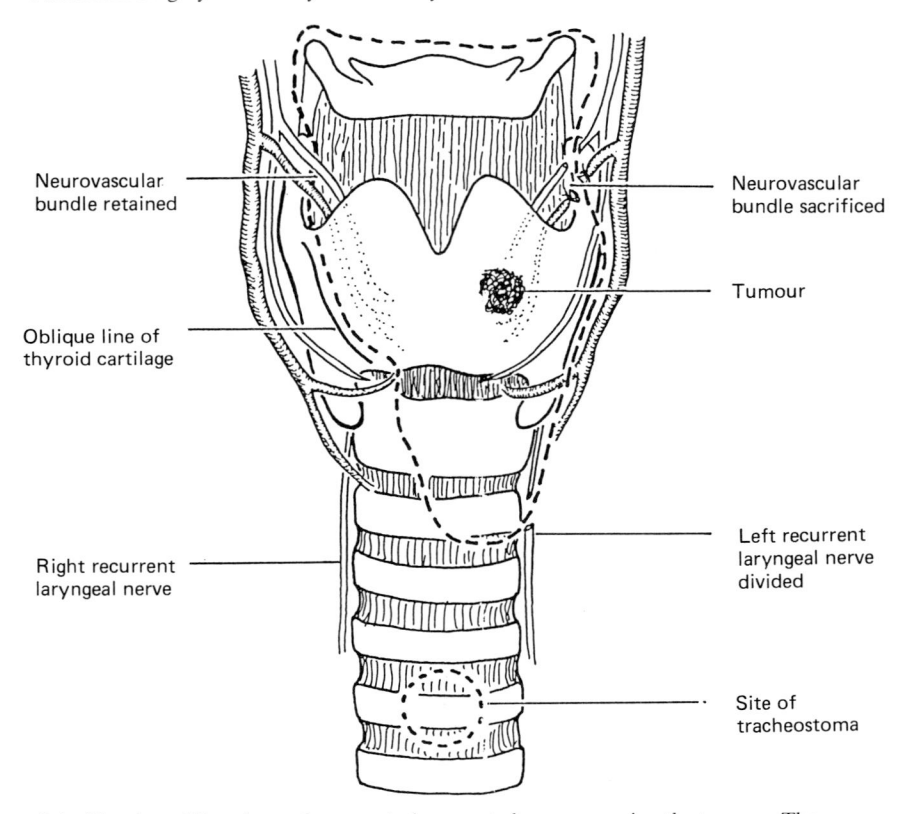

Figure 9.4 The dotted line shows the areas to be resected, encompassing the tumour. The neurovascular bundles supplying the larynx are removed on the tumour side and retained on the opposite side

in one stage; there should be no aspiration or stenosis problem; there should be no increase in morbidity or mortality; the procedure should not be lengthy; and it should not compromise voice production at the expense of total clearance of cancer from the larynx. Based on experience of more than 9 years with the technique of parsimonious laryngectomy (near-total laryngectomy with innervated myomucosal valved shunt, Figure 9.4), the author believes that this procedure meets all the aforementioned requirements. It is indicated in advanced cases of layrngeal cancer. It is proposed that parsimonious laryngectomy should be the standard treatment for all cases of T3 glottic carconoma (Figure 9.5), piriform sinus cancer (Figure 9.6), supraglottic cancer and transglottic carcinoma, where a small tumour-free strip of laryngeal mucosa can be identified and spared to form a sphincteric speaking tube. Where this is not possible, total laryngectomy should be carried out. In cases where the laryngeal mucosa is not sufficient to form a sphincteric speaking tube, a tracheal flap based inferiorly can be sutured to the posterior margin of the remnant laryngeal mucosa to help in forming the tube.

Near-total or parsimonious laryngectomy 129

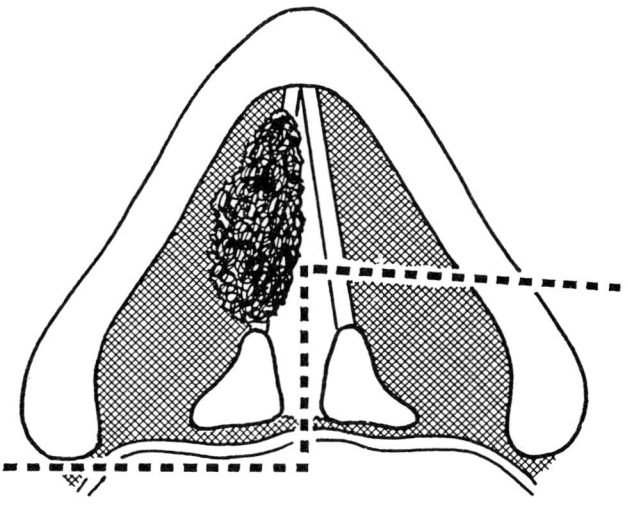

Figure 9.5 Line of resection of T3 glottic tumour

Operative technique

Preliminary endoscopy is performed to reassess the site and size of the growth, before proceeding with the operation. With the patient under anaesthesia and the muscles relaxed, the neck is palpated again for any missed nodes.

Position of the patient
The anaesthetized patient lies supine on the operating table, with a sandbag or pillow under the shoulders to extend the neck (Figure 9.7). This position helps to make the

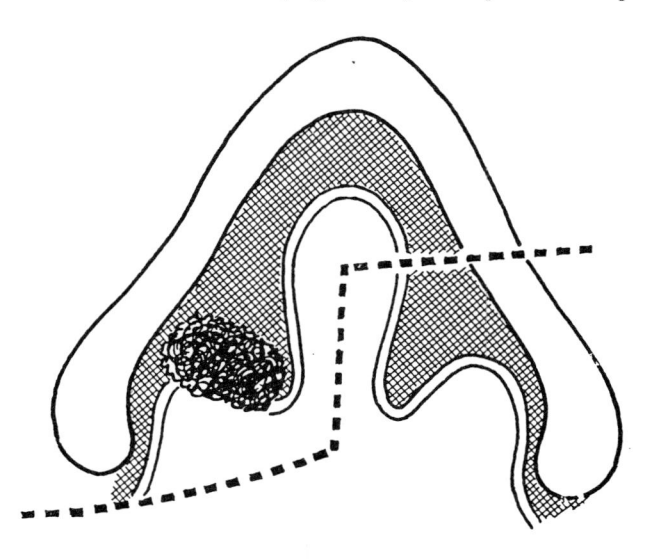

Figure 9.6 Line of resection of piriform sinus tumour

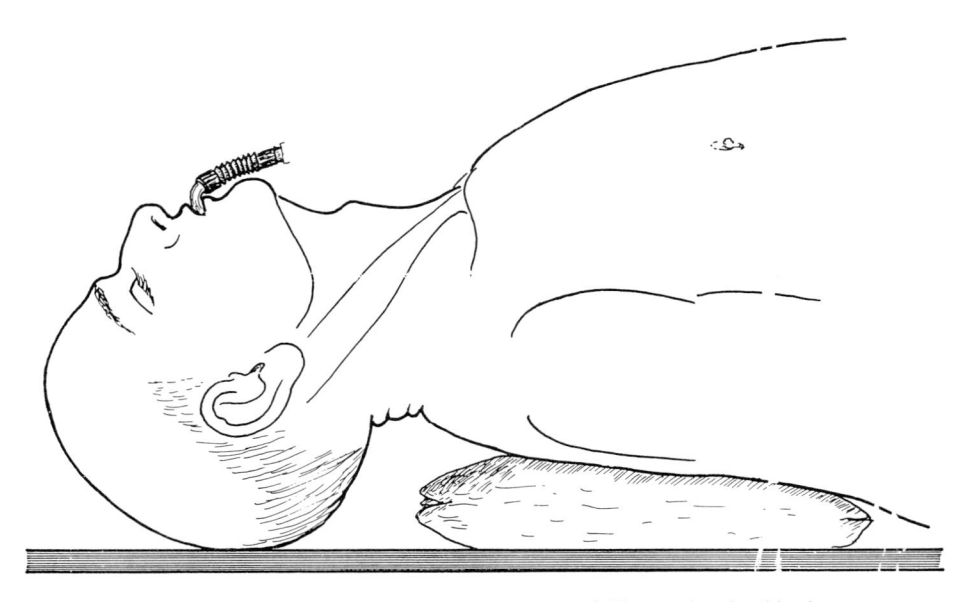

Figure 9.7 Position of patient for parsimonious laryngectomy (pillow under shoulders)

larynx, trachea and sternomastoid muscles prominent as landmarks for skin incision, and also facilitates execution of the surgical procedure.

Skin incision
A U-shaped skin incision is made, with each vertical limb starting at the anterior border of the sternomastoid muscle, at the level of the tip of the greater cornua of the hyoid bone and running down along the anterior border of the respective muscle to the level of the upper border of the cricoid arch (Figure 9.8). At that level the vertical limbs are joined by an incision with a smooth downward convexity. This incision provides good access to the tumour and good skin cover for the suture line of the repaired pharynx and speaking tube. The skin incision is deepened to include the platysma in the apron flap.

If a radical neck dissection is to be performed at the same time, the incision can be extended, above to the ipsilateral mastoid bone and below to the middle of the clavicle. An elective neck dissection is never performed for occult cervical nodes.

Raising of skin flaps
The apron flap of skin with platysma is raised upwards till the hyoid bone and suprahyoid musculature are in view (Figure 9.9) The flap is sutured temporarily to the head drapes to economize on the services of an assistant to hold it. The lower skin flap is undermined up to the suprasternum, to expose the lower parts of the strap muscles, the thyroid gland and its isthmus.

Dissection of infrahyoid muscles
The following description presumes that the tumour is on the left side.

On the left (tumour) side (Figures 9.10 and 9.11) the sternohyoid and sternothyroid muscles are divided inferiorly above the sternum, while the omohyoid is divided near

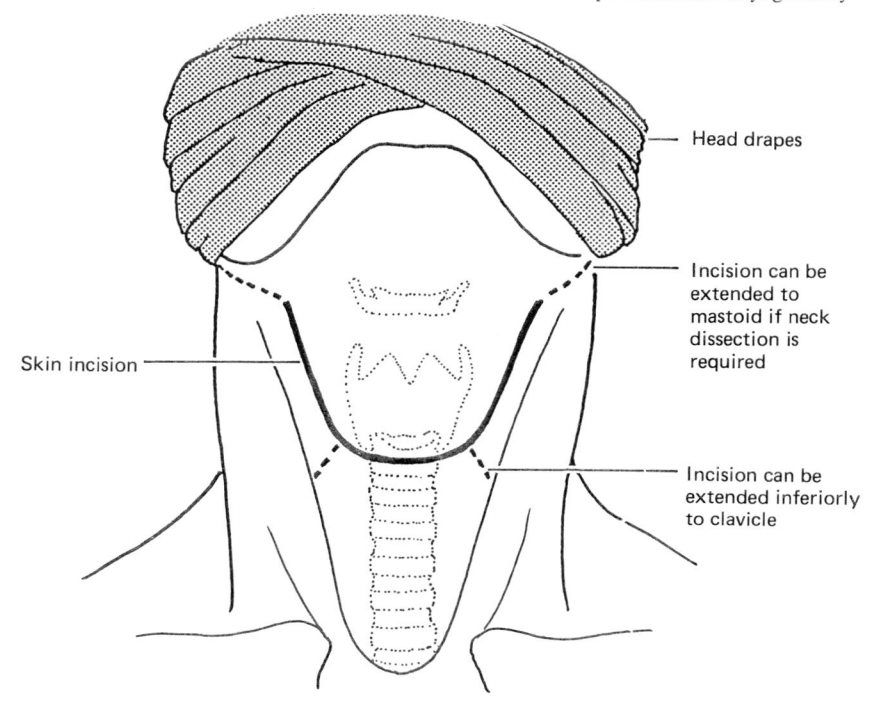

Figure 9.8 Skin incision for parsimonious laryngectomy

its insertion into the hyoid bone. The thyrohyoid muscle is left intact and is removed as such with the rest of the tumour-bearing larynx.

On the right (non-tumour) side (Figure 9.11) the sternohyoid muscle is divided at the level of the lower border of the thyroid cartilage and its upper divided part is reflected to its hyoid attachment. The omohyoid is divided near its insertion into the hyoid bone. The thyrohoid muscle is divided at its attachment from the oblique line and reflected up to the hyoid bone, to expose the right thyroid lamina and right thyrohyoid membrane with the superior neurovascular bundle piercing it. The sternothyroid muscle with its attachment to the oblique line is left intact. A small strip of thyroid lamina posterior to the oblique line and in the region of the cricothyroid joint is ordinarily not removed as it would involve risk of damage to the right recurrent laryngeal nerve. If the posterior part of the lamina in the region of the cricothyroid joint is affected by tumour, then the whole of the thyroid cartilage has to be removed. In this case it is advisable to proceed to total laryngectomy.

Division of thyroid isthmus
The isthmus of the thyroid gland is divided at its junction with the right thyroid lobe (Figure 9.12). The cut ends of the isthmus and the right thyroid lobe are tied by transfixation sutures (medium chromic atraumatic catgut size 0 on a round-bodied needle). The left thyroid lobe with the whole of the isthmus is removed later with the tumour-bearing surgical specimen.

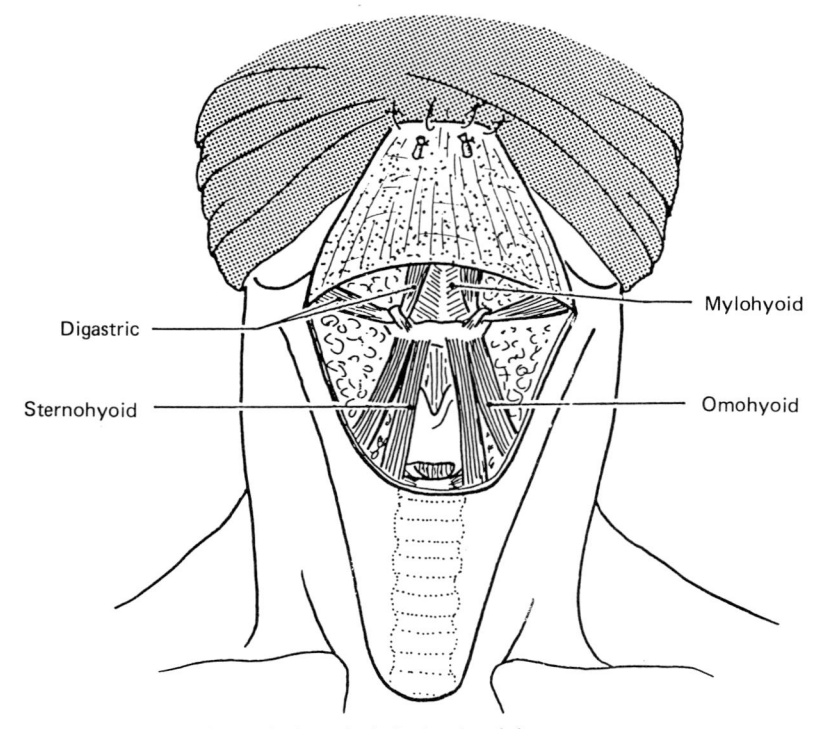

Figure 9.9 Skin flap reflected superiorly and stitched to head drapes

Neurovascular bundle
The superior neurovascular bundle perforating the left thyrohyoid membrane is divided and the vessels ligated (Figure 9.12). Similarly the inferior neurovascular bundle on the left side is divided and the vessels ligated. The superior and inferior neurovascular bundles on the right side are preserved.

Suprahyoid muscles
The suprahyoid muscles are dissected from the hyoid bone (Figure 9.13) until the vallecular mucous membrane is exposed and the tip of the epiglottis (suprahyoid) is visible through it.

Inferior constrictor muscle
The inferior constrictor muscle on the left side is divided along the posterior border of the thyroid lamina till the underlying hypopharyngeal mucosa is visible (Figure 9.13).

Thyrocricotracheal incision
The thyrocricotracheal (TCT) incision is shown in Figures 9.14 and 9.15. The oblique line on the right thyroid lamina (already exposed by reflecting the thyrohyoid muscle upwards) is identified. The perichondrium along the upper border of the right lamina is incised and the inner thyroid perichondrium is separated from the cartilage using a Freer's elevator. The thyroid lamina and its outer perichondrium are cut (by Bard-Parker knife or Heymann's saw) with an incision starting at the upper end and carried downwards parallel to and just in front of the upper part of the oblique line. In its

lower part the knife blade is turned slightly backwards just below the inferior tubercle, so that the plane of incision lies between the vertical and oblique fibres of the ipsilateral cricothyroid muscle. Thence the incision is extended downwards and forwards, cutting through the right arch of cricoid (lateral to its midline) and first tracheal ring. At the lower border of the first tracheal ring the incision is carried horizontally to the left so as to meet the posterior midline incision on the ventral surface of the cricoid lamina. The TCT incision is selected to give good exposure of paraglottal tissue and a clear, direct view of subglottis and trachea, without molesting the median cricothyroid ligament which may contain tumour in its overlying lymphatic network. The retained posterior part of the cricothyroid muscle is functional as it receives its nerve supply from behind. Even if the nerve to this muscle is injured it does not affect significantly the sphincteric control of the neoglottis. The laryngeal framework is inspected by retracting the margins of the TCT incision with hooks. In the upper thyroid part the paraglottal tissue is palpated and also inspected with a magnifying loupe or spectacles. In the lower cricotracheal part of the incision the mucosa may be cut, as it is quite adherent, and the subglottis and upper trachea may be seen directly. If all looks well, and on palpation is normal, a provisional decision is made to go ahead with parsimonious laryngectomy. If the tumour extends below the

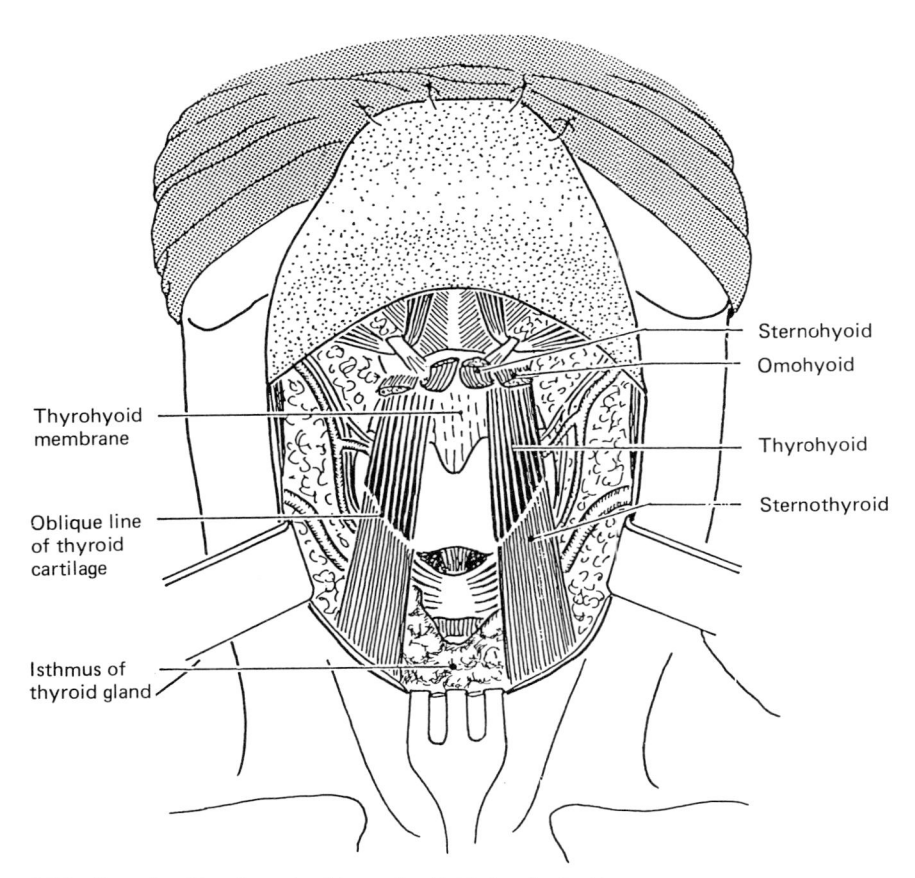

Figure 9.10 Sternohyoid and omohyoid muscles divided on both sides

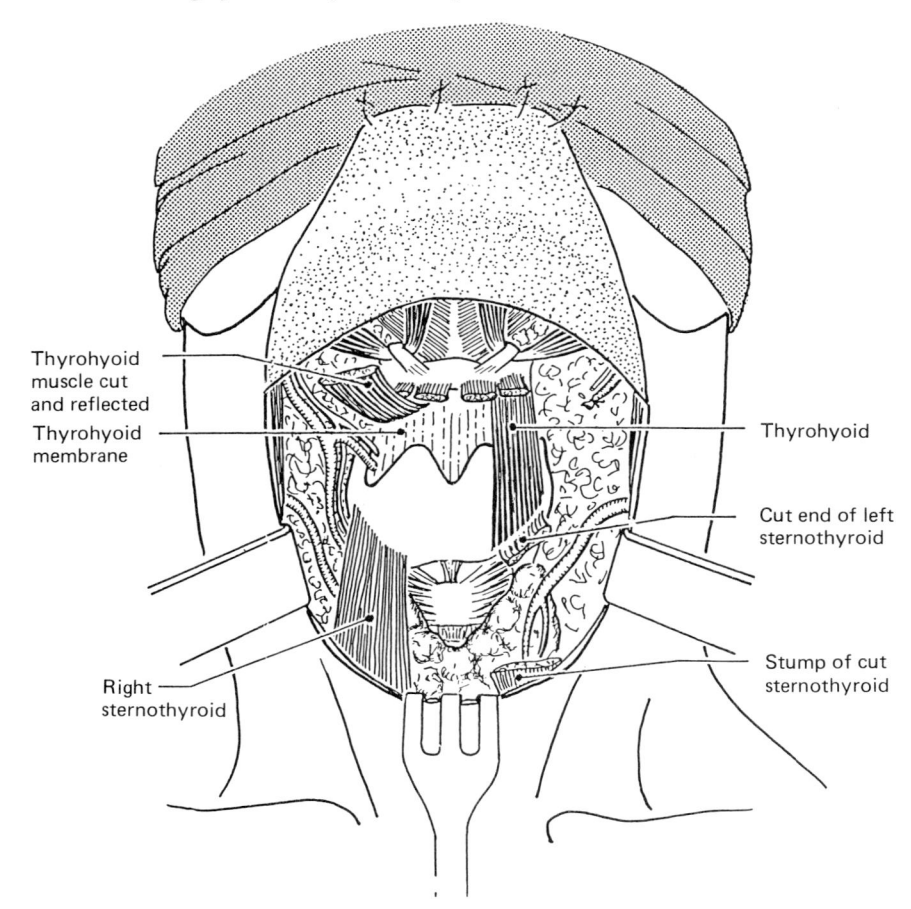

Figure 9.11 Left sternothyroid muscle divided and right thyrohyoid muscle reflected upwards

inferior border of the cricoid cartilage, the parsimonious laryngectomy must be abandoned and a total laryngectomy performed.

Vallecular incision
If the posterior third of tongue is tumour-free, the vallecular mucosa is incised to expose the epiglottis. The epiglottis is held with Allis forceps and pulled downwards and anteriorly and the larynx is examined again.

The final decision (to do or not to do parsimonious laryngectomy)
With the epiglottis held by Allis forceps, the hypopharyngeal mucosa is incised along the posterior border of the left thyroid cartilage, thus removing the whole of the left piriform sinus mucosa with the surgical specimen. The hypopharyngeal incision gives a better view for reassessing the extent of the growth inside the larynx, both visually by magnification loupes and by bimanual palpation. This additional information assists in the final decision, whether to go ahead with parsimonious laryngectomy or to proceed with the alternative of total laryngectomy. Presuming that the TCT

incision below the first tracheal ring is clear of subglottal tumour, the tracheostoma opening is made at the fourth tracheal ring, through the inferior skin flap, and the tracheal margins are sutured to the skin, using Dexon atraumatic size 1 sutures on a trocar-pointed needle. The endotracheal tube is removed via the mouth, a Portex tracheostomy tube inserted into the newly created tracheostoma and its cuff inflated. A nasogastric tube (16 FG) is inserted through the left side of the nose and its outer end is taped or transfixed to the left ala of the nose to prevent accidental extrusion.

While the epiglottis is held with Allis forceps the inside of the larynx (endolarynx) is inspected again, this time unobstructed by the endotracheal tube. This is the last opportunity to confirm the clinical decision, based on previous findings, to go ahead with parsimonious laryngectomy. In parsimonious laryngectomy the mucosal incision starts at the aryepiglottic fold. It runs from above downwards, behind the epiglottis, in front of and parallel to the mucosal fold formed by the underlying cuneiform cartilage, and reaching below to the posterior end of the ventricle. If the ventricle is clear, as anticipated, the incision is slanted slightly anteriorly, dividing the vocal cord and the thyroarytenoid muscle between the two blades of the scissors. This incision is extended to meet the previously incised right cricoid arch and first tracheal ring. This incision does not injure the nerve supply to the retained posterior part of the thyroarytenoid muscle which contributes sphincteric function to the neoglottis, as the muscle receives its nerve supply from behind.

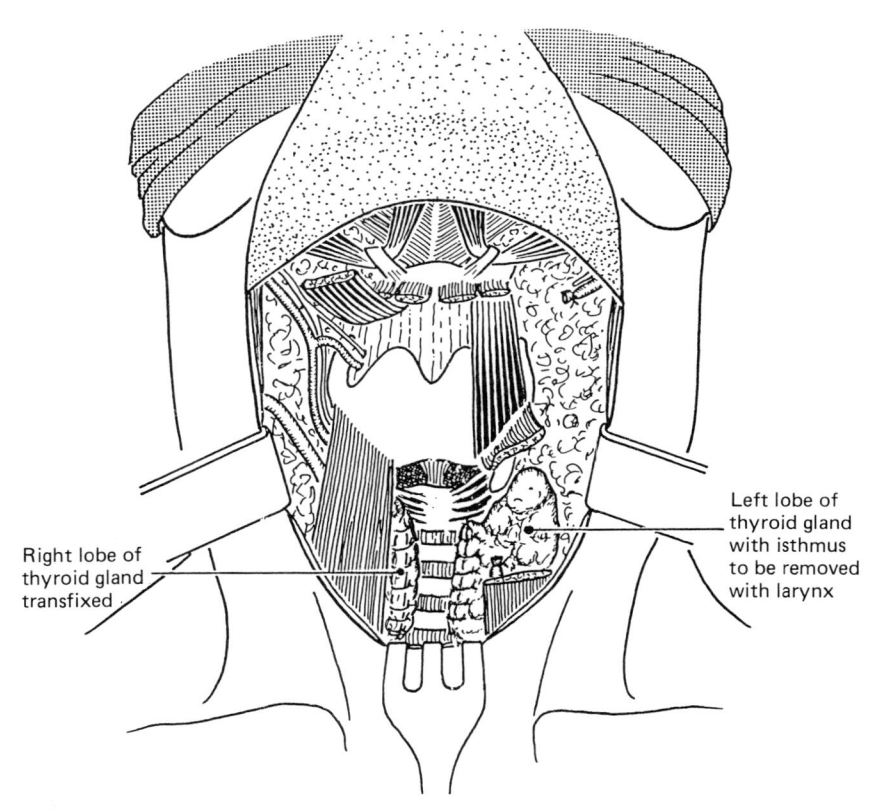

Figure 9.12 Isthmus of thyroid gland divided; thyroid stumps are transfixed and trachea exposed

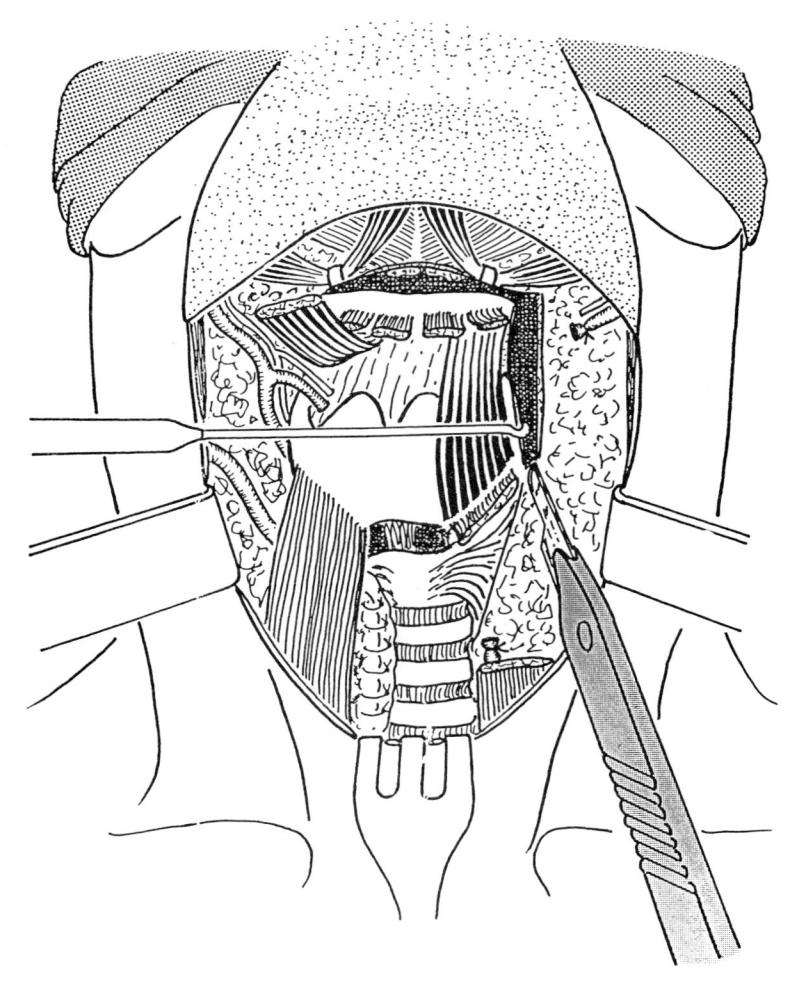

Figure 9.13 Suprahyoid muscles divided and left inferior constrictor muscle being separated from posterior border of thyroid cartilage

The interarytenoid myomucosal fold is incised with a Bard-Parker knife. Thence the incision is extended vertically downwards in the midline, incising the mucosa, the underlying ventral surface of the lamina of the cricoid cartilage and the first tracheal ring, where it joins the previous TCT incision. When the two incisions meet, the tumour-bearing larynx opens like a book. Above, the vertical cricoid incision joins the lower end of the left hypopharyngeal incision which encircles and excises the left piriform sinus. Thus the tumour-bearing surgical specimen is removed along with the ipsilateral thyroid lobe and isthmus. By prior arrangement with the pathologist, the surgical specimen is sent for frozen-section examination of the margins to confirm histological clearance of tumour. If histological clearance is obtained, parsimonious laryngectomy can be performed.

Sphincteric speaking tube

A nasotracheal catheter (ureteric catheter 8 FG) is inserted through the tracheostoma upwards (Figure 9.16); the smooth tip is brought out through the right nostril and taped or transfixed to the right ala, while the lower end is fixed to the chest wall by a silk suture. The mucosa covering the laryngotracheal remnant (Figure 9.17) above the stoma is dissected from the underlying cartilage and fashioned into a tube (approximately 5–6 mm in diameter) by using medium chromic atraumatic catgut (3/0 on a round-bodied needle). Subglottal pressure studies performed in the voice research laboratory show that neoglottal patients need approximately 5–6 mm diameter of speaking tube for effortless and fluent speech. The nasotracheal catheter is of lesser diameter, not to act as a stent for the speaking tube; it helps in orientation and suturing during the fashioning of the myomucosal tube. In the postoperative period the catheter keeps the tube clear of any thick mucus, and discourages blood from entering, clotting, organizing and thus blocking the tube. When the nasotracheal catheter is removed (in 8–10 days) and healing has been attained, the patient is capable of speaking immediately. This is a great morale booster for the otherwise depressed patient. The function of the neoglottis is depicted in Figure 9.18 which shows that on placing the finger on the stoma, the expired air passes into the pharynx producing speech, but on swallowing the neoglottis closes, preventing aspiration. For 'hands free' speech the Singh tracheostoma valve (Singh, 1985, 1987a, 1988a, 1989a, 1990) has been used successfully by our patients.

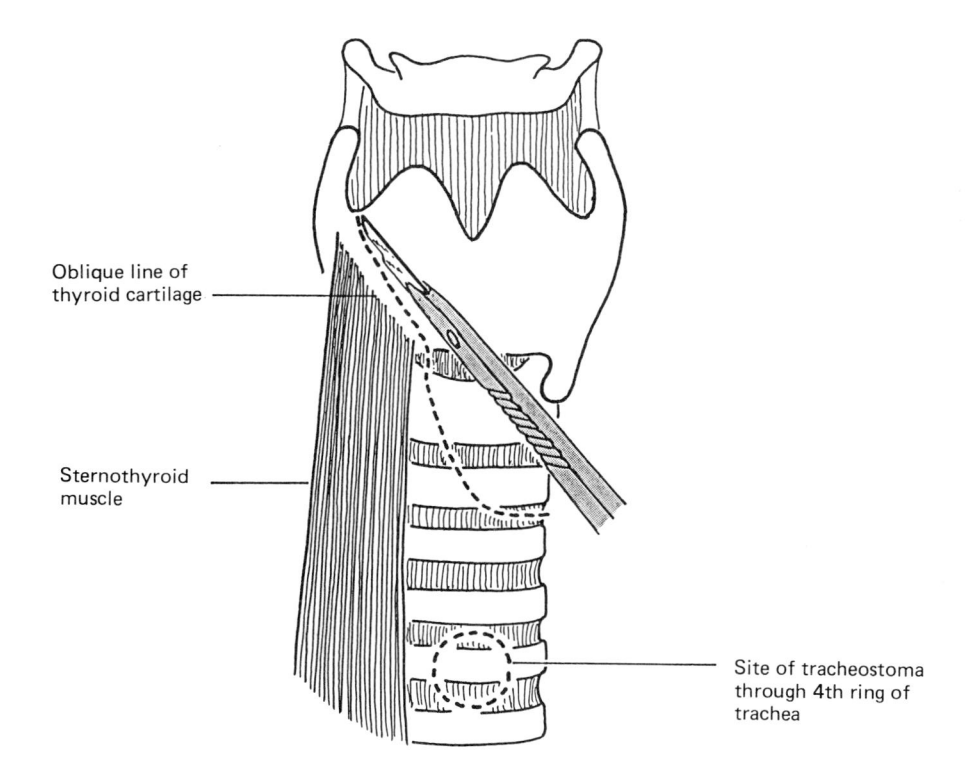

Figure 9.14 Thyrocricotracheal (TCT) incision on non-tumour side

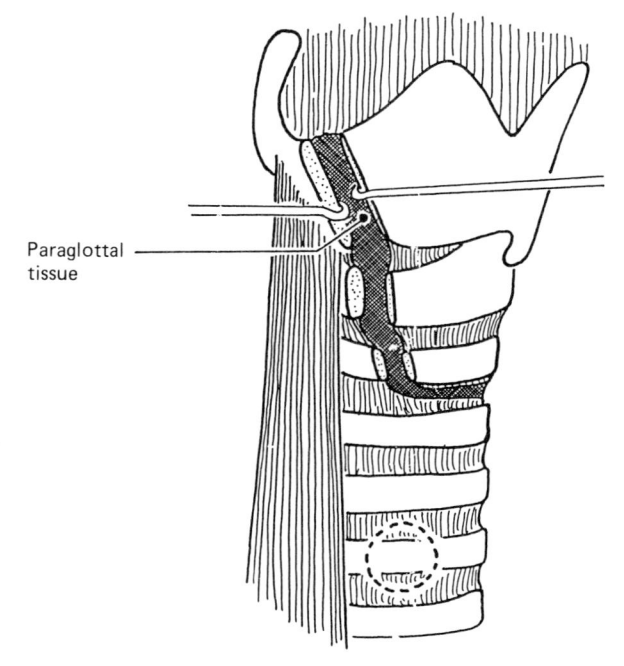

Figure 9.15 Exposure of interior of the larynx

Repair of pharynx
The pharyngeal remnant is repaired around the upper end of the tracheoarytenoid shunt (speaking tube) by catgut suture. The rest of the mucous membrane of the pharynx above it is either sutured by catgut (Figure 9.19) or by Auto Suture clamp (Figure 9.20) in a vertical fashion. The inferior constrictor muscle is sutured transversely, with atraumatic Mersilk on a 30-mm round-bodied needle, and surrounds the already repaired pharyngeal mucosa. It should be appreciated at this stage that no laryngeal framework is left for upward movement of the larynx or laryngeal remnant during swallowing. Any attempt at reconstruction will raise the intact piriform fossa only, not the laryngeal remnant. Raising the level of the piriform fossa above that of the neoglottis during swallowing may encourage spill-over and aspiration into the trachea. To avoid this, any infrahyoid muscle remnants should not be sutured to the suprahyoid musculature, directly or indirectly.

Cricopharyngeal myotomy
Myotomy of the cricopharyngeal muscle and about 1 cm of the oesophagus below it is performed in all cases of parsimonious laryngectomy, but there is no myotomy above the cricopharyngeal muscle. Any myotomy of the inferior constrictor muscle above the cricopharyngeal muscle will be counterproductive, for the following reasons.

(1) Myotomy will decrease the force of the peristaltic squeeze of food downwards during the pharyngeal phase of deglutition, because of insufficient force exerted by the divided muscle fibres.
(2) Incoordination (or lag period) between the relaxed sphincter and the decreased

force of propulsion by the muscle fibres above it will further aggravate the difficulty in swallowing and hence increase spill-over and aspiration.
(3) Because of weak pharyngeal muscular wall support, the patulous pharynx will contribute to a weaker voice.

Skin closures and drains
Before skin closure and drainage, the tracheostoma is completed by applying further Dexon sutures. The neck is flexed and the skin flap returned to its preincision position. Subcutaneous continuous suction drainage is attained by connecting the suction tubes, on either side of neck, to low-pressure suction. Subcutaneous interrupted or continuous medium chromic atraumatic catgut sutures on a 30-mm needle are followed by interrupted 3/0 silk sutures on a cutting needle for skin closure; alternatively, Auto Suture Premium 35 skin clips are used. The platysma is included in skin sutures. The closure should be airtight.

Site and mechanism of phonatory function

Electrolaryngography (electroglottography) (see Figures 6.1 and 6.2) is used as an adjunct to other methods of assessing vocal cord function (e.g. phonetography, spectrography) in voice disorders. To study the site and function of the neoglottis in speech production, electrolaryngography was performed on some of the patients who had undergone near-total laryngectomy and who began speaking with finger

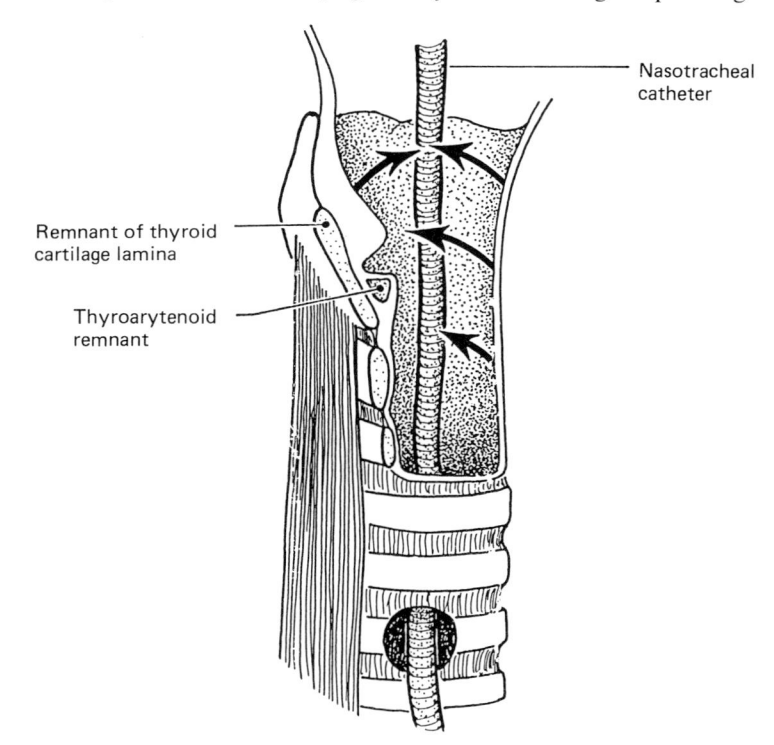

Figure 9.16 Formation of laryngotracheal tube (sphincteric speaking tube) around the catheter

140 Functional Surgery of the Larynx and Pharynx

Nasotracheal catheter — Nasogastric tube

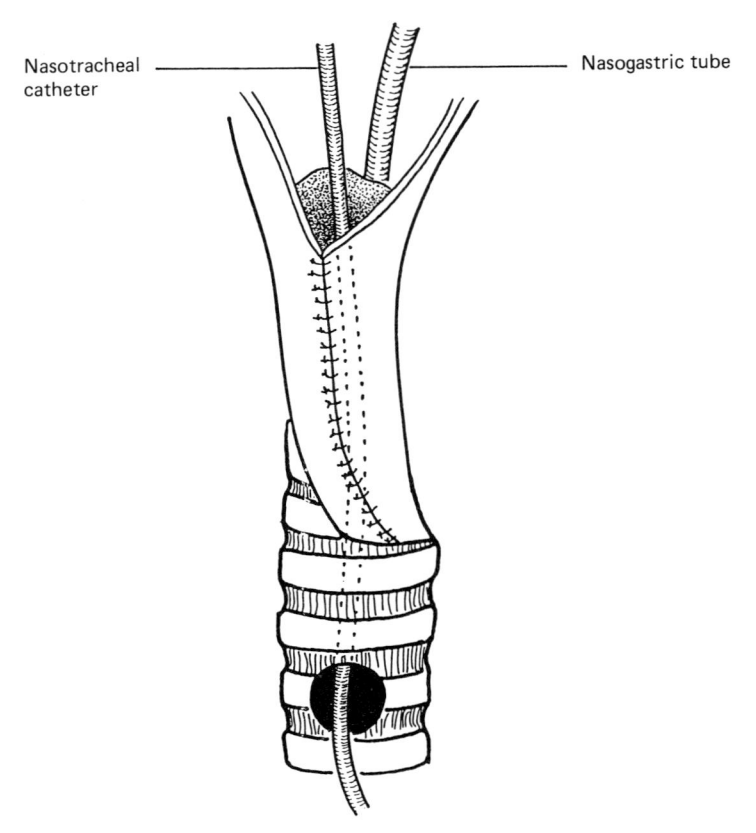

Figure 9.17 Laryngotracheal tube formed around small nasotracheal catheter

occlusion of the tracheostoma. Approximately 1 month after the operation, when the neck wound had healed completely, two circular gold-plated guard-ring electrodes were placed on the skin of the neck of the patient, on either side of the neoglottis and held in place by a neck band (Singh, 1987b, 1988b, 1989b, 1992). The laryngograph monitored the varying electrical conductance between the electrodes in terms of current flowing between them on the application of a constant voltage (Abberton et al., 1989). The patient was asked to read aloud the Rainbow passage (Fairbanks, 1940) and then phonate the vowel 'ah' by manual occlusion of the stoma. The electrolaryngographic output was displayed on the oscilloscope and on the computer monitor as a waveform (L_x). The wave pattern showed that the neoglottis not only controlled the airflow through it, it also vibrated, thus acting as a source of phonation. The different phases of the waveform showed whether the neoglottis was open or closed. The varying degree of neoglottal vibratory activity was represented by the amplitude variation of the waveform (L_x). Direct visualization through the Olympus flexible fibre-optic nasopharyngolaryngoscope confirmed the myomucosal neoglottis as the source of vibration (Figure 9.21).

Neoglottal voice analysis

Electrolaryngography (electroglottography) is used in the voice research laboratory in conjunction with other vocal efficiency measurements. In normal and in neoglottal speakers there is a high degree of correlation between the L_x wave from the electrodes at the level of the normal vocal cords or neoglottis and the acoustic signal picked up by a microphone placed 30 cm from the patient's mouth. The fundamental frequency of the neoglottal speaker is somewhat higher than that of the normal speaker and the range of fundamental frequency is wider, especially at the upper end. The neoglottal speaker can control both the direction of the fundamental frequency and can change the direction of fundamental frequency movement. Fundamental frequency movements of this kind are important in a number of ways. A rising fundamental frequency can be used to distinguish phrases intended as questions, which have a rising frequency, from phrases intended as statements of fact, which are typically pronounced with a falling frequency. Fundamental frequency movement is also one of the factors that distinguishes such phrases as '*black*board' (as found in classroom) from 'black*board*' (a board that is black). Clearly, the ability of neoglottal speakers to produce such fundamental frequency movements will contribute a great deal to the naturalness and overall intelligibility of their speech. Electrolaryngography (electroglottography) in neoglottal patients showed that they are capable of producing the desired fundamental frequency movements, although the electrolaryngography traces are not as smooth or as regular as those produced by the normal speakers.

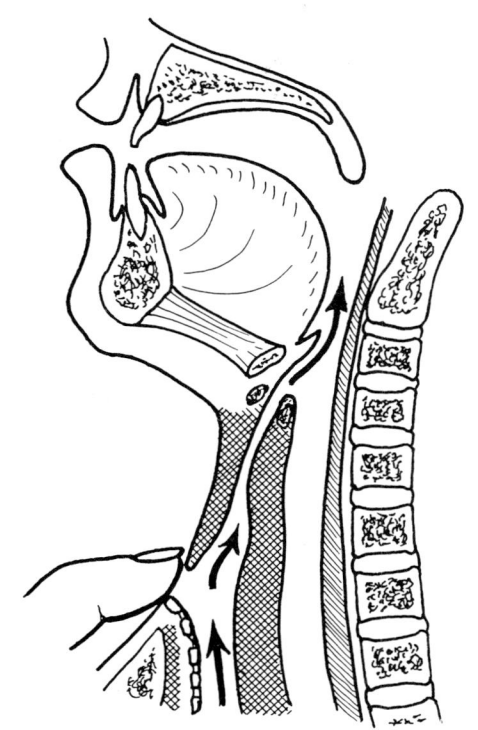

Figure 9.18 Mechanism of sphincteric speaking tube (neoglottis)

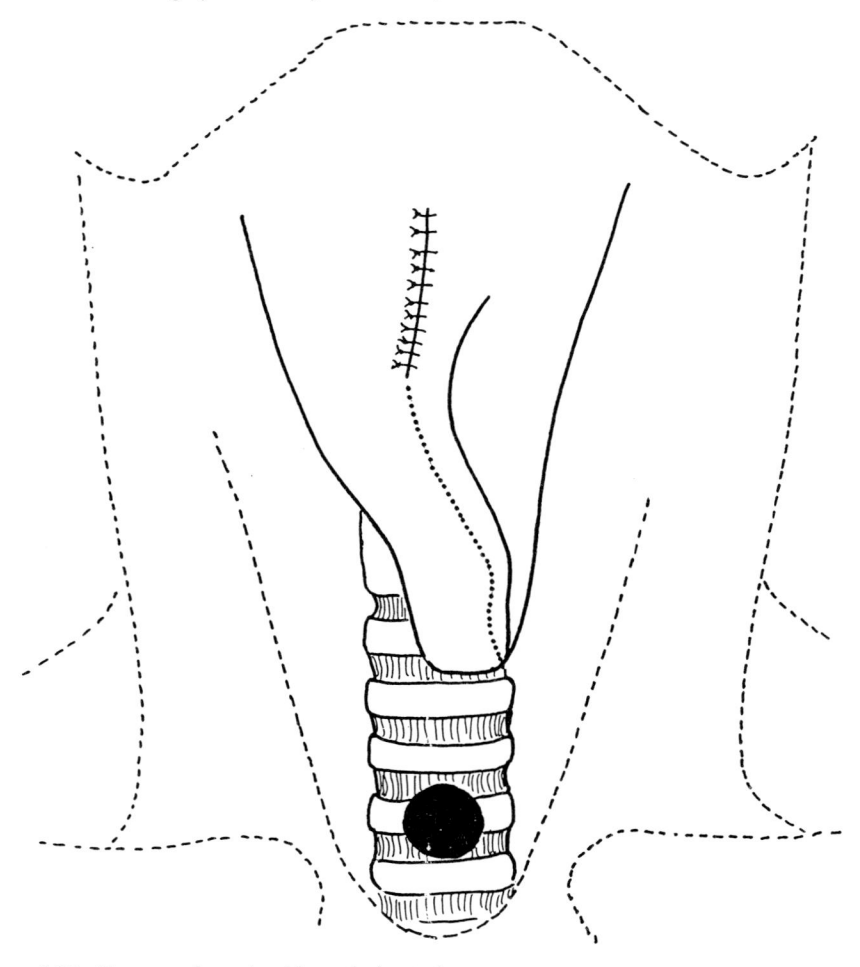

Figure 9.19 Pharyngeal repair with vertical suturing

Subglottal pressure studies

The comparative dearth of aerometric studies over the last decade is somewhat surprising in view of the relevance of this kind of investigation. Air flow through the vocal tract is a function of the subglottal pressure created by the air supply and the resistance offered by (mainly) the voicing source. Subglottal pressure is here taken to mean the pressure below the voicing source (neoglottis in parsimonious laryngectomy). Obviously, the greater the resistance of the voicing source the greater is the subglottal pressure required to produce a sound of given intensity, and in consequence there is increased stress on the cardiopulmonary system. This is of great clinical importance in neoglottal patients where most of the speakers are 50–70 years old. Measurement of the subglottal pressure can therefore provide valuable information about the resistance of the voicing source, and this has implications concerning the degree of effort required of the speaker for phonation.

Subglottal pressure is measured routinely in all our neoglottal patients in follow-up

Near-total or parsimonious laryngectomy 143

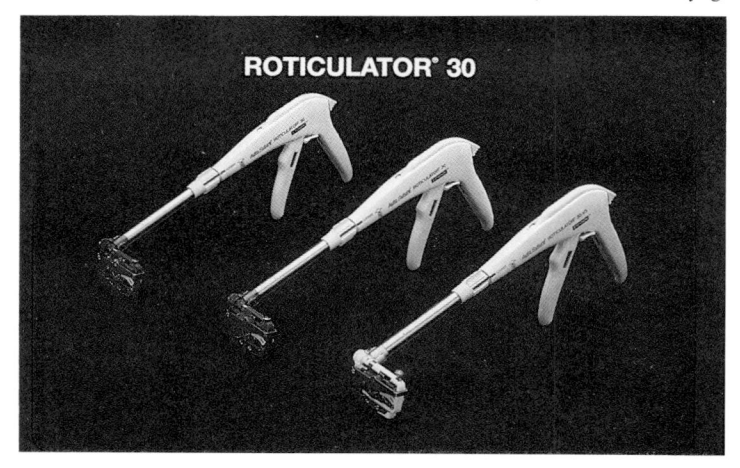

Figure 9.20 Auto Suture clamp for pharyngeal repair

clinics (see Figure 6.21). The pressure below the voicing source in neoglottal patients is around 15 cmH$_2$O (in normal laryngeal speakers the pressure is 6–10 cmH$_2$O). An increase in pressure is immediately investigated to rule out local recurrence, a second primary in the same region or secondaries in the neck pressing on the neoglottis. Measurement of subglottal pressure is easy and takes a few minutes to perform. It requires a mercury electromanometer, a modified Singh tracheostoma valve, a microcomputer with a monitor and software (Singh program). It is recommended that all surgeons performing parsimonious laryngectomy should have this facility in their clinic.

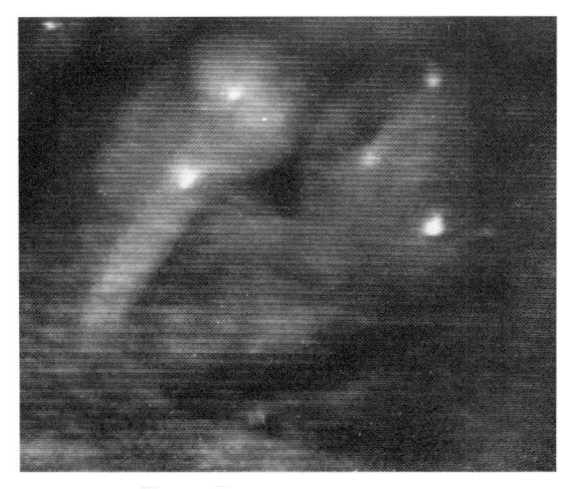

Figure 9.21 Vibrating neoglottis seen through flexible nasopharyngolaryngoscope when patient phonates 'ah'

Results and comments

All 25 patients (24 male and 1 female) who underwent parsimonious laryngectomy have achieved good, intelligible speech. Four of the male patients and the only female patient had unsuccessful preoperative radiotherapy, and parsimonious laryngectomy was performed as a secondary procedure; the rest were treated by primary surgery. There was no aspiration in the men, but the woman complained of some aspiration of fluids; she was relieved of aspiration by the use of a Singh fistula valve (large size), but an extremely sensitive stoma caused excessive coughing. There has been no local recurrence so far. The longest follow-up has been over 9 years.

These observations, in 25 patients, when compared with total laryngectomy encourage more widespread use of a conservative procedure (parsimonious laryngectomy) which has equally good results in terms of cancer clearance and control with the added advantage that the patient acquires a good voice. The small number of cases and short duration (maximum 9 years) precludes absolute certainty in recommending that this should be the standard procedure to replace total laryngectomy in selected cases; however, the initially good results in cancer control with voice preservation justifies a wider and closely critical assessment in more cases. Because of the results achieved by parsimonious laryngectomy, this procedure is preferred in St John's Hospital as a routine procedure, where appropriate, for advanced laryngeal cancer.

Future developments

Knowledge of partial laryngeal surgery has expanded since the first laryngofissure was performed by Buck in 1851. Partial laryngectomy (parsimonious laryngectomy) is based on scientific investigation of the paths of spread of laryngeal cancer and improved understanding of the mechanism of human voice production. Although it is an advance in laryngeal surgery, it is still far from satisfactory. Our ultimate aim should be elimination of the tracheostoma and restoration of an intact airway. Though the solution does not seem near, hopefully our interest and efforts will eventually lead us to our goal in the 1990s.

References

Abberton E., Howard D., Fourcin A. (1989). Laryngographic assessment of normal voice: a tutorial. *Clin. Ling. Phon.*, **3**, 281–96.
Ardran J., Kemp F. (1951). The mechanism of swallowing. *Proc.Roy.Soc.Med.* **44**, 1038.
Baclesse F. (1949). Carcinoma of the larynx. *Br.J.Radiol.* (suppl.) **3**, 1–62.
Buck G. (1853). On the surgical treatment of morbid growths within the larynx, illustrated by an original case and statistical observations, elucidating their nature and forms. *Trans. Am. Med. Assoc.*, **6**, 509–35.
Czigner J. (1972). Vertical subtotal laryngectomy. *Laryngoscope*, **82**, 101–7.
Fairbanks G. (1940). *Voice and Articulation*. Drillbook. New York: Harpers, p. 168.
Hajek M. (1932). *Pathologie und Therapie der Erkrankungen des Kehlkopfes der Luftrohre und der Bronchien*. Leipzig: Georg Thierne Verlag p. 23.
Hofmann Saguez R. (1951). Nouveau cas de laryngectomie subtotale. *Ann. Otol.*, **68**, 736.
Iwai H., Koike Y. (1973). Primary laryngoplasty. *Arch. Otorhinolaryngol.*, **206**, 1–10.
Kirchner J.A. (1975a). Pyriform sinus cancer: a clinical and laboratory study. *Ann. Otol.*, **84**, 793–803.
Kirchner J.A. (1975b). Staging as seen in serial sections. *Laryngoscope*, **85**, 1816–21.

Kirchner J.A. (1977). Two hundred laryngeal cancers. Patterns of growth and spread as seen in serial sections. *Laryngoscope*, **87**, 474–82.

Kirchner J.A. (1984a). Pathways and pitfalls in partial laryngectomy. *Ann. Otol. Rhinol. Laryngol.*, **93**, 301–5.

Kirchner J.A. (1984b). Invasion of the framework by laryngeal cancer. *Acta Otolaryngol.* (Stockholm), **97**, 392–7.

Kirchner J.A., Cornog J., Holmes R.E. (1974). Transglottic cancer: its growth and spread within the larynx. *Arch. Otolaryngol.*, **99**, 247–51.

Kleinsasser O. (1988). Anatomy of the larynx and tumour growth. In *Tumours of the Larynx and Hypopharynx* (Kleinsasser O., ed.) Stuttgart & New York: Georg Thieme Verlag, p. 75.

Le Roux-Robert J. (1936). *Les Épitheliomas Intralarynges*. Thesis. Paris: Gaston Doin.

Majer E.H., Reider W. (1958). Über eine Modifikation der laryngektomien unter Ehraltung der Luftwege. *Arch. Ohrenheilk.*, **173**, 422.

McGavran M.H., Bauer W.C., Ogura J.H. (1961). The incidence of cervical lymph node metastases from epidermoid carcinoma of the larynx and their relationship to certain characteristics of the primary tumor. *Cancer*, **14**, 55–66.

Michaels L., Hassmann E. (1982). Ventriculosaccular carcinoma of the larynx. *Clin. Otolaryng.*, **7**, 165–73.

Micheau C., Luboinski B., Sancho H., Cachin Y. (1976). Modes of invasion of cancer of the larynx. *Cancer*, **38**, 346–60.

Mittal B., Marks J.E., Ogura J.H. (1984). Transglottic carcinoma. *Cancer*, **53**, 151–61.

Mozolewski E.S., Zietek R., Wysocki K., Jach W. (1975). Arytenoid vocal shunt in laryngectomised patients. *Laryngoscope*, **85**, 853–61.

Myers E.M., Ogura J.H. (1979). Stomal recurrence: a clinicopathological analysis and protocol for future management. *Laryngoscope*, **89**, 1121.

Negus V. (1949). The second stage of swallowing. *Acta Otolaryngol.*, **78** (suppl.), 75.

Ogura J.H., Dedo H.H. (1965). Glottic reconstruction following subtotal glotticsupraglottic laryngectomy. *Laryngoscope*, **75**, 865–78.

Olofsson J., Van Nostrand A.W.P. (1973). Growth and spread of laryngeal and hypopharyngeal carcinoma with reflections on the effect of pre-operative irradiation. 139 cases studied by whole organ serial sectioning. *Acta Otolaryngol.*, (suppl.) **308**, 1–84.

Pearson B.W. (1981). Subtotal laryngectomy. *Laryngoscope*, **91**, 1904–11.

Pittam M.R., Carter R.L. (1982). Framework invasion by laryngeal cacinomas. *Head Neck Surg.*, **4**, 200–8.

Pressman J.J. (1956). Submucosal compartmentation of larynx. *Ann. Otol. Rhinol. Laryngol.*, **65**, 766–71.

Pressman J.J., Simon M.B., Morell C.M. (1961). Anatomic studies related to the dissemination of cancer of the larynx. *Cancer*, **14**, 1131–8.

Robbins K.T., Michaels L. (1985). Feasibility of sub-total laryngectomy based on whole-organ examination. *Arch. Otolaryngol.*, **111**, 356–60.

Shaheen O.H. (1959). Two cases of laryngeal carcinoma at the posterior commissure. *J. Laryngol. Otol.*, **73**, 838–42.

Singh W. (1985). New tracheostoma flap valve for surgical speech reconstruction. In *new Dimensions in Otorhinolaryngology — Head and Neck Surgery* (Myers E.N., ed.) Amsterdam: Elsevier, pp. 480–1.

Singh W. (1987a). Tracheostoma valve for speech rehabilitation in laryngectomees. *J. Laryngol. Otol.*, **101**, 809–14.

Singh W. (1987b). Electrolaryngography in near-total laryngectomy with myomucosal valved neoglottis. *J. Laryngol. Otol.*, **101**, 815–18.

Singh W. (1988a). Valvula fonatoria de Singh. In *Recuperacion de la Voz en los Laryingectomizados. Fistuloplastias y Protesis Fonatorias* (Algaba J., ed.) Madrid: Garsi, pp. 331–3.

Singh W. (1988b). Clinical application of electrolaryngograph for speech rehabilitation in near-total laryngectomy with myomucosal valved neoglottis. *J. Laryngol. Otol.*, **102**, 335–6.

Singh W. (1989a). Singh tracheostoma valve. In *Proceedings of the International Voice Symposium*, Edinburgh (Singh W., ed.) pp. 81–2.

Singh W. (1989b). Near-total laryngectomy. In *Proceedings of the International Voice Symposium*, Edinburgh (Singh W., ed.) pp. 53–8.

Singh W. (1990). Singh tracheostoma valve. In *Proceedings of XXIst International Congress of the International Association of Logopedics and Phoniatrics*, Prague, pp. 435–7.

Singh, W. (1991). Preservation of voice in laryngectomy. *Acta Phoniatrica Latina*, **13**, 302–4.

Singh, W., Ainsworth, W. (1992). Computerised measurement of fundamental frequency in Scottish neoglottal patients. *Folia Phoniatr.*, **44**, 231–7.

Singh W., Hardcastle P. (1985). Near-total laryngectomy with myomucosal valved neoglottis. *J. Laryngol. Otol.*, **99**, 581–8.

Singh W., Kaur A. (1987). Laryngeal carcinoma in a six year old with a review of the literature. *J. Laryngol. Otol.*, **101**, 957–8.

Stell P., Bowdler D. (1988). The T3 glottic cancer — diagnosis and management. In *Dilemmas in Otorhinolaryngology* (Harrison D.F.N., ed.) Churchill Livingstone, Edinburgh, p. 275.

Vermund H. (1970). Role of radiotherapy in cancer of the larynx as related to the TNM system of staging. *Cancer*, **25**, 484–504.

Chapter 10

The carbon dioxide laser in laryngeal and pharyngeal surgery

G. Motta, G. Villari, G. Salerno, F.A. Salzano, L. D'Angelo, E. Esposito and S. Motta

Since Jako first used the carbon dioxide laser to remove small lesions of the vocal cords in 1972, technology has advanced and these instruments have proved to be safe and effective surgical tools. The indications for laser microsurgery remain a subject of intense debate and this has, to a certain extent, limited its diffusion into surgical practice and perhaps led to the underestimation of the real advantages of laser surgery.

The senior authors' experience of 777 patients treated for various laryngeal pathologies has shown that accurate preoperative evaluation of the laryngeal disease and the adoption of the correct surgical technique are essential to obtain successful results and avoid predictable failures which might decrease the validity of laser surgery.

The CO_2 laser can be used for simple vaporization or as an instrument for resection. Surgeons advocating the CO_2 laser point to its advantages in performing more rapid and precise surgery with a remarkable decrease in tissue trauma, local oedema and postoperative pain and a reduction in hospital stay (Andrews and Moss, 1974; Jako, 1977; Strong et al., 1979a, b; Tucker, 1979; Dedo and Jackler, 1982; Motta et al., 1984, 1986; Nishimura et al., 1988; Rontal and Rontal, 1990; Zeitels et al., 1990; Rudert, 1991; Friend, 1992).

The CO_2 laser can be used in benign lesions, premalignant lesions and in frank malignancy; moreover, it can be advantageously utilized for the treatment of bilateral abductor cord paralysis and laryngotracheal stenoses.

Laryngeal surgery

The CO_2 laser is not uniformly better than traditional surgical techniques and the results, as mentioned previously, are dependent upon accurate preoperative evaluation.

Benign lesions

Nodules and small polyps
Simple vaporization is the technique of choice when using the laser but it offers little advantage over traditional surgical techniques. Great care must be taken when using the CO_2 laser to protect neighbouring structures from accidental combustion. Sometimes only the outer part of the laser beam is used to complete excision of these small nodules or polyps, which allows the margins to be made more regular. The remaining beam is dispersed on to a small saline-saturated gauze introduced into the hypoglot-

tic region to protect neighbouring structures as mentioned above. Care must also be taken to preserve the elastic lamina intact. Normally the elastic lamina is separated from the overlying mucosa by only a thin, loose connective tissue layer. Injury to the elastic lamina during vaporization can result in reactive nodules or small scars in the treated areas. Although these may be noted on microscopic examination, they seldom impair the quality of voice.

Pedunculated polyps
The CO_2 laser offers little advantage in the treatment of pedunculated polyps over traditional surgical techniques and the difficulties mentioned above should be borne in mind.

Voluminous polyps and oedemas of Reinke
In cases of voluminous polyps or oedemas of Reinke the CO_2 laser can be used to perform a submucous resection, and here the gross oedema of the mucosa usually protects the elastic lamina from harmful heating caused by the laser beam. Asymptomatic mucosal irregularities are observed in about 10% of cases and this is similarly found when traditional surgery is performed. These irregularities from laser treatment are reputedly due to unpredictable tissue reactivity or to vocal distress, especially in the immediate postoperative period. In cases of bilateral oedema of Reinke it is important to avoid damage to the anterior commissure. In such cases, it is advisable to remove the lesion in two different stages separated by an interval of approximately 2 months. This allows the cord treated first to re-epithelialize and so limits the formation of troublesome synechiae.

Laryngeal papillomatosis
Simple vaporization is the technique of choice for small papillomata. Larger lesions sometimes require resection of the pedicle or submucous dissection of their base. It is important to remove the endotracheal tube at the end of surgery to inspect the posterior commissure and the tracheal wall in order to eliminate residual papillomata. In cases of tracheal papillomatosis a special tracheoscope (Motta et al., 1986), which is longer than the traditional laryngoscope, has proved useful.

It is imperative to perform serial endoscopic examination in the early postoperative period (4–5 days after the operation) and in the subsequent few weeks. This allows the re-epithelialization process to be monitored, enabling the detection and removal of fibrin clots from the anterior commissure which otherwise would tend to promote the formation of synechiae. Further endoscopies every 1–3 months are required to identify and eliminate recurrences.

Following this rigorous regimen, very satisfactory anatomical and functional results can be achieved. The age of onset and course of the disease remain important prognostic factors. Papillomatosis in children tends to involve more circumscribed areas and show a lower incidence of recurrence. In the authors' series of 30 cases, complete remission generally occurred at puberty and was maintained as demonstrated by repeated endoscopies carried out over subsequent years. Multiple papillomatosis in adults who previously suffered from the disease in childhood tended to recur and often involved the trachea and main bronchi. Despite this, in the authors' experience, the majority of cases were free from the disease at the 3-year follow-up. It is unusual to observe recurrence of a solitary adult papilloma if the mucosa at the base of the lesion is excised.

Many authors have similarly reported the advantages of treating laryngeal papillo-

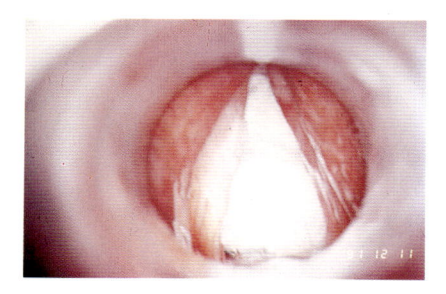

Figure 10.1 Keratotic lesion of the left vocal cord: preoperative view

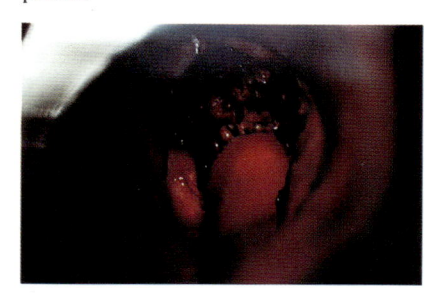

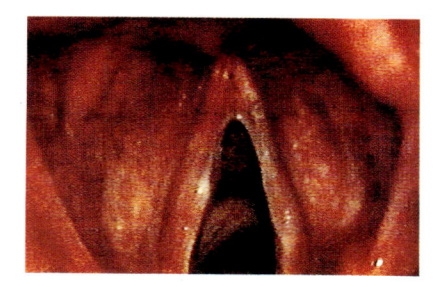

Figure 10.2 Endoscopic appearance of the larynx 6 months after laser surgery

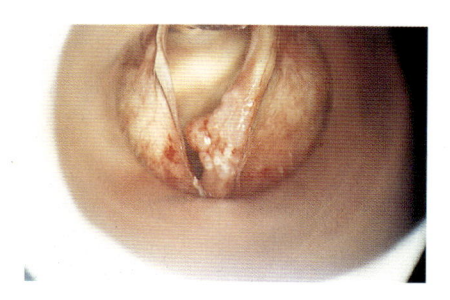

Figure 10.3 Preoperative aspect of a T1a carcinoma of the left vocal cord

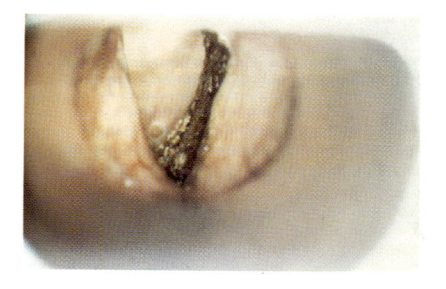

Figure 10.4 After the CO_2 laser cordectomy

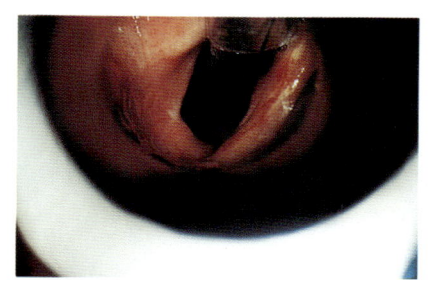

Figure 10.5 Endoscopic control 4 months after surgery: a good re-epithelization occurs and no evidence of the disease is present

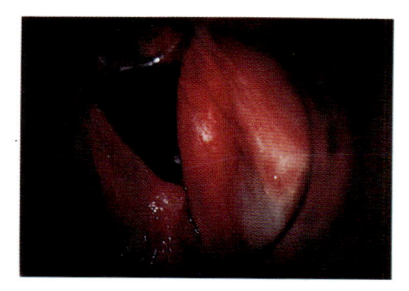

Figure 10.6 T1b carcinoma of the right vocal cord involving the anterior commissure and the controlateral cord

Figure 10.7 At the end of laser surgery

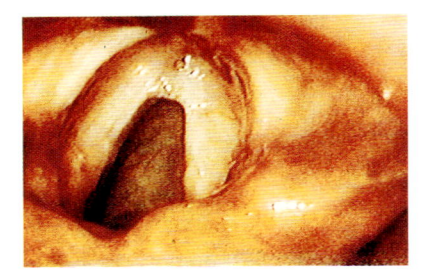

Figure 10.8 Larynx appearance 5 months after the operation

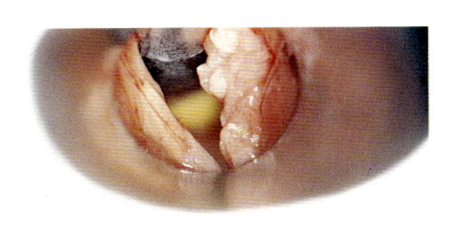

Figure 10.9 T2 Left vocal cord carcinoma extending to the anterior commissure and the anterior third of the controlateral cord: mobility of the left cord was reduced

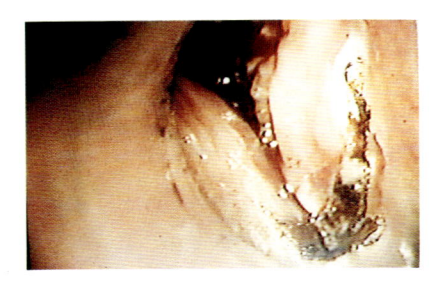

Figure 10.10 A bilateral cordectomy is carried out with the CO_2 laser: first incision on the involved left vocal cord

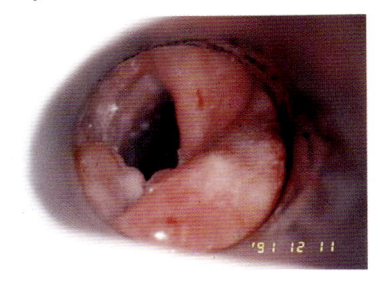

Figure 10.11 Clinical picture 5 months after surgery: no recurrence of the disease is noted

Lines of incision adopted for the removal of:

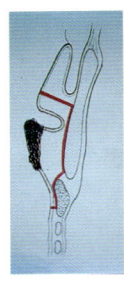

10.12 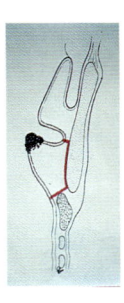 10.13 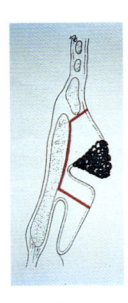 10.14 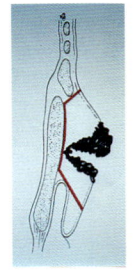 10.15 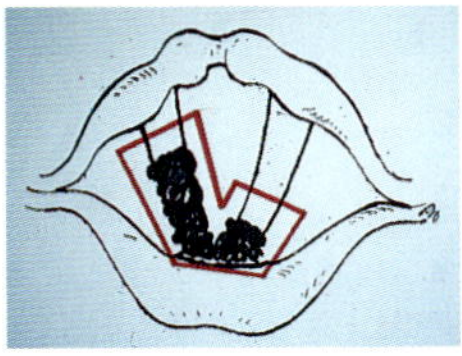 10.16

Figure 10.12 Glottic tumour extending to the hypoglottis

Figure 10.13 Vocal cord localized neoplastic lesion

Figure 10.14 Glottic tumour involving the ventricle

Figure 10.15 Vocal cord tumour extended to the false cord

Figure 10.16 Glottic tumour involving the anterior commissure and the controlateral cord

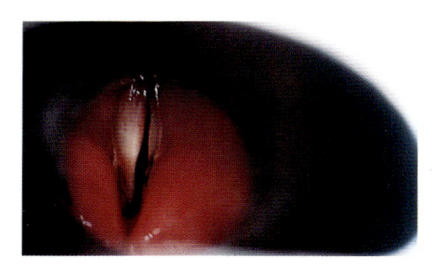

Figure 10.17 Preoperative view of a bilateral abductor vocal cord paralysis

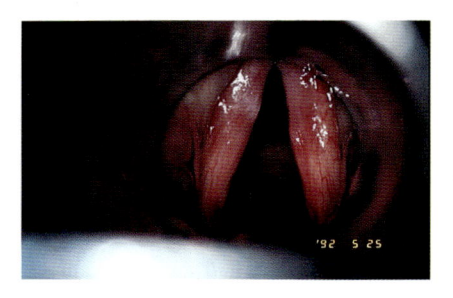

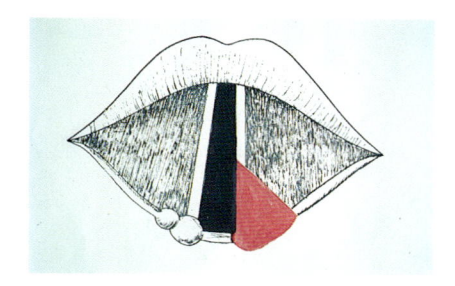

Figure 10.18 The arytenoid and the posterior or half third of the vocal cord are removed with the CO_2 laser

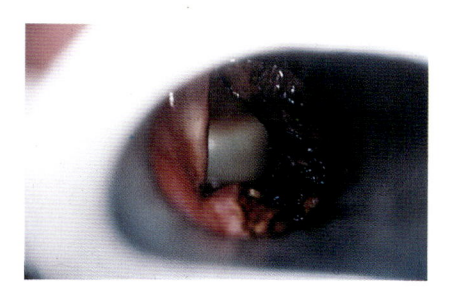

Figure 10.19 At the end of the laser surgery

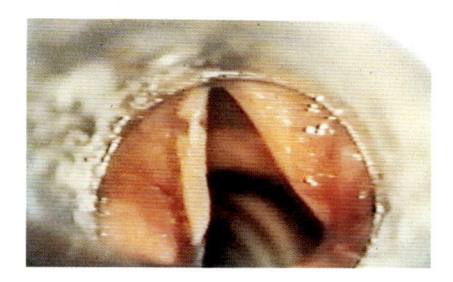

Figure 10.20 Endoscopic control 4 months after the operation: the respiratory space is sufficiently wide

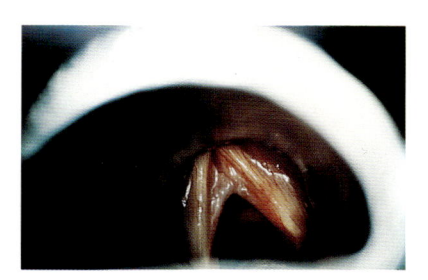

Figure 10.21 Small glottic synechia subsequent to the excision of a polyp of the anterior commissure

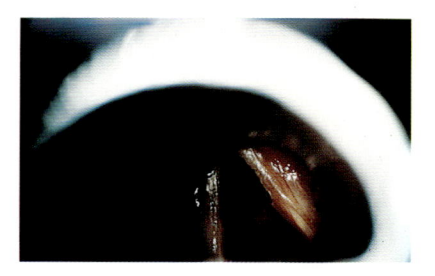

Figure 10.22 After the CO_2 laser vaporization

Figure 10.23 Endoscopic larynx appearance 6 months after surgery

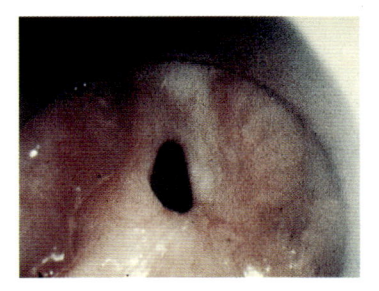

Figure 10.24 Post-traumatic cicatricial diffuse laryngotracheal stenosis

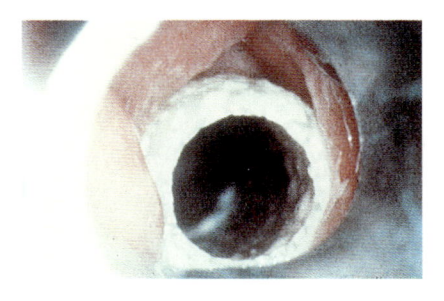

Figure 10.25 Insertion of the silastic Montgomery T-tube after CO_2 laser vaporization of the endoluminal scar tissue

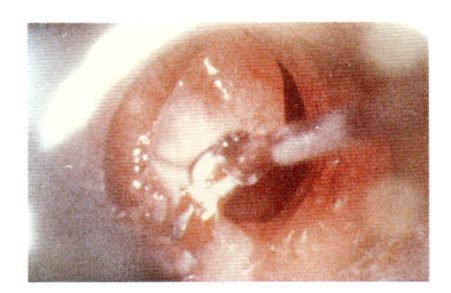

Figure 10.26 The tube once removed, granulations are noted

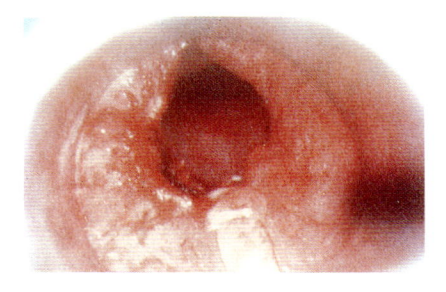

Figure 10.27 Traditional technique is employed to excise the granulation tissue

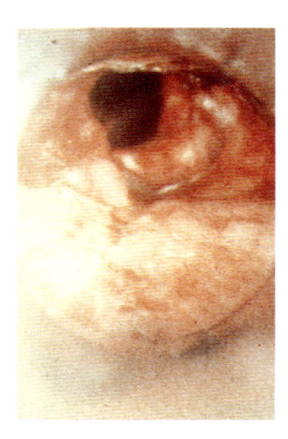

Figure 10.28 Endoscopic larynx appearance 4 months after the surgery: a sufficiently wide respiratory space has been restored

matosis with the CO_2 laser (Strong and Jako, 1972; Andrews and Moss, 1974; Jako, 1977; Steiner et al., 1980; Dedo and Jackler, 1982; Krajina, 1982; Steiner, 1982; Motta et al., 1984; Friend, 1992). The main advantages are the ease with which radical removal can be performed with minimal bleeding and a reduction in tissue trauma and local oedema, avoiding the necessity to perform a tracheostomy. Distortion of anatomy and functional impairment are minimized, and repeated endoscopies with further laser treatment allow the disease to be controlled. The hospital stay is usually shorter when compared with traditional techniques, and also allows more rapid decannulation of previously tracheostomized patients.

Premalignant lesions (keratoses)

The CO_2 laser provides a useful alternative to traditional surgery for premalignant lesions. The relatively bloodless field allows accurate removal of these lesions, and by limiting oedema and allowing the areas to re-epithelialize, good functional results can be achieved. Submucous resection is usually the method of choice, avoiding damage to the elastic lamina (Figures 10.1 and 10.2). It is important to remove adequate margins of normal surrounding tissue since carbonization of the marginal areas caused by the CO_2 laser often makes accurate histological examination of the surgical specimen difficult for the pathologist. It is imperative that accurate preoperative histological studies are performed, particularly when neoplastic changes are suspected. Repeated endoscopies every 3–4 days in the immediate postoperative period and subsequently at longer intervals should be performed to remove fibrin layers and limit the formation of anterior synechiae.

The high incidence of recurrence and spread of keratoses further emphasizes the need for repeated investigations and prompt treatment. In the authors' series of 190 patients, recurrence of disease was observed in only 10% of the cases.

When the anterior commissure is involved, removal of the entire lesion in a single step helps avoid spreading of the disease from the unoperated cord to the denuded contralateral one. Provided accurate preoperative and intraoperative histological examination is performed, the CO_2 laser used for submucous resection should prove a worthwhile technique in dealing with keratoses.

Malignant lesions

Glottic cancers

Several reports indicating the advantages of the CO_2 laser when compared with traditional open surgical techniques have been published (Strong and Jako, 1972; Andrews and Moss, 1974; Jako, 1977; Steiner et al., 1980; Motta et al., 1984, 1986; Zeitels et al., 1990; Rudert, 1991; Friend, 1992). These authors pointed out the advantages of accurate endoscopic removal of tumour. Such an approach avoids the problems of external procedures which breach the laryngeal cartilages and might promote spread of disease into the soft tissues of the neck. Furthermore, the use of the laser in endoscopic surgery allows accurate excision with minimal bleeding and minimal local trauma and oedema. There is no need for a tracheostomy and the patient's stay in hospital is reduced to 2–4 days. Because of the accuracy of excision and the limit of surrounding damage, better functional results can be achieved and the quality of voice preserved.

There are, of course, limits to the usefulness of endoscopic laser surgery. Contraindications to such surgery as a radical treatment of glottic tumours include cartilage infiltration and involvement of the cricothyroid membrane. similarly, the presence of regional lymph nodes would favour a traditional external approach.

It is of fundamental importance to evaluate the extent of the tumour and accurately plan appropriate surgical treatment. The degree of deep infiltration is often difficult to assess, since apparently large lesions often extend only superficially without involvement of the inner perichondrium. Similarly, immobility of the vocal cords does not always indicate extensive infiltration. Involvement of muscle without involvement of the cartilage can itself be responsible for reduced motility. Histological aspects of the tumour and degrees of differentiation influence the natural history of the disease and the likelihood of metastasis to regional lymph nodes.

Experience has shown that the tumours most likely to be treated successfully with the CO_2 laser are:

T1a— lesions confined to one vocal cord, mobile (Figures 10.3–10.5)
T1b— tumours involving the anterior commissure and contralateral vocal cord (Figures 10.6–10.8)
T2 — selected tumours with limited extension to surrounding areas but without cartilage infiltration, e.g. laryngeal ventricle, false cords, hypoglottic region (Figures 10.9–10.11).

The plane of dissection for removal of glottic carcinomas is the same as that used in traditional open surgery, i.e. the inner thyroid perichondrium. In cases where the lesion extends to the hypoglottic region, dissection extends to the cricothyroid membrane and the cricoid perichondrium (Figure 10.12).

The incision margins will depend on the localization of the tumour. In cancers strictly confined to one vocal cord, the initial incision is on the lateral wall of the laryngeal ventricle (Figure 10.13). When tumour extends to the ventricle the initial incisions are placed between the inferior and middle thirds of the false cord (Figure 10.14). Where the false cord is involved, then the initial incision is placed on the ventricular fold (Figure 10.15).

Dissection is continued from the anterior commissure to the arytenoid region, extending deeply to reach the cleavage plane which is the inner thyroid perichondrium. The lesion is finally removed via an incision at the hypoglottic level.

Tumours involving the anterior third of both vocal cords including the anterior commissure require bilateral cordectomy. Two horseshoe-shaped incisions are made, the first in the region of the laryngeal aditus and the second on the cricoid cartilage. Dissection is completed via two vertical incisions on the middle or posterior third of both vocal cords (Figure 10.16).

In all cases, it is imperative to remove adequate margins of normal surrounding tissue and avoid intratumoural manoeuvres. As previously stated, a clear margin is essential to enable an accurate histopathological estimate of tumour clearance. Intratumoural manoeuvres including vaporization or morcellation should be avoided.

Tracheostomy is generally not required. In the immediate postoperative period there is often short-lived dysphagia, and the majority of patients can be discharged within a few days.

Remarkably good results can be achieved adopting the above precautions and techniques. The authors' experience of 360 cases with a 5-year follow-up are shown in Table 10.1. Good local control is achieved in the majority of cases provided the strict criteria mentioned above are adhered to. Local recurrence of the tumour usually requires total laryngectomy, often associated with bilateral neck dissection.

Table 10.1 Glottic cancers (360 cases)

Stage	Number of patients	Survival at 5 years (%)
T1a	146	97.3
T1b	107	91.2
T2	107	86.9

Supraglottic cancers
Tumours suitable for endoscopic removal with the CO_2 laser are those localized to:

(1) the free margin of the epiglottis, without pedicle involvement;
(2) the lateral margin of the aryepiglottic fold with extension to the laryngeal aditus, preserving the piriform sinus;
(3) the false cord without deep infiltration of the thyroid cartilage.

Contraindications to laser surgery include:

(1) lesions extending from the false cord to the aryepiglottic fold and to the piriform sinus;
(2) infiltration of the epiglottic pedicle;
(3) invasion of the thyroepiglottic space;
(4) cervical lymph node metastases.

In such cases, it is mandatory to perform a supraglottic laryngectomy associated with bilateral neck dissection. A traditional open surgical technique ensures radical removal of the tumour including the thyroepiglottic space. Accurate preoperative evaluation of the tumour is essential to plan radical surgery. Histology including the degree of differentiation and infiltration will indicate the likely behaviour of the tumour. Reduced mobility of the vocal cords does not *per se* demonstrate cartilage infiltration but can be due to a large tumour mass or to involvement of muscle.

The extent of excision is dependent on the site and size of the tumour and can vary from a simple epiglottectomy to wide excisions of the lateral margin of the aryepiglottic fold or removal of the false cord, extending where necessary to the superior aspect of the vocal cord. It is imperative, as mentioned previously, to include a large amount of normal surrounding tissue in the resection. The authors' results, from a series of 55 cases with a minimum of 5-year follow-up, are shown in Table 10.2.

Bilateral abductor cord paralysis

The treatment of bilateral abductor cord paralysis has been greatly improved by the use of the CO_2 laser when compared with traditional open surgery techniques such as cordopexy (King, 1939; Woodman, 1946; Rontal and Rontal, 1990) or arytenoidectomy. The ease of endoscopic surgery with the avoidance of tracheostomy has led to improved respiratory results and quality of voice.

Table 10.2 Supraglottic cancers (55 cases)

Site	Number of patients	Survival at 5 years (%)
Epiglottis or aryepiglottic fold	34	89.7
False cord	21	68.9

Two surgical approaches can be used in the treatment of bilateral abductor cord paralysis. The first is vaporization of the arytenoid vocal process, as reported by Krajina (1982). The second is total arytenoidectomy, where the surgeon makes an incision on the posterior portion of the aryepiglottic fold to expose the corniculate cartilage and the upper body of the arytenoid. The arytenoid is dissected along its perichondrium and then disarticulated from the cricoid cartilage (Figures 10.17–10.20). In both techniques, vaporization of the adjacent posterior third or half of the vocal cord is performed. Damage to the posterior commissure must be avoided to prevent the occurrence of troublesome synechiae or scars. As mentioned previously, repeated endoscopic examination is required in the early postoperative period to remove fibrin layers which might cause respiratory distress in untracheostomized patients.

In the authors' experience of 45 cases, successful restoration of the airway has always been achieved. Vaporization of the vocal process can promote the formation of granulation tissue in the area of exposed cartilage. In the authors' view, therefore, it is advisable to perform total arytenoidectomy to eliminate this problem. The functional results have also improved, with the early postoperative dysphonia reducing 5–8 months following surgery.

Laryngotracheal stenosis

Laryngotracheal stenosis most commonly occurs following cervical trauma, severe infections, ingestion of corrosive substances or after surgery to the larynx and trachea. It is often classified according to its site and extent:

(1) *Supraglottic stenosis* may present as a chronic oedema secondary to lymphatic stasis, which can occur after supraglottic laryngectomy. The other presentation is of a cicatricial lesion subsequent to corrosive ingestion, inflammatory disease, prolonged intubation or following supraglottic laryngectomy.
(2) *Glottic or hypoglottic stenosis* may also present as oedema, such as voluminous oedemas of Reinke, or as cicatricial stenosis subsequent to accidental damage to the anterior commissure which may occur during laryngeal surgery.
(3) *Tracheal stenosis* most commonly results from prolonged intubation or incorrectly performed tracheostomy.
(4) *Diffuse laryngotracheal stenosis* may result from partial laryngectomy or from severe trauma to the anterior cervical region. It poses a formidable problem for the reconstructive surgeon.

Accurate preoperative assessment is essential but is often quite difficult. Indirect laryngeal examination can yield useful information concerning laryngeal motility and can identify glottic and supraglottic stenoses. Various radiographic examinations including xeroradiography and computed tomography are useful diagnostic tools. Essentially, however, they give a two-dimensional assessment of the stenosis, and images may be impaired by overlapping and by the presence of a tracheal cannula. Photographic investigations are static and give no indication of dynamic problems during respiration and phonation. Direct laryngoscopy, on the other hand, performed under general anaesthesia, allows an accurate evaluation of laryngeal motility. Biopsies can also be performed to rule out any active inflammatory or neoplastic disease.

Supraglottic stenosis

Simple anterior cicatricial stenoses of the laryngeal aditus can be treated by simple laser vaporization, taking care to avoid damage to the posterior commissure mucosa. Where the interarytenoid region is involved, it is advisable to perform unilateral arytenoidectomy to ensure sufficient respiratory space in the posterior glottis. Oedematous stenoses such as chronic aditus oedemas are best treated by direct vaporization or by submucous dissection of the oedematous mucosa with vaporization of the wound margins to make them more regular.

As mentioned above, repeated endoscopies in the early postoperative period are essential to remove fibrin clots and assess healing.

More severe stenoses require the insertion of a Silastic Montgomery T-tube. A metallic tracheostomy cannula must always be inserted in the horizontal and descending branches of the Montgomery tube to prevent respiratory distress and allow easy aspiration of seromucous secretions which might otherwise require emergency treatment. The Montgomery tube can be safely left in place for several (4–12) months, since it shows good tissue tolerance.

Glottic or hypoglottic stenosis

The vaporization of webs and synechiae with the CO_2 laser has been widely reported in the literature (Andrews and Moss, 1974; Jako, 1977; Steiner et al., 1980; Shugar et al., 1982; Motta et al., 1984; Friend, 1992). The denuded surfaces should be coated with a cyanoacrylic glue to promote healing and prevent recurrence of the webs and synechiae (Figures 10.21–10.23).

Voluminous oedemas of Reinke, as mentioned previously, are best treated with accurate dissection in the submucous plane, taking care to protect the anterior commissure from accidental damage. Where there is an associated bilateral abductor cord paralysis it is advisable to perform a unilateral total arytenoidectomy to ensure sufficient respiratory space.

Tracheal stenosis

Tracheal stenosis can often be difficult to assess preoperatively, and as mentioned above the tracheoscope can be advantageously used to allow a clearer vision of the trachea. Stenoses involving half or two-thirds of the anterior wall are best treated by direct vaporization. Circumferential stenosis requires the insertion of a Montgomery T-tube once a new cavity has been created by vaporization.

Diffuse laryngotracheal stenosis

Laser surgery has proved useful in providing a simple and relatively effective treatment of diffuse laryngotracheal stenosis (Figure 10.24). The laryngotracheal lumen is enlarged by vaporization of the scar contracture. This is often difficult because of the distorted anatomy and requires a strict cooperation between surgeon and anaesthetist. Following the formation of a neocavity, a Montgomery T-tube is inserted, incorporating a metallic tracheostomy cannula as previously mentioned (Figure 10.25). The tube should be left in place for a minimum of 6–12 months. Following removal of the tube, repeated endoscopic examination is required to evaluate the healing process and to prevent recurrence of stenoses (Figures 10.26–10.28).

The authors have now treated 97 patients with laryngotracheal stenoses. All cases (38 with chronic aditus oedemas) were successfully treated. More severe lesions including supraglottic stenoses, large glottic stenoses and circumferential tracheal stenoses also gave good results, with 2 cases of recurrent stenosis in the 42 patients treated. The authors treated 17 patients with diffuse laryngotracheal stenosis; in the first 6 cases, a successful result was obtained in only 1. After adoption of the precautions and protocol described here, the next 11 cases showed improved results, with 5 cases being successfully treated.

Pharyngeal surgery

The CO_2 laser has been used in a variety of oropharyngeal pathologies (Lyons et al., 1976; Strong et al., 1979a, b; Tucker, 1979; Adams and Griebie, 1985; Nishimura et al., 1988; Oswal et al., 1988). These authors agreed on the possibilities that the CO_2 laser offers with regard to precision, oedematous reaction, tissue trauma and decrease in postoperative pain. As in laryngeal surgery, the CO_2 laser has been used for both benign and malignant conditions of the pharynx.

Benign lesions

Chronic tonsillitis
In 1988 Nishimura reported on 30 patients undergoing tonsillectomy with good results (Nishimura et al., 1988). To assess any advantages of this technique, the author carried out a trial in which one tonsil was removed using conventional techniques (blunt dissection with scalpel, scissors or electric knife) and the other with the CO_2 laser. In this way it was possible to carry out a direct comparison of results.

Intraoperative progress Compared with traditional techniques of surgical dissection, the CO_2 laser does not decrease bleeding and in the authors' experience the most effective tool appeared to be the electric knife. It should be remembered that larger vessels cannot be sealed by the laser; in addition, great care is required to avoid accidental damage or perforation to the tonsillar pillars.

Postoperative progress On the laser-operated side it was noted that pain was more severe. Fibrin clots were remarkably more abundant and healing tendency was delayed. The conclusion of this small study was that CO_2 laser in tonsillectomy was relatively inefficient and the risks were not justifiable.

Papillomas, granulomas
Lesions with a small pedicle or with a well-circumscribed base are relatively simply treated with the traditional techniques of surgery and healing is rapid. Use of the CO_2 laser in these situations offers no advantage.

Voluminous cysts
Large cysts included in the pharyngeal wall can be excised using the CO_2 laser with some degree of precision because of the reduced or absent bleeding. It should be remembered, however, that large vessels must always be electrocauterized or ligated.

The laser can be advantageous in the removal of localized cysts of the glosso-epiglottic vallecula. Once the cyst has been identified using a Boyle–Davis mouth gag or a Weerda laryngoscope the lesion can be excised under microscopic control. This allows a high degree of accuracy and preserves function.

Angiomatous lesions

It is not advisable to use the CO_2 laser for the removal of angiomas. Here intraoperative bleeding is diffuse and the precise cleavage plane is difficult to identify. The most useful instrument appears to be the electrocautery knife which provides adequate haemostasis during the dissection.

The use of the CO_2 laser for such pharyngeal lesions mentioned above poses no advantage in the postoperative course and the results have been similar to those observed following tonsillectomy. The laser is absolutely contraindicated if subsequent reconstructive surgery is required to repair loss of tissue.

Premalignant lesions (keratoses)

Premalignant lesions can be easily excised from the pharynx along the submucosal plane. Carbonization of the marginal areas of keratosis by the CO_2 laser should be allowed for so that an adequate margin of normal tissue is removed for histological examination. It is imperative to carry out several intraoperative biopsies to exclude neoplastic transformation.

Malignant lesions

Oropharyngeal carcinoma is a highly invasive condition which usually requires radical surgery. Only very rarely can limited surgery be performed satisfactorily. Adams in 1985 reported 10 recurrences in 12 patients treated with CO_2 laser for T1 and T2 carcinomas of the oral cavity (Adams and Griebie, 1985). It is the authors' view that the CO_2 laser is contraindicated in the treatment of malignant neoplasms of the oropharynx and that traditional techniques should always be preferred. Such techniques allow the excision of an adequate margin of apparently normal tissue. In addition, a neck dissection can be performed, and the majority of cases require reconstruction.

Conclusion

The precision of endoscopic laser surgery has significant advantages, particularly in the treatment of laryngeal disease. The absence of postoperative oedema facilitates recovery and avoids the need for tracheostomy in the majority of patients. The functional results are often superior to those that can be achieved by traditional surgery.

In the oropharynx, the CO_2 laser is less useful since the majority of lesions are readily treated by conventional surgical techniques. There appears to be little advantage in healing or in tissue preservation here, and in malignant disease radical surgery is usually required, negating any advantages of the CO_2 laser.

References

Adams G.L., Griebie M.S. (1985). Role of the CO_2 laser in the management of localized carcinoma of the oral cavity. Emphasis on second primary malignancies. *Minn. Med.*, **68**, 285–9.

Andrews A.H. Jr, Moss H.W. (1974). Experience with the carbon dioxide laser in the larynx. *Ann. Otol.*, **83**, 462–72.

Dedo H.H., Jackler R.K. (1982). Laryngeal papilloma: results of the treatment with the CO_2 laser and podophyllum. *Ann. Otol.*, **91**, 425–30.
Friend M.P. (1992). Laser surgery. *Otorhinol. Head Neck Surg.*, **106**.
Jako G.J. (1977). Carbon dioxide laser microsurgery and its applications in laryngology. *Trans. Laser*, Munich.
King B.T. (1939). A new and function restoring operation for bilateral abductor cord paralysis. *JAMA.*, **112**, 814.
Krajina Z. (1982). International symposium on laser in laryngology. *Acta Otorhinolaryngol. Ital.*, **2**, 113–19.
Lyons G.D., Lousteau R.J., Mouney D.F. (1976). CO_2 laser as a clinical tool in otolaryngology. *Laryngoscope*, **86**, 1658–62.
Motta G., Villari G., Ripa G. De Maio. (1984). *Il laser a CO_2 Nella Microchirurgia Laringea*. (G. Motta ed.) Milano: Libreria Scientifica gia Ghedini, pp. 39–55.
Motta G., Villari G., Motta G. Jnr, et al. (1986). The CO_2 laser in the laryngeal microsurgery. *Acta Otolaryngol.*, (suppl.), **433**, 5–30.
Nishimura T., et al. (1988). Laser tonsillectomy. *Acta Otolaryngol.* (suppl.) **454**, 313–15.
Oswal V.H., Kashima H.K., Flood L.M. (1988). *The CO_2 Laser in Otolaryngology and Head and Neck Surgery*. London: Wright.
Rontal M., Rontal E. (1990). Endoscopic laryngeal surgery for bilateral midline vocal cord obstruction. *Ann. Otol. Rhinol. Laryngol.*, **99**, 605–10.
Rudert H. (1991). Larynx and hypo-pharynx cancers. Endoscopic surgery with laser: possibilities and limits. *Arch. Otorhinolaryngol.*, **1**, 3–18.
Shugar J.M.A., Sonn P.M., Biller H.F. (1982). An evaluation of the carbon dioxide laser in the treatment of the traumatic laryngeal stenosis. *Laryngoscope*, **92**, 23–6.
Steiner W. (1982). International workshop on laser in laryngology. *Acta Otorhinolaryngol. Ital.*, **2**, 99–105.
Steiner W., Jaumann, M.P., Pesch H.J. (1980). Endoskopische Laserchirurgie in larynx. *Ther. Umsch./Rev. Therapeut.*, **37**, 1103–9.
Strong M.S., Jako G.J. (1972). Laser surgery in the larynx. Early clinical experiences with continuous CO_2 laser. *Ann. Otol.*, **81**, 791–8.
Strong M.S., Vaughan C.W., Healy G.B., et al. (1979a). Transoral management of localised carcinoma of the oral cavity using the CO_2 laser. *Laryngoscope.*, **89**, 897–905.
Strong M.S., Vaughan C.W., Healy G.B., et al. (1979b). Transoral resection of cancer of the oral cavity: the role of the CO_2 laser. *Otolaryngol. Clin. North Am.*, **5**, 207–18.
Tucker H.M. (1979). *Use of the CO_2 Laser in Treating Lesions of the Mouth and Larynx*. Cleveland, Ohio: Cleveland Clinic.
Woodman De Graaf (1946). A modification of the extra laryngeal approach to the arytenoidectomy for bilateral abductor paralysis. *Arch. Otolaryngol.*, **43**, 63.
Zeitels S.M. et al. (1990). Endoscopic management of early supraglottic cancer. *Ann. Otol. Rhinol. Laryngol.*, **99**, 951–6.

Chapter 11

Nursing care of the patient undergoing laryngectomy

J.M. Muir

Preparation of the patient for laryngectomy begins as soon as the decision for surgery has been made. The role of the nurse may be summed up as that of carer, counsellor and communicator. Good communication between the patient and every member of the clinical team is of paramount importance.

The aims of the nursing staff are:

(1) to prepare patients and their families physically, mentally and emotionally for surgery;
(2) to care for patients during the postoperative phase;
(3) to show patients how to care for themselves and for their altered airway.

The final aim is to rehabilitate the patients to a quality of life that is acceptable to them.

Preoperative preparation

There are several aspects to the preparation of a patient who is to undergo a laryngectomy.

Initial consultation

It is helpful if a nurse can be present at the interview between patient and doctor when the question of a laryngectomy is first raised. Patients rarely take in all that is said at this stage and the nurse frequently finds it necessary to reinforce or elaborate on what has been discussed. In the role of counsellor, a nurse may prove instrumental in helping a patient reach a positive decision for surgery, although it should be emphasized it is no part of a nurse's role to persuade a patient to undergo an operation that the patient does not want. There are few patients more difficult to rehabilitate successfully than one who has undergone this operation reluctantly.

Once a date has been set for the operation, probably within 7–10 days, the patient should be able to go home for a few days. This gives an opportunity for the patients to spend time with their families; they can then be readmitted a few days prior to surgery when physical and psychological preparation can be continued.

Admission to hospital

The admission procedure is carried out by the nurse who will assist with the preoperative preparation and who will care for the patient immediately following surgery. An effort is made to minimize the number of nursing staff caring for each patient and to provide nursing in the same physical environment; this all helps in reducing the stress and anxiety felt by the patient.

The admission procedure and nursing assessment is identical with that of any other patient undergoing elective surgery in an ear, nose and throat ward, although the more radical implications of this admission for the patient must always be borne in mind. It is helpful if a spouse or other significant person can be present during part of the admission as it provides a good opportunity for discussion and questions; since they may be closely involved with the patient following surgery it is as well that they are involved with the care from the beginning. Various forms of literature are available and are offered to the patient and the family as a resource for information, although written material is never regarded as a substitute for good communication from the clinical team.

Clinical investigation

Physical preparation of the patient will already have been started, usually during the previous admission for investigation and biopsy. Some clinical tests have to be performed nearer the time of the operation. Such investigations are performed for three main reasons:

(1) to assess the extent of the tumour;
(2) to assess the patient's general state of health;
(3) to allow for correction of any deficiencies or treatment of infection prior to surgery.

Clinical investigations for the prospective laryngectomy patient are shown in Table 11.1.

Prior to surgery, the patient is assessed by the anaesthetist who discusses this aspect of the operation and helps allay any fears regarding the anaesthesia. Some form of night sedation to be given the night before the operation, as well as a premedication to be given the following morning, is prescribed.

Psychological and emotional support

Knowledge is a key factor in reducing fear and anxiety, so much of the support given to patients at this stage is aimed at giving them as much knowledge as they want. Repeated explanations may frequently be necessary; the patients and their families need to know the following basic information.

(1) The stoma — how this will be the patient's only airway, that it is permanent and cannot close over.
(2) tracheal suction — the necessity for removing excess secretions, usually only necessary during the immediate postoperative period. The amount of secretions produced gradually diminishes.
(3) Loss of the sound source of communication — recovery of speech may well

Table 11.1 Clinical investigations for the prospective laryngectomy patient

Blood tests
    Full blood count
    Urea and electrolytes
    Liver function tests
    Erythrocyte sedimentation rate
    Blood group and cross-match

Radiographs
    Chest X-ray
    Computed tomography

Microbiological investigation
    Nose and throat swabs
    Sputum specimen
    Midstream urine specimen

Electrocardiogram
Dental assessment

depend on the type of operation proposed, e.g. neoglottis or tracheo-oesophageal prosthesis. Simple diagrams can be useful in explaining the surgery and how sound is produced postoperatively.

(4) Intravenous infusion is usually only necessary for the first 24–48 hours. The possibility of a blood transfusion should also be mentioned.
(5) Nasogastric tube — this is left in position for 8–10 days following the operation, during which time all the patient's dietary requirements are given via the tube. This avoids stress to the healing area and means the patient will not feel hungry or thirsty.
(6) Incision line and sutures — the incision is U-shaped following the natural creases in the neck, so that once healed it is not at all obvious. Skin sutures are removed at 7–8 days and the stoma sutures at 9–10 days postoperatively.

Other points of information such as pain control and humidification are also covered. It is essential that a patient has time to ask questions and express fears and anxieties. Communication is a two-way process and is the key to successful rehabilitation.

A visit by a former patient who has successfully undergone the same operation is arranged if the patient so desires. This can prove of enormous encouragement since the patient can actually see what can be achieved. Likewise the local laryngectomy club can be of great help and support preoperatively as well as following discharge from hospital.

Other members of the team who play a part in the rehabilitation of the patient are the social worker, physiotherapist and speech therapist. Even if the patient does not require actual assistance from the social worker at this stage, it is a good idea for them to be aware of each other's existence and of the help that is available should it become necessary. The physiotherapist initially has a high degree of involvement with the patient and it makes both of their tasks easier if each knows what is expected by the other. The speech therapist takes on a more prominent role in the care of the patient postoperatively, but plenty of contact from the beginning helps in building a good working relationship. The speech therapist can do much to boost patient morale and can prove invaluable in describing how speech may be regained following laryngectomy.

Preparation for theatre

The evening prior to operation, the patient's skin is shaved from neck to nipple line, and the patient is asked to shower the face and neck the following morning. Every effort is made by the nursing staff to ensure optimum conditions for a peaceful night's rest so that the patient goes to theatre in as relaxed a frame of mind as possible. The patient is given nothing to eat after 10 p.m. but is allowed a cup of tea at 5 a.m. the following day; most patients accept it, knowing it will be their last for several days. The patient is prepared for theatre, the premedication given and the patient left to rest. Patients are accompanied to theatre either by the nurse who cares for them during the preoperative stage or by the one who nurses them during the immediate postoperative period.

Postoperative care

Since infection is the cause of many of the problems that beset laryngectomy patients in the immediate postoperative phase, every effort is made to ensure a high standard of cleanliness in their immediate environment. Various nursing measures are taken to reduce the risk of cross-infection, such as the wearing of disposable aprons by all personnel who have contact with the patient, cleaning the room to which the patient will return from theatre, and adhering to a high standard of technique when suctioning or caring for the stoma or neck wound.

Early postoperative care

On arrival in the ward from theatre patients are handed over to the care of a nurse who will be involved in their constant care for the next 2–3 days. They are nursed in a semiprone or upright position with the head well supported at all times. Care is taken that the bedclothes do not occlude the newly formed airway. A cuffed tracheostomy tube is in position with the cuff inflated and left so until the following morning. A humidifier and filter are attached to make respiration easier.

An intravenous infusion is in progress and continues for the next 24 hours. A nasogastric tube is in position but this is spigoted and left alone until the patient is able to start taking fluids down it. There are two drains in position, one on either side of the neck wound; and exuded fluid is observed for its quality and quantity. The drains are usually removed between the third and fifth postoperative day.

Where a neoglottis has been fashioned, a second tube inserted into the nose in a similar fashion to the nasogastric tube is in position with the distal end emerging through the tracheostoma. This tube goes through the fistula which is part of the reconstruction and is removed on the eighth to tenth postoperative day. Extreme care must be taken that this tube does not become dislodged before then.

Vital signs are recorded by an automatic recording machine which is less disruptive to the patient than manual recording by the nursing staff. The signs are noted at gradually increasing intervals over the first 24 hours and thereafter recorded every 4 hours. Tracheal suction is carried out as necessary, and oral or nasal suction may also be required to cope with any copious production of secretions. Oral hygiene, nasal toileting and stoma care are carried out every 4 hours to keep those areas clean and prevent the formation of crusts which might predispose to infection. Urine output is carefully monitored and noted as part of maintaining an accurate fluid balance; catheterization may sometimes be necessary for a few days. Analgesia is provided either as intramuscular injections or by way of a syringe driver.

For the first 2–3 days, a nurse is allocated to the care of the patient 24 hours a day. For both physical safety and psychological support the patient is not left alone during this difficult period. As few nurses as possible share this care; this provides continuity for the patient's well-being and minimizes the effort of getting to know strange staff at a time when familiar faces are most appreciated.

Nasogastric feeding can usually begin on the first postoperative day, once it has been ascertained that bowel sounds are present. An intake of 2.5 litres of fluid containing 2000 calories in 24 hours is generally an adequate amount, although this will vary according to the patient's preoperative dietary requirements and an assessment of present needs. The patient is weighed weekly to detect any change and dietary adjustments are made accordingly. It is as well to ensure that constipation does not develop since this can become a major problem in these patients.

Humidification of the patient's airway is continued for most of the stay in hospital, as the patient's body learns to adjust to the absence of the humidifying function of the nasal passages. The patient is taught how to provide humidification at home and the importance of this in keeping the stoma clean and healthy.

On the second postoperative day the tracheostomy tube is changed for a plain one, and thereafter each subsequent tube change becomes a learning opportunity for the patient, so that by the time of discharge the patient is proficient in the full care of the stoma.

The first 5 postoperative days are some of the busiest for these patients. They are encouraged to move about from the very first morning and, as drips and drains are removed, this gradually becomes easier. Getting dressed by day and mixing with other patients helps them become part of the ward community even where there may be difficulty in communicating. Feelings of depression and withdrawal often occur while the patient is in hospital, and may recur weeks or months later. Patients need support and understanding from carers and family in adjusting to a new self-image and an altered life.

As physical recovery progresses, tubes and sutures are gradually removed. On the eighth to tenth postoperative day, a contrast test is carried out to ensure that internal healing is complete. If this is successful, the nasogastric and pharyngeal tubes are removed and the patient may begin to drink and eat again.

Rehabilitation

Patients are encouraged to carry out more and more of their own care as their condition improves. They learn how to manage their altered airway in the outside world, and speech therapists work hard at achieving sound as the patient looks forward to going home. The community nursing service and the patient's own family doctor are advised of the pending discharge, and often the community nurse will visit the patient prior to going home so that maximum continuity of care may be achieved. It should be emphasized that laryngectomy patients are never sent home until they feel ready to go. Some patients need longer than others before they feel able to cope. Support continues after discharge through the community services, the laryngectomy club and the outpatient clinic. Rehabilitation is very much a team effort, and the well-adjusted patient is a member of a team in which the patient's role and involvement is as necessary as that of anyone else.

Part Four

Voice Rehabilitation

Chapter 12

Oesophageal speech

P.H. Damsté

As long as laryngectomies have been performed patients have searched for a new voice and some have found out by themselves the use of oesophageal voice. At the first International Congress of Otolaryngology in 1908 in Vienna, H. Gutzmann demonstrated 25 patients who had learned to speak after laryngectomy. Since then it has become customary in most centres to teach oesophageal speech. It is, however, not the only way towards voice rehabilitation. Since the beginning of major laryngeal surgery there have been attempts at surgical restoration of the vocal function; also a never-ending series of external voice prostheses of various designs have been available for the laryngectomized patient.

The three methods of vocal rehabilitation are not always in competition with each other. Depending on the communicative situation a person may choose one method or another: for instance, fistula speech normally and oesophageal speech when the patient needs the use of both hands, or oesophageal speech normally and an electric voice prosthesis when making a telephone call. Recently patients with fistula speech or neoglottal speech (Singh, 1989b) can speak with both hands free if fitted with a tracheostoma valve (Singh, 1989a).

Aerodynamics of oesophageal speech

A look at Figure 12.1 explains the change in the vocal organs brought about by total laryngectomy. The pharynx has become a narrow funnel that converges into the entrance to the oesophagus. The transition of the pharynx and the oesophagus has regularly been indicated as the pharyngo-oesophageal segment. This area can be constricted by the hypopharyngeal and cricopharyngeal musculature and the oesophageal sphincter. When moderately narrowed, it can be brought into vibration by an air stream passing through it.

Since the oesophagus can only contain a limited amount of air the emission of sound can only be of short duration. Still, considering that an average oesophageal speaker can phonate for 2–3 seconds on one oesophageal load of air of 40–60 ml, oesophageal voice is extremely efficient when compared with a normal male voice which uses an air volume of 140 ml/s.

The way in which the air volume in the oesophagus is constantly replenished is crucial for the quality of oesophageal voice. There are two main ways.

(1) *Inhalation or suction.* During inspiration the negative pressure in the oesophagus

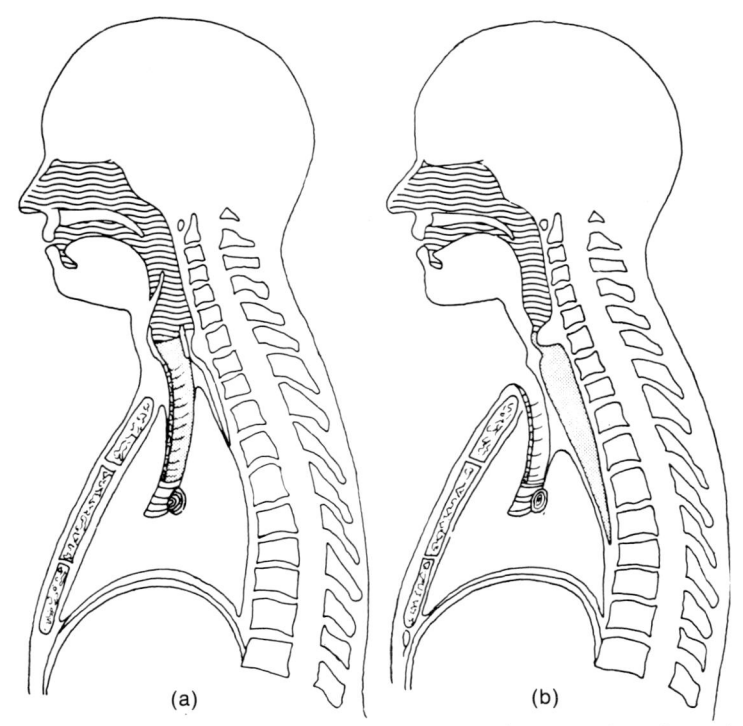

Figure 12.1 Vocal tract: (a) normal anatomy: the air for phonation comes from the trachea; (b) the situation after laryngectomy: the air supply for voice production is in the oesophagus. From Damsté (1958).

is lowered still further. By opening the pharyngo-oesophageal segment simultaneously, air is drawn into the oesophagus.
(2) *Injection*. When the oropharyngeal cavity is shut off by closed lips or when the tongue makes occlusion against the palate, the air in the cavity is compressed by elevating the base of the tongue. When the oesophageal sphincter is released the compressed air is allowed to escape in the oesophagus.
(3) *Swallowing*. Actual swallowing is rarely done and is more cumbrous than the glossopharyngeal pump described in (2) above.

Practising oesophageal speech

Early stages

The first session of practising the new voice can take place as soon as the surgical wound has healed completely. The feeding tube will have been removed a few days before, there should be no sign of any leakage and there should be no traces of fibrin visible in the hypopharyngeal area.

First, the student should learn how to move air in and out of the mouth, by pumping with the tongue; the correct movement can be checked by applying two fingers to the floor of the mouth. The pumping motions result in little puffs of air escaping between the lips. This is a familiar feeling, like pronouncing the 'p' sound, because plosive consonants always increase the air pressure in the mouth.

The patient will learn to direct the air into the oesophagus instead of through the lips, concentrating on a wide and relaxed throat while repeating the pumping manoeuvre with lips closed. Soon this will be followed by a soft clucking sound of air entering the oesophagus. After repeating this several times the collected air will find its way out of the oesophagus and the first oesophageal voice sound is born.

In the session just described the injection method or plosive consonant method was employed to initiate oesophageal voice. If the expected result is not achieved, other methods or devices to produce the first oesophageal sound should be attempted, e.g. inhaling or swallowing air or the use of carbonated water.

Obstacles to learning oesophageal speech

Preconditions for achieving results without delay are that students can learn to produce these unusual sounds, and that they are encouraged by their environment. If a spouse, for example, is scared of the patient's tracheostomy tube and is disgusted by the first attempts to speak, this can be a serious handicap. It can lead to involuntary avoidance behaviour: a tightly constricted pharynx and pharyngo-oesophageal segment. If this is allowed to persist it may result in a pharyngeal voice: a pinched, high-pitched voice of short duration which is quite unsuitable for fluent speech. It is important to recognize this immediately and correct the habit by proper remedial teaching (Keith and Darley, 1986).

Another essential for an unhindered course toward speech rehabilitation is that there is no organic obstacle, such as a pouch or diverticulum in the pharyngo-oesophageal segment. This can be found out by lateral X-rays of that part of the neck. In the example shown in Figure 12.2 the origin of a shallow diverticulum could be traced back to a fistula where a suture had broken down. It shows the importance of expert nursing during the postoperative period. Irregular shape of the pharyngo-oesophageal segment can have an adverse affect on the quality of phonation by causing stagnation of secretions.

Advanced stage

When, after a few weeks or months, patients have reached a degree of proficiency that has restored their confidence and removed much of the initial post-surgery depression, it is time to attend to the finishing touches in their speech. The following qualities should be aimed for:

(1) voice always available on request;
(2) reduced interval between the intake of air and the emission of sound;
(3) increased duration of the sound, and the number of syllables on one intake of air;
(4) no audible 'clunk' on injection;
(5) no unnecessarily repeated injections or surplus movements;
(6) reduction in noise from the stoma during speech if possible;
(7) improved articulation;
(8) overall intelligibility.

These and other items can be worked into a checklist or score card with which the progress can be monitored.

At this stage it is recommended to work in group sessions. It accustoms the timid not to fear speaking clearly in the presence of others, and for some the competition is stimulating.

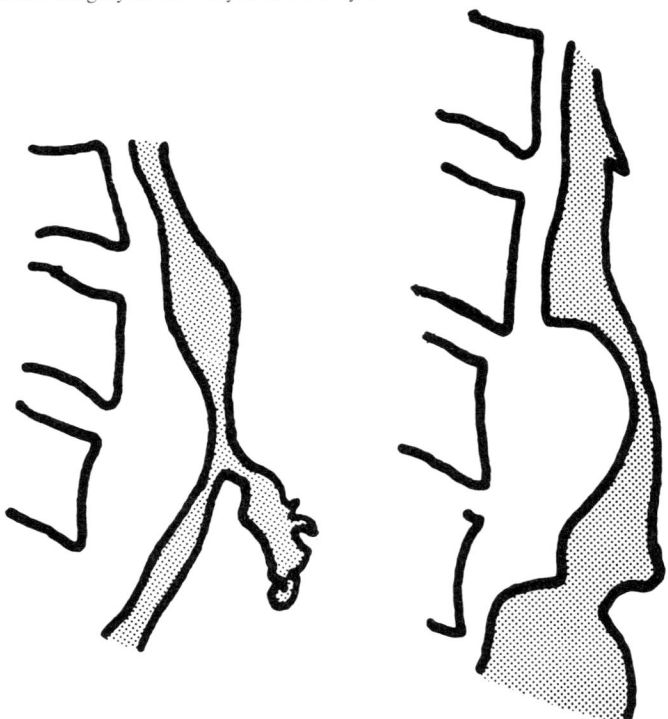

168   Functional Surgery of the Larynx and Pharynx

Figure 12.2   Pouch or diverticulum (right) that has remained as a consequence of a broken-down suture of the anterior pharyngeal wall (left). From Keith and Darley (1986) with permission.

The patient is encouraged to establish contact with a regional chapter of the association for laryngectomized patients. These societies have provided invaluable support to patients who enter a new phase in their lives as a handicapped person. Notable exceptions are those successfully rehabilitated patients who do not consider themselves handicapped. They prefer not to maintain relations with the hospital and with fellow patients.

Some patients have very soft voices. Even if they have mastered the correct technique they cannot produce a sufficiently loud and clear voice. The explanation is that the pharyngo-oesophageal segment is wide and lax, and does not offer enough resistance to the air. These patients can sometimes be helped by an elastic neckband that exerts pressure on the skin exactly above the pharyngo-oesophageal segment. A custom-made Plexiglass strip that fits the hollow above the stoma gives the best results.

A rehabilitation programme is not complete without restoration of the capacity to smell. After laryngectomy the sense of smell is apparently lost. The olfactory sense as such is usually intact; however, the lack of air stream through the nose means that odorous vapours cannot reach the sensory epithelium. The air stream through the nose is re-established by the same pumping action as is taught in the first stage of oesophageal speech training. By moving the bottom of the mouth it is possible to displace enough air to cause a good ventilation of the nose. The main difference with the glossopharyngeal action during speech is that the air is allowed to pass the velopharyngeal isthmus. During air injection for speech the velum is closed.

For laryngectomized patients who used to enjoy swimming there is no reason to give up this healthy activity. With simple equipment and sufficient practice it is quite safe to take to the water. A tracheal cannula of the correct size with an inflatable cuff is inserted into the tracheostoma. Initially a surface anaesthetic and a few practice sessions are needed to become accustomed to this device. The cuff is then gently inflated by means of a syringe, and a check is made by closing the cannula with a finger to determine if the seal is airtight. If it is, a flexible tube carrying a snorkel can be fitted to the cannula and the snorkel attached to the head with a headband. The swimmer will first have to adjust to the dead space for breathing being larger than usual. Being able to swim again reduces the sense of being handicapped considerably.

Quality of life after laryngectomy

Postoperative depression has already been mentioned as a serious impediment to successful rehabilitation. In voice therapy it is particularly obvious that results depend in large measure on the motivation to work for progress. Not all patients have this motivation. There are those who cling to an attitude of 'you know what is best for me, doctor'. In so doing patients save themselves the anguish of having to make a choice in full freedom, and the doctor saves time that is otherwise spent in informing and counselling the patient. This helpless attitude that many patients are still accustomed to and which their doctors expect from them, can be the basis of a reactive depression. There is every reason to train doctors in a less authoritarian attitude and to educate patients towards a less submissive and more responsible state of mind.

Already many doctors respect the patient's autonomy in making decisions that affect the course of treatment. No longer is the mode of rehabilitation determined entirely by the doctor on the basis of personal preference and the tradition of the clinic. The medical team should give full information on the possibilities of speech: oesophageal speech, tracheo-oesophageal fistula speech or tracheopharyngeal shunt speech in near-total laryngectomy (Singh, 1989b). A personal bias will influence the outcome when counselling a hesitant patient, but the therapist should not force a choice upon the patient.

Growth towards more self-determination on the part of the patient is related to more openness with regard to the diagnosis and prognosis of throat cancer. Death will eventually come to all our patients, to some sooner than to others. An inevitable part of the quality of life after laryngectomy is the quality of death. It is normal that the mind of every patient is now and then occupied by thoughts of death and dying. The subject should not be avoided in pretreatment deliberations. The expected quality of death may weigh heavily in the choice between alternative courses of treatment. Patients have reason to expect that in the case of an untreatable recurrence, they will become the battleground of a heroic but futile combat by the hospital staff to prolong life. Faced with this prospect they have serious doubts about the quality of life in its terminal stage, in the intensive care unit of a surgical ward. For a patient with cancer of the throat, it is reassuring to know that, when the time arrives, there will be assistance in the home or a place in a hospice. The prospect of good terminal care is important for the laryngectomy patient who is about to be rehabilitated. It relieves anxiety about the future. This is a propitious starting point for rehabilitation.

References

Damsté P.H. (1958). *Oesophageal Speech*. Dissertation, University of Groningen.
Keith R.L., Darley F.L. (1986). *Laryngectomy Rehabilitation*. San Diego: College Hill Press.
Edels Y., ed. (1983). *Laryngectomy; Diagnosis to Rehabilitation*. London: Croom Helm.
Laryngectomy rehabilitation Seminars, Poole 1987, Abingdon 1980. A Macmillan report. London: National Society for Cancer Relief.
Singh W. (1989a). Singh tracheostoma valve. In *Proceedings of the International Voice Symposium*, Edinburgh (Singh W., ed.) Edinburgh: Singh, pp. 81–2.
Singh W. (1989b). Near-total laryngectomy. In *Proceedings of the International Voice Symposioum*, Edinburgh (Singh W., ed.) Edinburgh: Singh, pp. 53–8.

Chapter 13

Fistula speech

W. Singh

It may be possible for speech to be produced after laryngectomy, but the production mechanism will obviously be different from that of normal speech. There are a number of mechanisms which might be employed depending upon whether total or partial laryngectomy was performed and whether any prostheses are employed to assist speech production. (Ainsworth and Singh, 1990).

Approximately 180 cases of cancer of the larynx occur in Scotland each year (Scottish Cancer Registration Scheme, 1981). In the UK about 2000 cases occur every year and about 300 laryngectomies are performed; the majority of these patients are 50–70 years old. Cancer of the larynx rarely occurs in children (Singh and Kaur, 1987). There is a high probability of cure following surgery, but at the cost of severely impaired speech and consequently great emotional distress. Many of these patients are potentially able to return to full-time employment provided they can communicate. Loss of speech may not only disrupt the patient's livelihood, but also produce serious psychological stress and behaviour changes. In the USA approximately 11 700 new cases of laryngeal cancer in 1986 were reported by the American Cancer Society, and approximately 2500 laryngectomies are performed every year (Barria, 1985).

After surgical extirpation of cancer of the larynx, there are three main avenues available for voice production mechanism: surgical reconstruction, e.g. parsimonious laryngectomy (near-total laryngectomy with myomucosal valved neoglottis) or fashioning of a tracheo-oesophageal fistula and fitting a voice prosthesis (Staffieri, 1976; Singer and Blom, 1980; Singh, 1988a, b, 1990, 1991); oesophageal speech training; or an artificial larynx. Probably the three most commonly used artificial laryngeal devices are those made by Servox (Figure 13.1), Cooper-Rand (Figure 13.2) and Tokyo (Figure 13.3). However, their conspicuously artificial sound and appearance limit their acceptance by the patient.

Although oesophageal speech still remains the preferred method of communication in laryngectomized patients, only about 25% of these patients are able to communicate effectively (Ryan, 1979). The speaker swallows air into the oesophagus and brings it out in small volumes for speech production; a fresh intake of air is required after every four to five words (Snidcor and Curry. 1959). Oesophageal voice is low-pitched, usually between 60–80 Hz with reduced intensity and rate of speech compared with normal speakers (Snidcor and Curry, 1959; Robbins et al., 1984), with resultant poor intelligibility and acceptability. The voicing also contains comparatively large amounts of 'jitter' (cycle-to-cycle pitch perturbation) and 'shimmer' (cycle-to-cycle amplitude perturbation). Oesophageal speakers find it extremely difficult to communicate, especially in noisy surroundings such as large social events

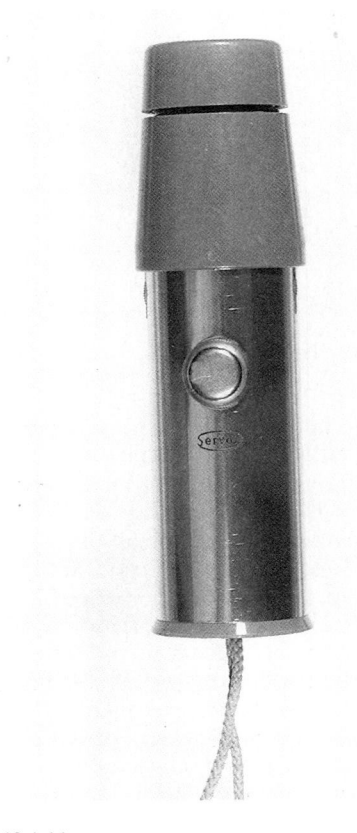

Figure 13.1 The Servox artificial larynx

or pubs. Failure to communicate effectively leads to withdrawal from society, sometimes leading to suicide.

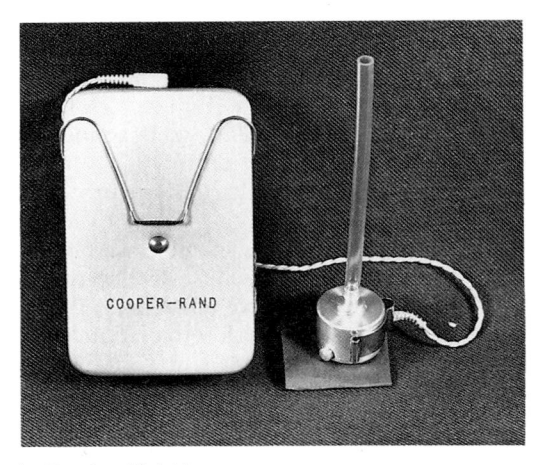

Figure 13.2 The Cooper–Rand artificial larynx

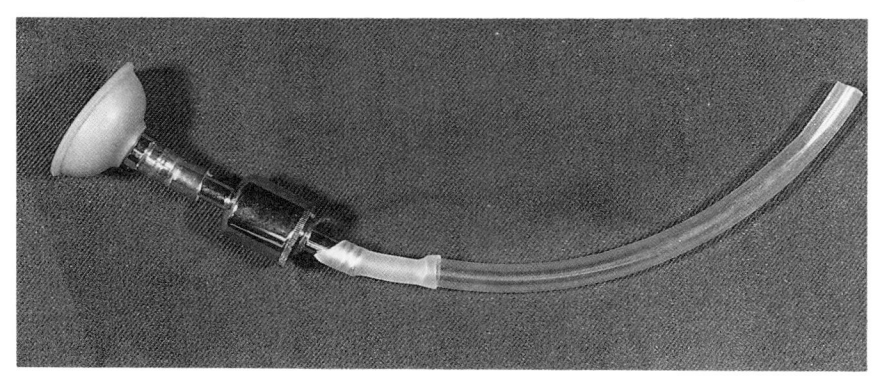

Figure 13.3 The Tokyo artificial larynx

The addition of a pulmonary air supply in tracheo-oesophageal speech brings the acoustic quality of speech closer to normal. The introduction of the tracheo-oesophageal puncture technique with the fitting of a voice prosthesis (Singer and Blom, 1980), thereby achieving fluent, intelligible speech without the aspiration of saliva or food, has brought about a dramatic change in the life-style of laryngectomy patients who cannot speak effectively. This technique permits the patient to use the greater volume of pulmonary air rather than being restricted to the much smaller capacity of oesophageal air (about 75 ml) used in conventional oesophageal speech. The prosthesis-free procedure of parsimonious laryngectomy (near-total laryngectomy with preservation of voice mechanism) has been developed (Singh, 1985, 1989, 1991; Singh and Hardcastle, 1985) as an alternative to total laryngectomy. Details are described in Chapter 9. This chapter deals with surgically reconstructed tracheo-oesophageal fistula speech only.

Historical perspective

Ever since the first total laryngectomy was performed by Professor Theodor Billroth in 1873, in Vienna, attempts to provide good, intelligible speech by a surgical technique that connects the trachea with the oesophagus or pharynx have exercised generations of surgeons.

It was well known in the nineteenth century that if a vibrating column of exhaled air is introduced into the oesophagus or pharynx the resultant voice produced is subsequently modulated into intelligible speech by the intact articulators of the vocal tract. However, all such attempts have been beset by two major complications; aspiration of saliva and food, and stenosis of the shunt between the trachea and the pharynx or oesophagus.

There have been several attempts at surgical reconstruction of the vocal mechanism. Gussenbauer (1874) and Park (1886) made the earliest attempts to create a tracheopharyngeal fistula, and to maintain it they employed mechanical devices. Gussenbauer designed a Y-shaped metallic device (Figure 13.4) connecting the tracheostoma and pharyngeal fistula. The establishment of the tracheopharyngeal communication resulted in good, intelligible speech, but the problems of leakage and stenosis were never overcome. In 1928 Scuri reported a case of spontaneous fistula between the tracheostoma and oesophagus with good, intelligible speech (quoted by Briani, 1959).

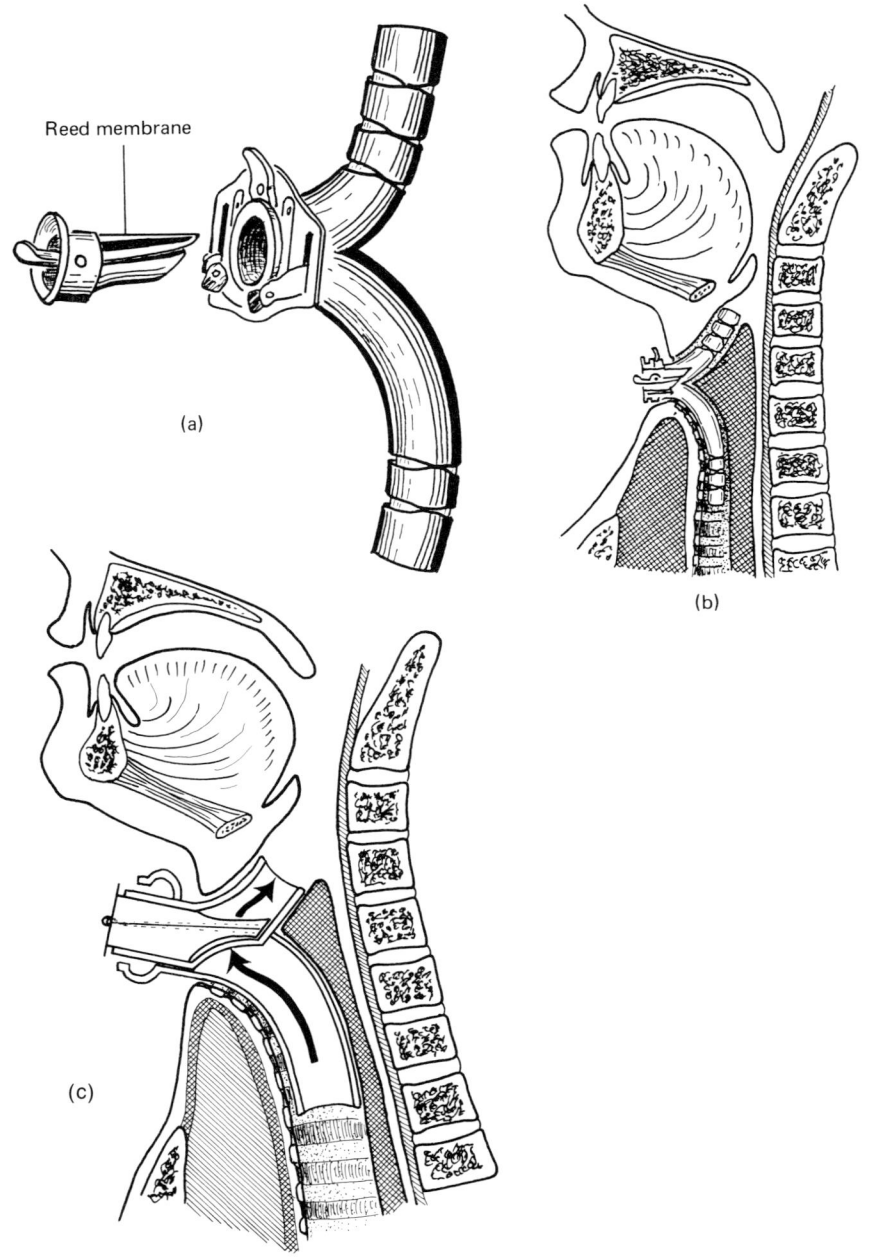

174 Functional Surgery of the Larynx and Pharynx

Figure 13.4 Gussenbauer's prosthesis: (a) component parts; (b) prosthesis in situ; (c) metallic reed vibrator producing sound

In 1927 at the meeting of the American College of Surgeons in Chicago, Dr Joseph C. Beck demonstrated a self-operated case of tracheohypopharyngeal fistula. A desperate laryngectomy patient, who hated using the artificial larynx, passed the point of a red-hot ice pick through the tracheostoma upwards and backwards to the hypopharynx. He repeated this heroic procedure on two more occasions until a permanent tracheohypopharyngeal fistula was created. By occluding his tracheostoma with a finger, he was able to direct the exhaled air to the pharynx through the fistula with subsequent production of loud, intelligible speech. Motivated by the experience of his patient, Guttman, in 1931, operated on a laryngectomized patient who was unable either to use an artificial larynx or to learn oesophageal speech effectively. A puncture needle was passed a few millimetres behind the uppermost part of the tracheostoma, in the midline, and pushed upwards and backwards to the hypopharynx. The needle was connected to a diathermy apparatus. The current was then switched on and the puncture needle withdrawn so as to ensure an electrocoagulated tract. A definite fistula was formed within 2 weeks. In 1935, Guttman described two more cases of tracheohypopharyngeal fistula, and mentioned stenosis in one and aspiration in the other as complications. Though the results were variable, Guttman had established the model for the present day tracheo-oesophageal puncture procedure half a century ago (Guttman, 1935).

In 1952 Briani in Italy created a pharyngostoma in the lateral neck region just below the base of the tongue, and connected it to the tracheostoma with a plastic and rubber cannula device (Briani, 1952). This valved prosthesis allowed for good, intelligible speech, and prevented aspiration of saliva and liquids into the trachea. These developments showed that voice could be achieved without the need for a reed as an external vibrating sound, as had been described by Gussenbauer.

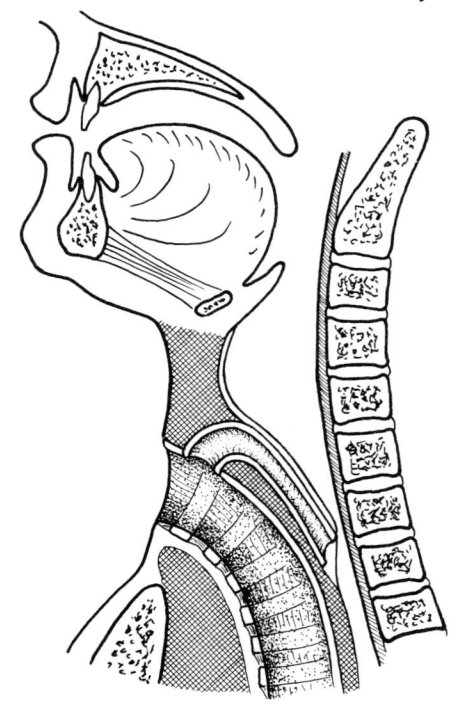

Figure 13.5 Conley's tracheo-oesophageal shunt

In 1958 Conley et al. created a tracheo-oesophageal shunt by a mucosal tube from the oesophagus to the trachea just above the level of the stoma (Figure 13.5) (Conley et al., 1958). In 1959 Conley used an 8-cm autogenous saphenous vein graft to connect the trachea and oesophagus. He reported three complications: stenosis, aspiration and the lack of a satisfactory speech mechanism to control the air flow for speech production (Conley, 1959).

In 1960 Asai in Japan described his now well-known staged method of using a buried skin tube, formed from local cervical skin, to join the trachea and pharynx (Asai, 1960) (Figure 13.6). In 1972 he reported rupture of the dermal tube, stenosis and salivary leakage as complications in some patients who had undergone this procedure (Asai, 1972). Miller (1967, 1971) developed Asai's technique of cutaneous shunt to connect the trachea with the pharynx, and popularized it in the USA. He reviewed his experience of 30 cases in 1971 and reported 5 cases of stenosis. Aspiration of saliva and food was a more frequent complication. In 1968 Montgomery and Toohill described a buried dermal tube technique, almost similar to that originally described by Asai for the patients who were already alaryngeal (Montgomery and Toohil, 1968). As the skin tube was flaccid, a silicone T-tube was inserted into the tracheostoma with the upper part extending into the lower part of the buried dermal tube to keep it patent. Four years later Montgomery modified his earlier technique. Regarding late stenosis and aspiration, no specific documentation was reported.

In 1971 McGrail and Oldfield described a one-stage modification of the Asai technique (McGrail and Oldfield, 1971). They used a skin tube formed from the medially based deltopectoral flap. This was especially useful in patients who had received a high dosage of radiation to the neck. In 1971 Calcaterra and Jafek experimented with 10 dogs, modifying Conley's technique by using a full-thickness cervical oesophageal wall flap which was tubed and sutured end-to-side to a fistula in the posterior membranous portion of the trachea (Calcaterra and Jafek, 1971). They reported no stenosis or aspiration problems using this full-thickness oesophageal flap. Komorn (1974) and Zwitman and Calcaterra (1973) adapted this technique to humans with a significant improvement in surgical success. In 1972, Taub and Spiro described a one-stage operation, after laryngectomy, in which a secondary fistula is created in the lateral side of the cervical oesophagus (Taub and Spiro, 1972). An external air bypass prosthesis called the VoiceBak (Figure 13.7) is interposed between the tracheostoma and the lateral cervical oesophageal fistula created earlier. The prosthesis works without manual occlusion and is regulated by exhaled lung air pressure. The most significant disadvantages of Taub's air bypass prosthesis are that it involves a delicate surgical procedure and needs a bulky, costly external apparatus (Dworkin and Sparker, 1980). Of the 26 laryngectomy patients who underwent the procedure, the subsequent increased pressure on the carotid vessels led to carotid rupture and death in 2 patients.

In 1972 Arslan and Serafini proposed the concept of joining the remnant of the subtotal laryngectomy to the trachea (Figure 13.8) to reconstitute the airway, phonatory mechanism and protection of the airway from aspiration (Arslan and Serafini, 1972). A temporary tracheostoma was fashioned on the pretext that the patient might eventually be decannulated and achieve good respiration by the natural air passages after the closure of the temporary tracheostoma. The high failure rate for decannulation (70%) and frequently occurring aspiration of saliva and food after this operation brings into question the advisability of performing this procedure. Moreover, the surgical principles of cancer clearance seem to have been sacrificed in some cases, as local recurrence occurred with time, and the wisdom of preserving the hyoid bone and suprahyoid part of the epiglottis was questioned.

In 1976 Mario Staffieri and associates reported the technique of tracheohypopharyngeal shunt (Figure 13.9) after total laryngectomy, which they developed in 1970 (Staffieri, 1976). The postcricoid flap is developed and placed over the top of the transected trachea. A phonatory tracheohypopharyngeal shunt of about 5 mm in length is created by pulling the hypopharyngeal mucosa through the incision in the postcricoid flap and suturing it to the external muscle. The postcricoid flap containing the phonatory fistula is sutured to the top of the tracheal stump. Voice is produced by occluding the tracheostoma with a finger, thus diverting the exhaled air into the hypopharynx for speech production. The Staffieri procedure can be performed on all cancerous lesions of the larynx that require total laryngectomy with or without neck dissection. Surgical principles of adequate tissue removal for tumour clearance are not sacrificed (Gatti et al., 1981). Bruce Leipzig (1980) reported aspiration as a nearly constant feature of the procedure. In 1980, Amatsu from Japan proposed the removal during laryngectomy of the anterior cartilaginous part of the trachea from the first to the fourth ring, and the formation of a tube from the remnant of the posterior membranous part of the trachea (Amatsu, 1980). A side-to-side tracheo-oesophageal anastomosis was established (Figure 13.10). Aspiration is a limiting factor. Amatsu suggested slight percutaneous digital pressure on the shunt during swallowing to avoid this difficulty. In 1985, Li from China described a tracheo-oesophageal shunt procedure after total laryngectomy, in which a tongue-like tracheo-oesophageal flap is created and transposed into the oesophageal lumen in a downward direction (Li, 1985). Occlusion of the tracheostoma directs the expired air flow into the oesophagus, producing voice. During deglutition the tongue-like flap covering the fistula prevents aspiration of saliva or food into the trachea. Fifteen of 19 patients operated on by Li developed good speech (78%). In 1989 Saito et al. described a mucodermal tracheo-oesophageal shunt technique for voice restoration in which a small U-shaped cervical skin flap is fashioned to form the anterior wall of the tracheo-oesophageal shunt. Digital pressure on the flap is used to avoid leakage from the shunt (Saito et al., 1989).

Fistula speech procedures and prostheses

In 1980, Singer and Blom, having considered the success or failure of past techniques, developed an endoscopic procedure for the restoration of voice after laryngectomy (Singer and Blom, 1980). Under general anaesthesia, a tracheo-oesophageal puncture is created by inserting a 14-FG needle through the posterosuperior membranous wall of the tracheostoma, 5 mm inferior to the mucocutaneous junction, into the lumen of a rigid oesophagoscope. A disposable intravenous catheter is inserted through the needle, and the needle is withdrawn. The tracheo-oesophageal puncture tract is dilated until a 14-FG urethral catheter can be inserted in the tract as a stent. Two days later, the urethral catheter is replaced by the Blom–Singer silicone voice prosthesis. This acts as a one-way valve directing the exhaled air to the oesophagus, when the tracheostoma is occluded with a finger, while preventing aspiration. The original Blom–Singer prosthesis is a hollow tube made of medical-grade silicone, 3 cm long with an outside diameter of 5.4 mm and is attached to thin flanges. The stomal end of the tube consists of a port, 3.5 mm × 7 mm, through which exhaled air enters the prosthesis on its way to the oesophagus.

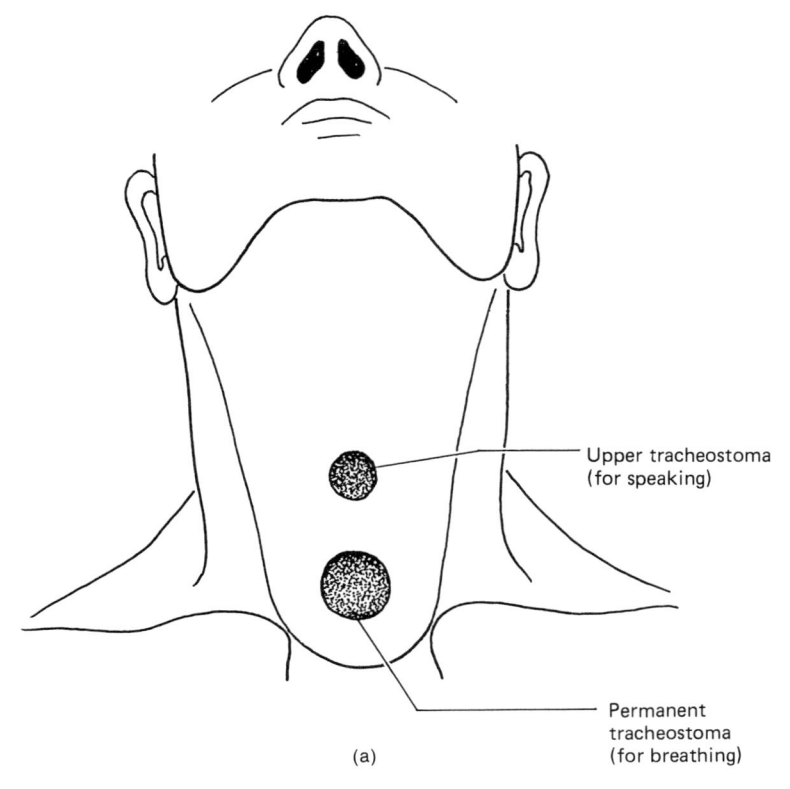

Figure 13.6 Asai's three-stage technique of creating a tracheopharyngeal shunt: (a) first stage — the upper tracheostoma is fashioned; (b) second stage — formation of pharyngostoma (i), shown in section (ii); (c) third stage — preparation of skin tube (i), skin tube sutured, ready to be buried (ii), median section to show connection of pharyngostoma and upper tracheostoma by means of skin tube (iii)

The oesophageal end of the tube has a single slit valve (duckbill) which opens by the exhaled pulmonary pressure, thus achieving speech. The valve closes when air flow stops on cessation of speech, and remains closed during swallowing. The Blom–Singer tracheo-oesophageal technique is simple, and easy to perform. The complications associated with this technique include closure of the fistula tract, tracheal mucositis, tracheostomal stenosis, aspiration of the prosthesis, oesophageal tear and aspiration from the oesophagus (Wetmore et al., 1981a, b). A second prosthesis was designed by Blom and Singer to solve the problem of increased resistance to air flow and inadvertent dislodgment of the prosthesis. This has a trap valve with a retention collar at the oesophageal wall. In 1982, Blom et al. described a tracheostoma valve which closed with the increased exhaled pressure during speaking and reopened when the patient stopped speaking (Blom et al., 1982). The prosthesis required the application of adhesives which gave way under the back pressure of speech, leading to air leakage. The most common problem was leakage of air from the valve housing due to an inadequate seal between the peristomal skin and the valve. The valve is less likely to maintain a seal when exposed to excessive heat or perspiration (Zanoff et al., 1990). Singer and Blom described the role of pharyngeal constrictor myotomy in (b)(i)

Pharyngostoma

Upper tracheostoma (for speaking)

Permanent tracheostoma (for breathing)

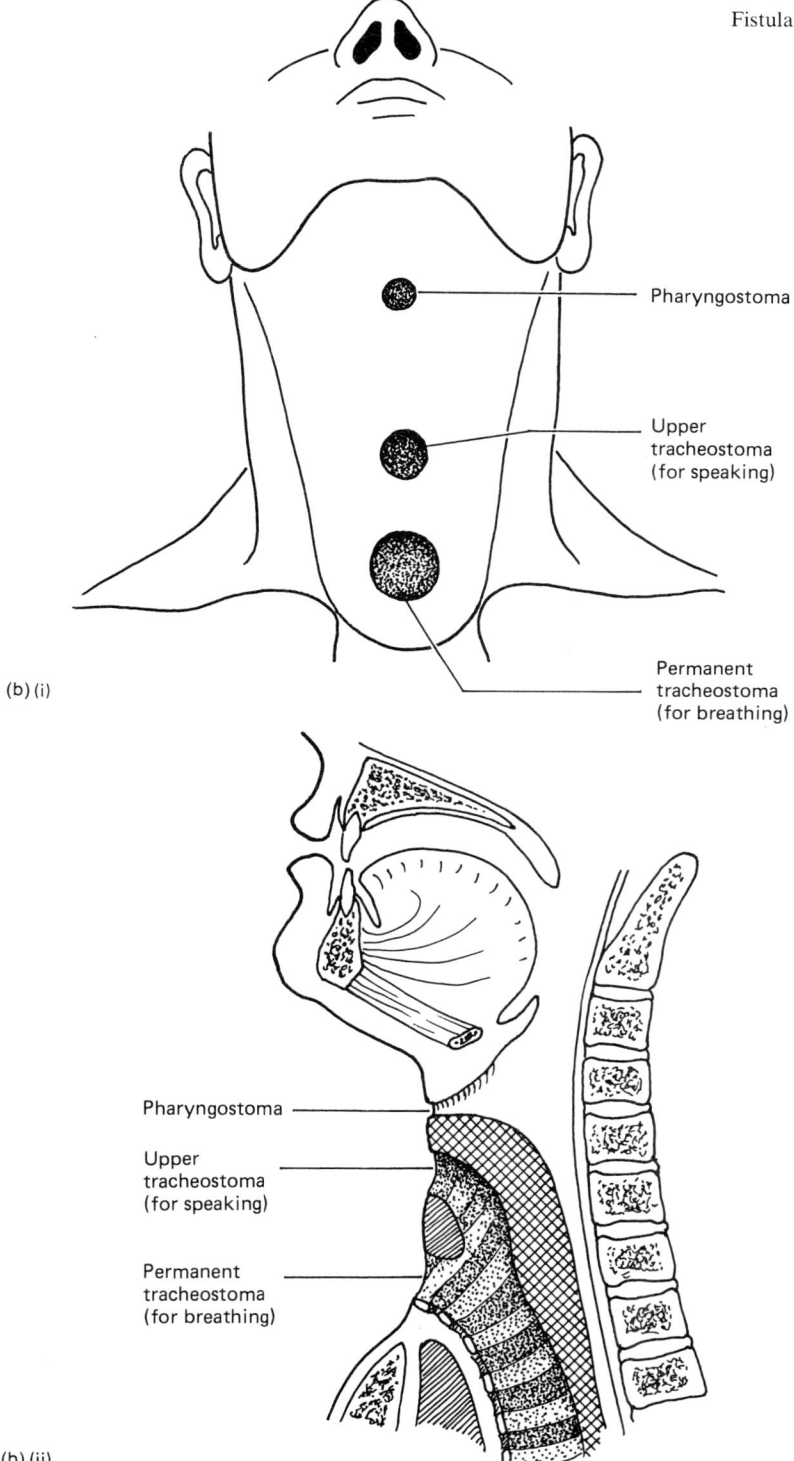

(b)(ii)

Pharyngostoma

Upper tracheostoma (for speaking)

Permanent tracheostoma (for breathing)

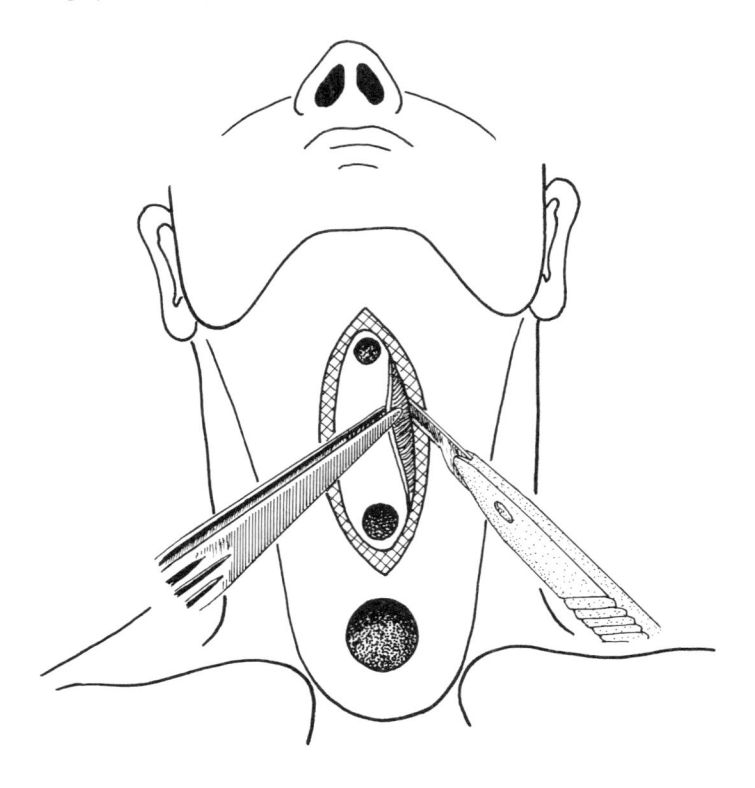

(c)(i)

cases in which the pharyngo-oesophageal spasm caused significant resistance in voice production. Recently Singh suggested that the pharyngeal constrictors should be left unsutured after total laryngectomy. In none of these cases did any mucocutaneous fistulae develop, and it is suggested that this technique avoids the need for a subsequent pharyngeal myotomy to facilitate fistula speech.

In 1981 Panje reported a tracheo-oesophageal fistula procedure for the insertion of a biflanged voice button (Panje, 1981). The tracheo-oesophageal fistula is stented by a 14-FG rubber catheter for approximately 7–14 days, when the catheter is removed and the voice button is inserted. Weinberg and Moon (1984) reported that the Panje voice button offers substantial opposition to air flow and is least efficient in relation to speech production.

In 1982 Nijdam et al. reported a silicone biflanged voice prosthesis which was inserted via the mouth and oesophagus with the help of a specially developed instrument (Nijdam et al., 1982). The thickness of the voice button is chosen according to the thickness of the tracheo-oesophageal wall. Recently deposits of *Candida albicans* on the oesophageal surface of the Groningen prosthesis were reported to cause leakage of the valve (Mahieu et al. 1989). A number of other prosthetic devices (Henley–Cohn, Traissac, E.S.K. Hermann, Staffieri, Blaise–Raphael, Algaba and Provox) have been developed for use after the creation of a tracheo-oesophageal fistula to produce fistula speech.

(c)(ii)

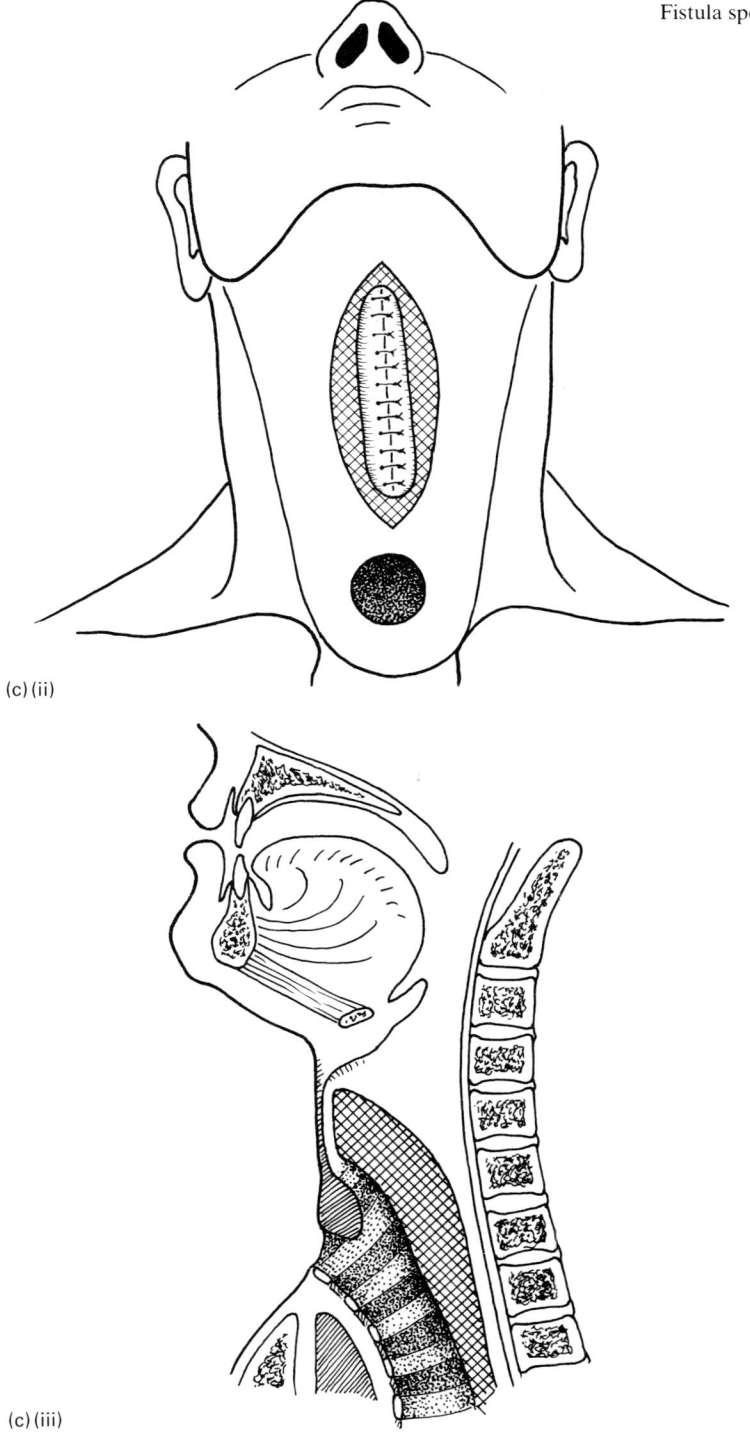

(c)(iii)

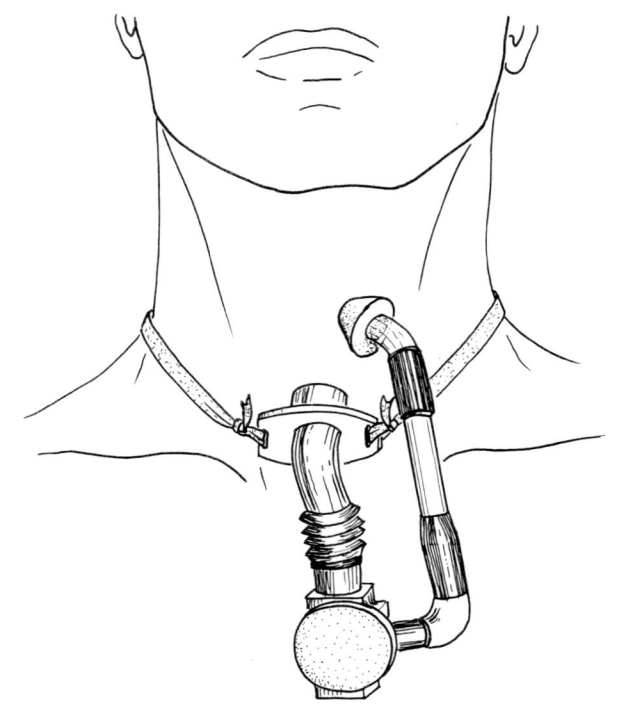

Figure 13.7 The VoiceBak prosthesis

Singh speech system

In an effort to avoid the problems encountered with various fistula techniques and voice prostheses, a simple surgical procedure was developed whereby a self-retaining fistula valve (Figure 13.11) is inserted. This has been designed to attain good, fluent and intelligible speech, without aspiration of saliva or food (Singh, 1988a, b). To eliminate manual occlusion of the stoma a recently designed Singh tracheostoma valve has been used with equally good results (Singh, 1985, 1987, 1988a, b, 1989, 1990).

The Singh fistula valve and dummy

Patients to be considered for the Singh fistula valve after secondary tracheo-oesophageal puncture are evaluated by both the otolaryngologist and the speech therapist. Special consideration is given to the patient's overall state of health, speech, manual dexterity to close the tracheostoma, stoma size, personal hygiene and the presence of any cardiovascular or pulmonary disorder. Taub's insufflation test is done to estimate the patient's response in terms of voice production and speech fluency.

Minimal instrumentation is needed for the secondary tracheo-oesophageal puncture technique. All the components are standard, readily available items: Vigon stomach tube (33 FG), Foley urinary catheter (18 FG) with a 30–45 ml balloon and a

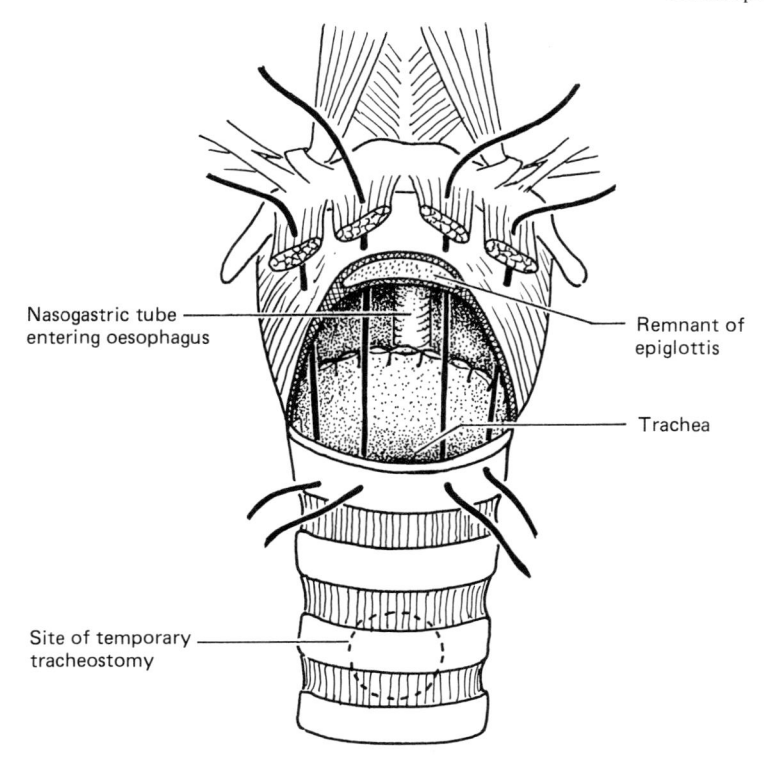

Figure 13.8 Tracheohyoidopexy technique of Arslan and Serafini

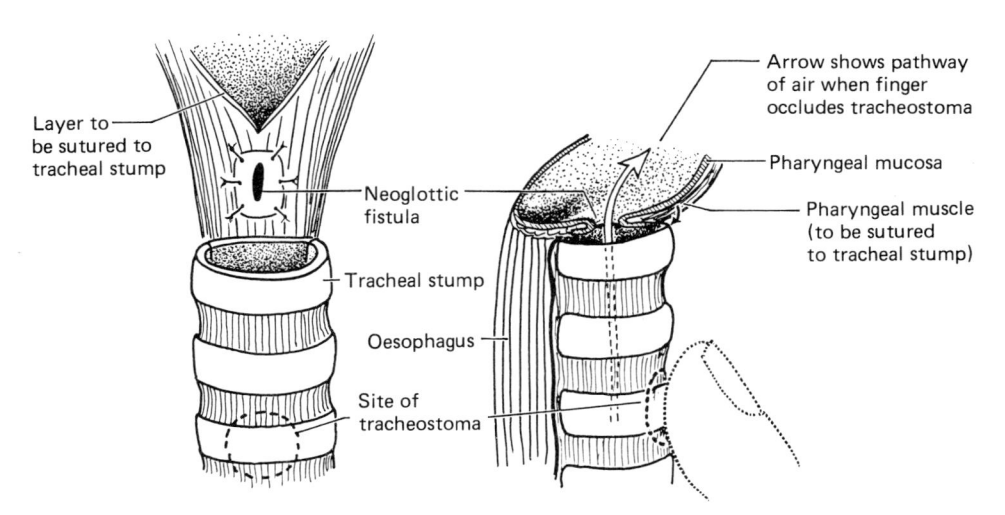

Figure 13.9 Construction of neoglottis by the technique of Staffieri and Serafini

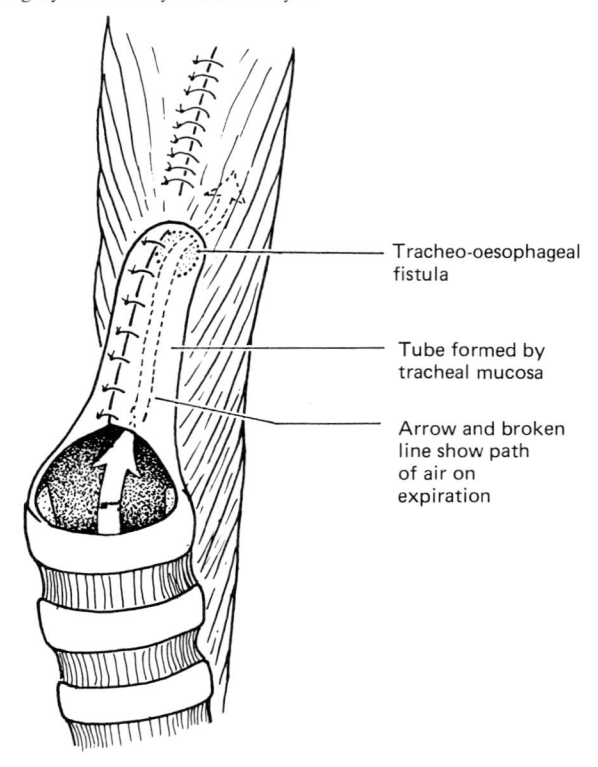

184   Functional Surgery of the Larynx and Pharynx

Figure 13.10   Amatsu's technique of one-stage laryngectomy with the creation of a tracheal tube shunt

30 cm³ syringe, curved haemostat, flexible nasopharyngolaryngoscope (optional) and a Singh fistula dummy.

Secondary tracheo-oesophageal puncture technique

The patient is anaesthetized and placed in a supine position on the operating table. Since the upper aerodigestive tract is surgically violated the patient is given a week's course of prophylactic antibiotics. Although the prophylactic use of antibiotics remains controversial, evidence supporting their efficacy in reducing the incidence of postoperative wound infection is compelling. A 33-FG Vigon stomach tube (outer diameter 11 mm) is selected. An additional hole of 15 mm × 15 mm is cut into the top of the tube 15 cm from the most proximal hole (fourth eyelet). The fourth eyelet is enlarged to 15 mm × 10 mm. An 18-FG Foley urinary catheter, marked 15 cm from the balloon, is lubricated and passed into the lumen of the Vigon stomach tube via the top hole and the balloon is brought level with the enlarged fourth eyelet of the stomach tube (Figure 13.12a). This tube, with the Foley catheter in its lumen, is passed through the mouth, keeping the top hole (which is aligned with the enlarged fourth eyelet housing the balloon) facing anteriorly (Figure 13.12b).

The progress of the stomach tube can be visualized down the pharynx by its bulge and the displacement of the anterior pharyngo-oesophageal wall forwards. When the bulge is seen at the level of the tracheostoma, 15–20 cm³ of air is injected into the

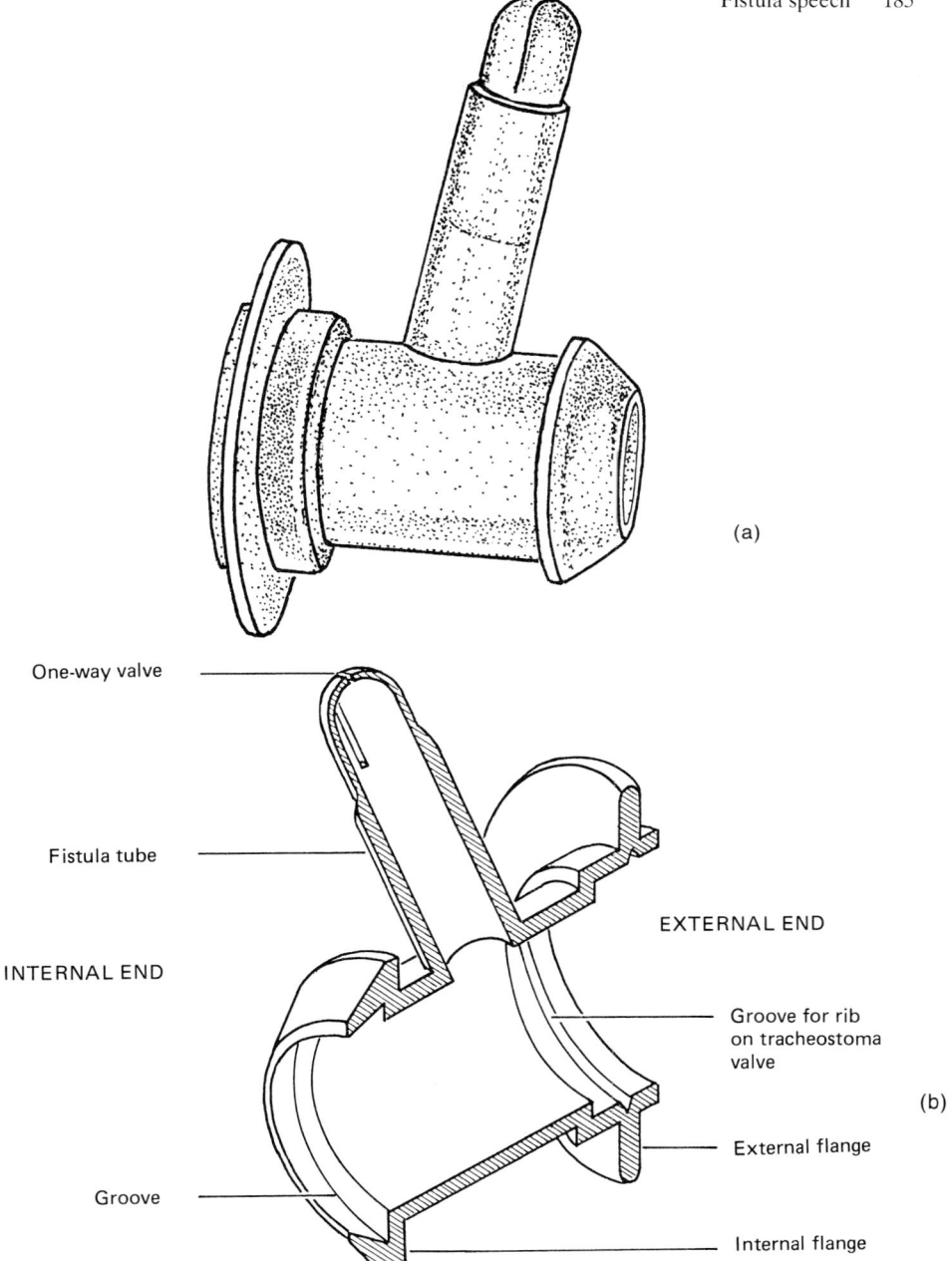

Figure 13.11 Singh fistula valve (a), also shown in section (b)

non-return valve of the catheter balloon. This injected air pushes the balloon through the enlarged fourth eyelet of the stomach tube, resulting in a bulge of the posterosuperior wall of the stoma forwards and downwards. A small, sharp horizontal incision of about 3–4 mm is made 5 mm from the mucocutaneous junction of the upper border of the tracheostoma, using the balloon bulge as a guide. The incision is stretched with a curved haemostat until the balloon is seen; care is taken not to puncture the balloon. The solid arm of the Singh fistula dummy (the size of button selected depends upon the size of the tracheostoma) is gently inserted in the newly fashioned tracheo-oesophageal fistula with the help of a curved haemostat. The fistula dummy (Figure 13.13a) is non-irritant, soft and compliant, and consists of radiopaque medical-grade silicone rubber containing flesh-toned pigment and barium sulphate salts.

The air is slowly withdrawn from the balloon and the arm of the fistula dummy is introduced further into the correct midline position in the oesophageal lumen. The Foley catheter is withdrawn as the dummy arm is inserted. The position of the dummy arm can be visualized through a flexible nasopharyngolaryngoscope passed via the stomach tube. Once the position of the dummy arm is satisfactory, the stomach tube is withdrawn and the outer flange of the fistula dummy may be sutured to the skin to avoid accidental dislodgement (Figure 13.13b). The patient is discharged home; after a week, the fistula dummy is removed (Figure 13.13c, d) and the one-way fistula valve is inserted (Figure 13.14). This procedure can be done in the outpatient department. Sometimes leakage of fluid around the dummy arm is noticed by the patient. In that situation the patient should be advised to take fluids along with solid foods for a couple of days. Usually the leakage stops by that time.

The simple procedure of secondary tracheo-oesophageal puncture described above may not be so easily accomplished in cases where the posterior tracheal wall and the anterior oesophageal wall were not tacked together at the time of previous surgery. In those cases the bevelled open end of the oesophagoscope or bronchoscope is inserted down the pharynx to stretch the common tracheo-oesophageal wall at the level of the tracheostoma for secondary puncture. To facilitate tracheo-oesophageal puncture the posterior wall of the trachea and the anterior wall of the oesophagus should be tacked together (using 3/0 chromic catgut) if the party wall gets separated during total laryngectomy or pharyngolaryngectomy. This is also done where pharyngeal reconstruction is achieved by myocutaneous flaps, free skin flaps or a free jejunal flap. The author's practice is to close the mucosal edges of the pharynx and bury them by means of interrupted submucosal stitches of 3/0 chromic catgut, or close the pharyngeal defect by Auto Suture clamp. The Auto Suture clamp has been found to be safe, quick and easy to use in pharyngeal mucosal closure after total laryngectomy (Singh, 1989). In order to avoid future myotomy the constrictor muscles are left unsutured.

Primary tracheo-oesophageal fistula procedure

Secondary tracheo-oesophageal puncture procedure has become well established since it was first described by Singer and Blom (1980). Later they found that if this technique was applied at the time of the original operation for removal of cancer it gave better results in speech production (Hamaker et al., 1985). The primary tracheo-oesophageal fistula procedure has recently been introduced in the author's practice, and the initial success rates seem encouraging.

After the total laryngectomy or pharyngolaryngectomy with reconstruction of the

Fistula speech 187

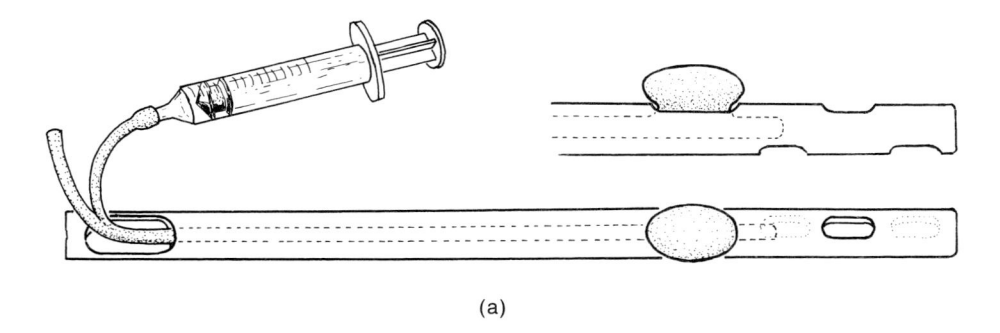

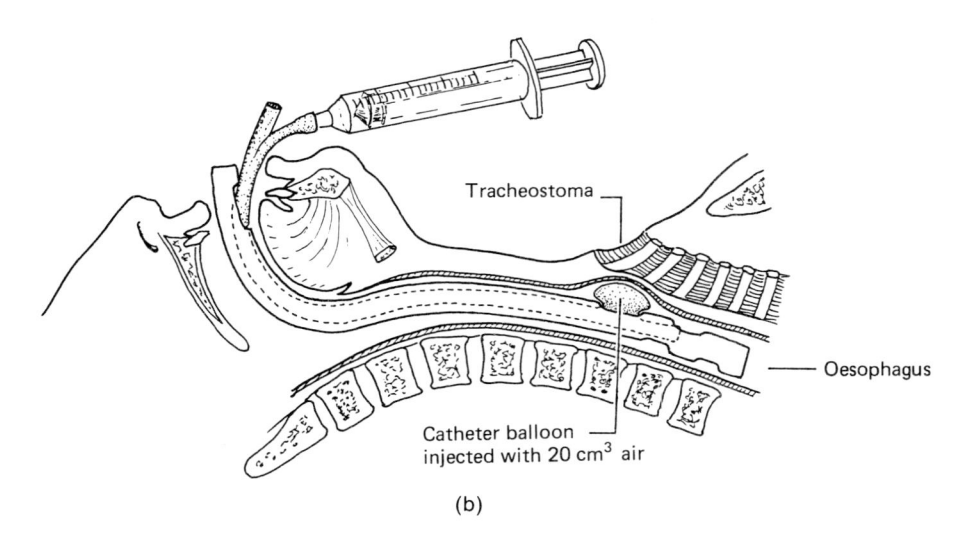

(a)

(b)

Figure 13.12 Vigon stomach tube (a) showing additional top hole and housing a Foley urinary catheter, with the balloon bulging through the enlarged fourth eyelet; (b) patient with the Vigon stomach tube lying in the lumen of the oesophagus, the distended balloon of the Foley catheter pushing the tracheo-oesophageal wall forwards (site of puncture)

Labels in (b): Tracheostoma; Oesophagus; Catheter balloon injected with 20 cm^3 air

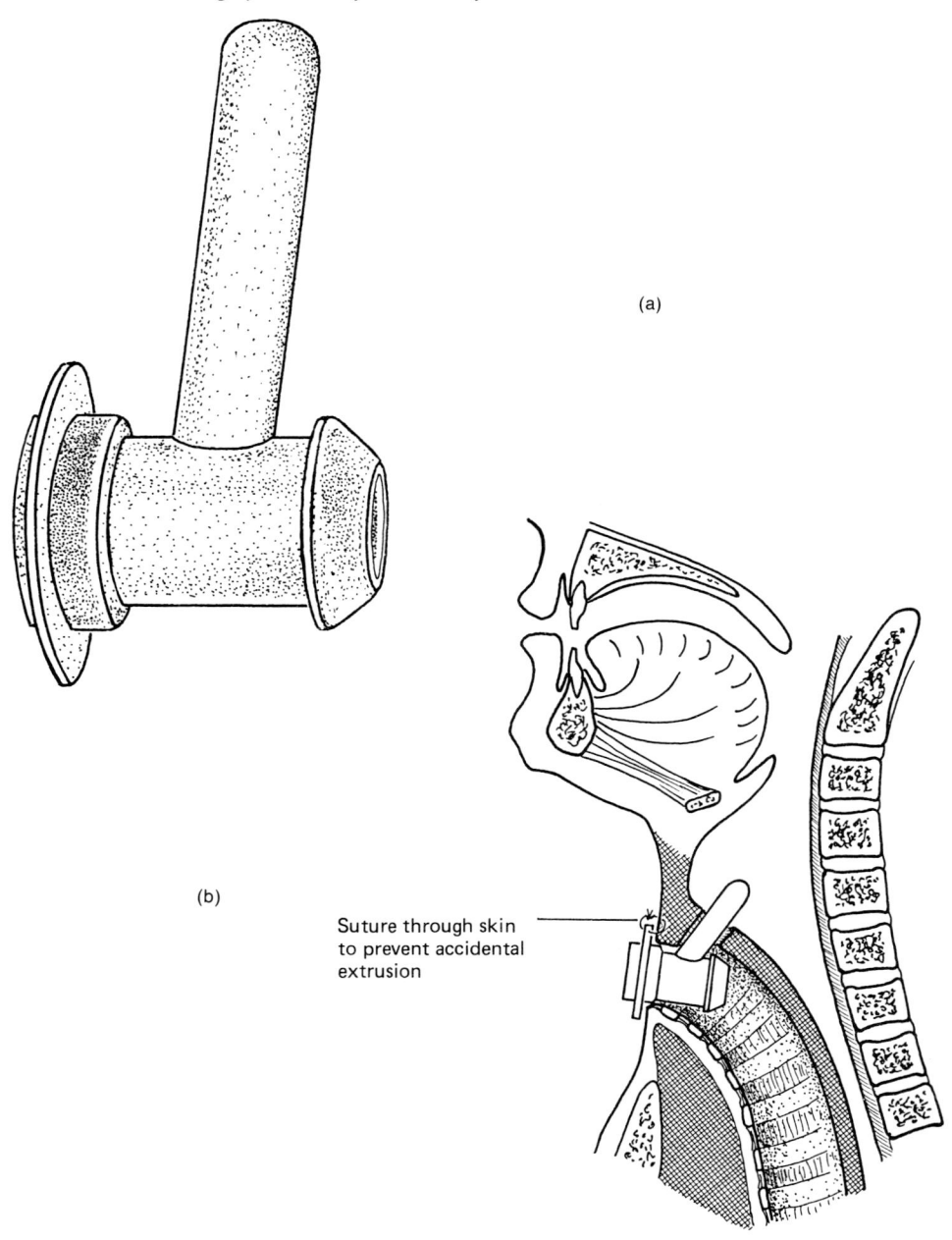

Figure 13.13 Singh fistula dummy (a); (b) fistula dummy in situ; (c,d) removal of fistula dummy by grasping the lower edge of the rim and pulling upwards (the same technique is used for removing the Singh fistula valve)

Fistula speech   189

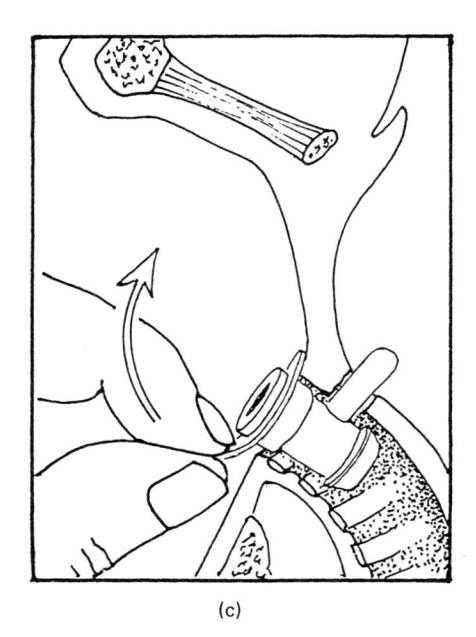

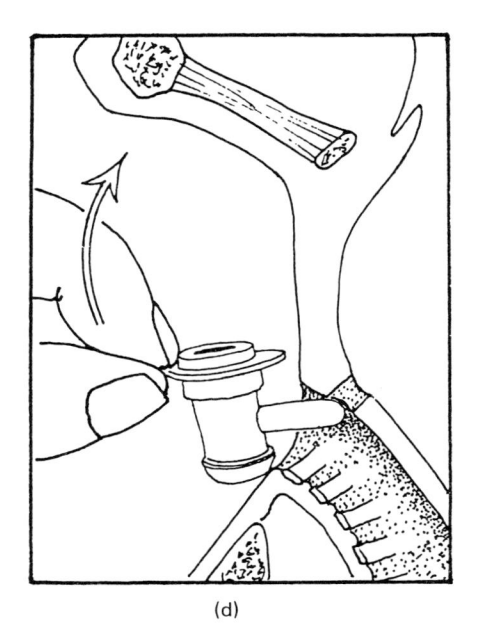

(c)

(d)

pharynx by myocutaneous flap or a free jejunal flap, the party wall between the trachea and oesophagus is approximated by 3/0 chromic catgut sutures. The tracheostoma is fashioned in the lower skin flap, by excising a circular piece of skin. With the index finger of the left hand inside the exposed oesophagus from above, the party wall is pushed forward so as to make a bulge to be seen through the stoma. With the knife (Bard–Parker blade 15), a horizontal 3–4 mm sharp incision is made in the posterior wall of the trachea 5 mm below the superior mucocutaneous junction, until the gloved left index finger is just visible. The incision is stretched with a curved haemostat. A large catheter (18-FG nasogastric tube) is inserted through the newly created fistula. The upper end is brought out of the nose and sutured (or taped); the lower end is sutured or taped to the skin lateral to the stoma. The nasogastric tube (size 16) is inserted into the stomach and the outer nasal end is taped beside the nose to avoid inadvertent removal by the patient. More recently we insert one large catheter (18 FG nasogastric tube) through the newly created fistula into the stomach and use it both for stenting and for feeding. The mucosa and submucosa are approximated in two layers with inverting 3/0 chromic catgut sutures. The pharyngeal constrictor muscles are left unsutured. The nasogastric tube is removed after 2 weeks and the patient is started on oral feeds. The tracheostomy tube is removed and replaced by the Singh fistula valve which acts as a miniature tracheostomy tube and also valves the tracheo-oesophageal fistula for phonation.

The primary tracheo-oesophageal fistule is becoming more popular universally. It is simple, because of improved surgical exposure; it adds little to the operating time, and the patient can start speaking quickly and return to work; it avoids long hours of speech therapy sessions; and it eliminates the need for a second operation to perform the tracheo-oesophageal puncture. The author has not observed any specific complication after this procedure. Both Maniglia et al. (1989) and Wenig et al. (1989) reported that the complication rate was higher after primary tracheo-oesophageal puncture compared with the secondary tracheo-oesophageal puncture.

The Singh fistula valve

Commonly used fistula voice prostheses have a number of disadvantages. The Blom–Singer voice button demands the use of adhesives for fixation, in a wet field around the stoma; there is also the possibility of accidental dislodgment. The Panje voice button suffers from very high opening pressure and difficulty in speech initiation. The Singh fistula valve (Figures 13.11, 13.14) is designed to overcome these problems.

The button part of the fistula valve is constructed of medical-grade silicone rubber; it is attached to a hollow tube 2.5–3.5 cm long, the tip of which enters the oesophageal lumen and has a single slit valve. This acts as a one-way valved fistula tube; it is made of a medically approved grade of silicone rubber containing a white pigment and barium salts. The size of the tracheostoma button depends upon the size of the tracheostoma. One week after the secondary tracheo-oesophageal fistula is created, the Singh fistula dummy is removed and the fistula valve is fitted. Because the fistula is created by stretching rather than cutting the tissues, it is very tight. Whenever patients want to remove and clean the fistula valve, they are advised to insert the fistula dummy, otherwise the fistula may close. Patients are given detailed instructions regarding the insertion of the fistula valve. The fistula valve should be cleaned regularly by the patient. Fluent, intelligible speech is produced when the patient occludes the stoma. So far, 80–90% success has been achieved in voice

Fistula speech 191

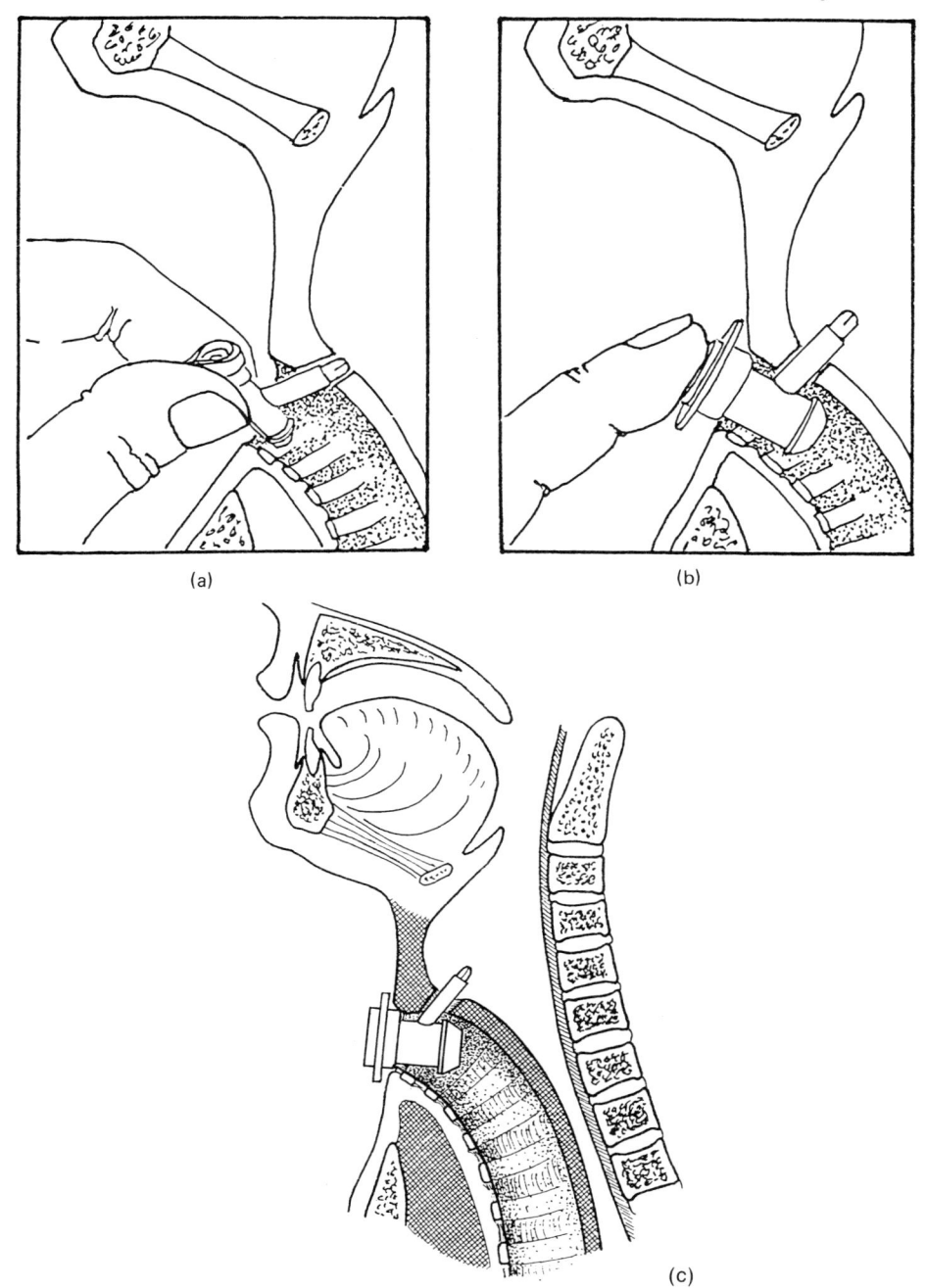

Figure 13.14 Insertion of Singh fistula valve: (a) folded valve partially inserted; (b) fistula valve pushed completely home with finger; (c) valve in position. The same technique is used to insert the dummy

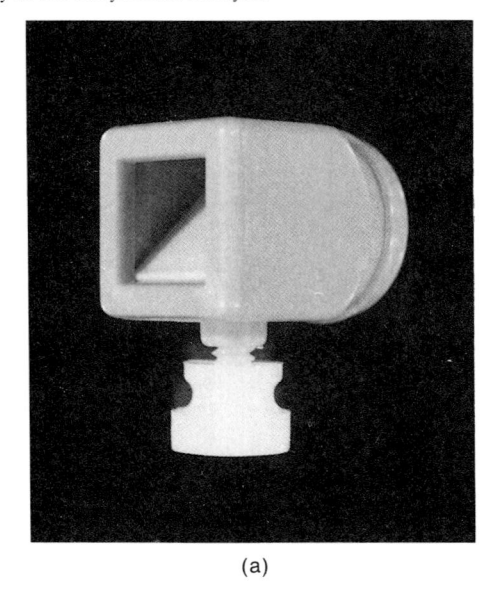

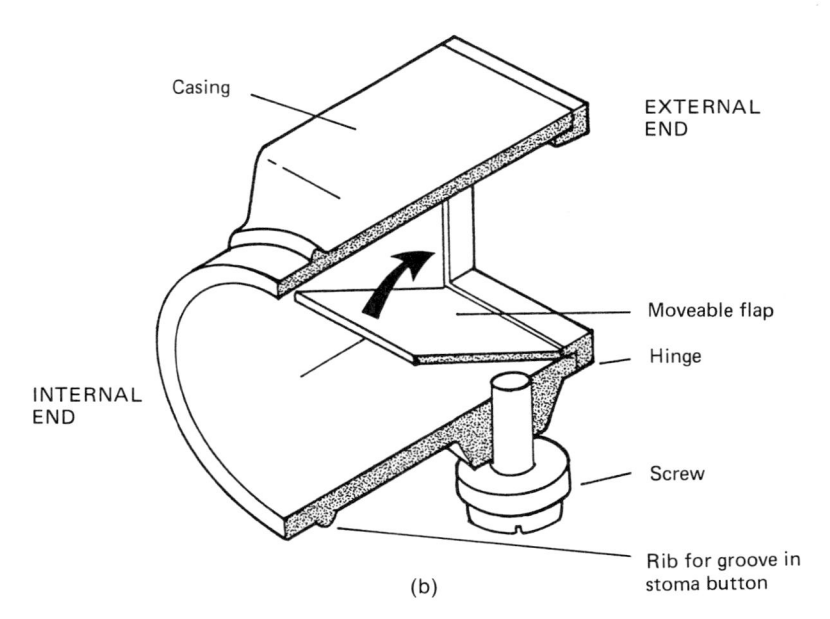

192 Functional Surgery of the Larynx and Pharynx

(a)

Casing
EXTERNAL END
Moveable flap
Hinge
INTERNAL END
Screw
Rib for groove in stoma button
(b)

Figure 13.15 The Singh tracheostoma valve (a); (b) longitudinal section; (c) fitting the tracheostoma valve — the inset shows how the ridge on the tracheostoma valve engages in the groove on the fistula valve; (d) adjusting the tracheostoma valve — the inset shows how the screw adjusts the angle of the flap; (e) removing the tracheostoma valve

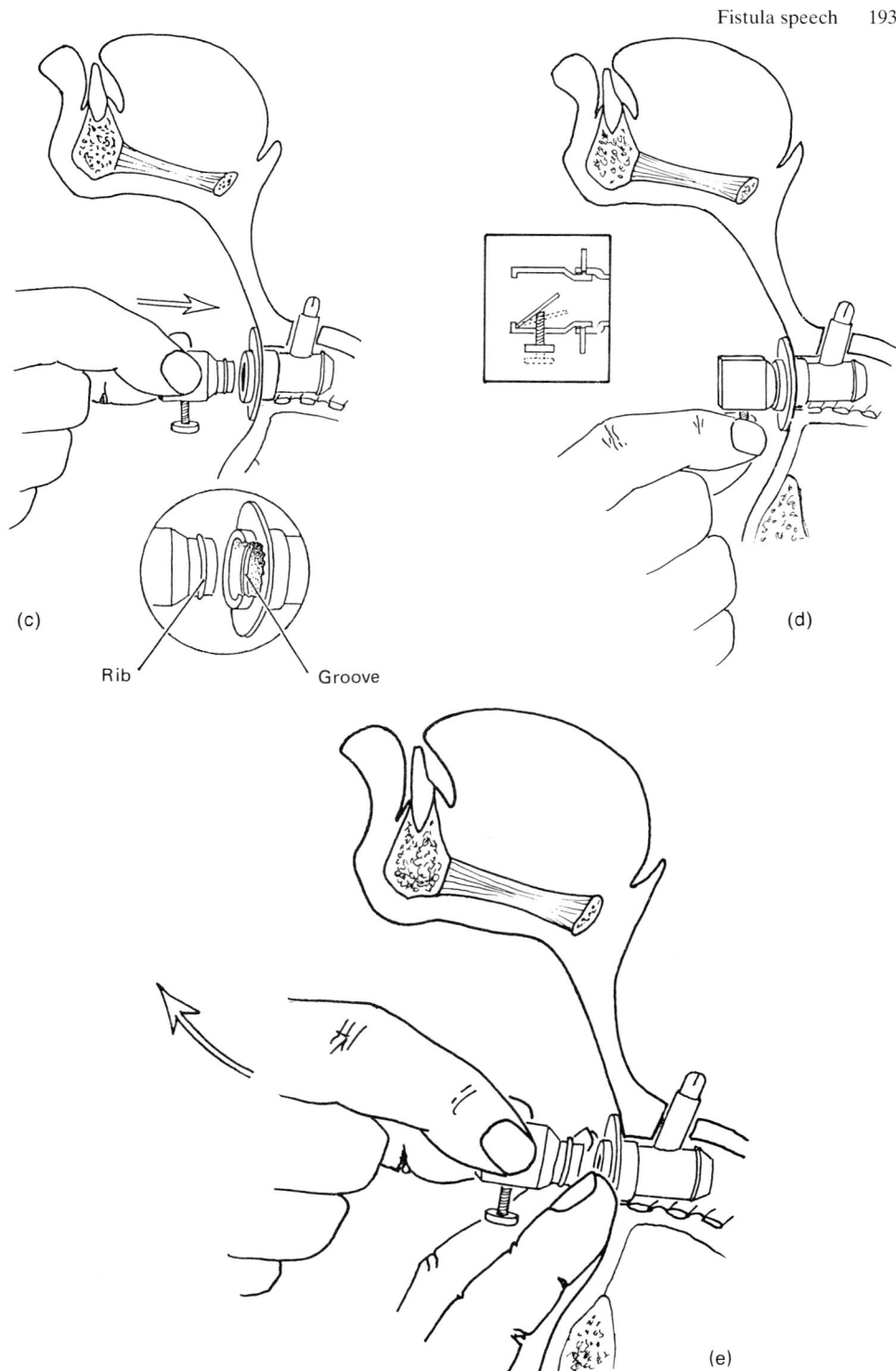

Fistula speech 193

(c)

Rib   Groove

(d)

(e)

production after secondary fistulization and fitting of the Singh fistula valve. However, the number of cases is small and demands a wider assessment in the future.

The Singh tracheostoma valve

In the newer surgical procedures for fistula speech, manual occlusion of the tracheostoma is necessary for the production of speech. This can be embarrassing, as it draws attention to the patient's stoma. The presence of the tracheostoma is considered generally by many people as the stigma of laryngeal cancer. Patients are hesitant to talk with finger occlusion as it tends to produce social embarrassment.

A questionnaire was sent to all patients with fistula speech asking them to record, each day for 2 weeks, the reason for every occasion on which they have not used a finger to occlude the stoma for speech. The hesitancy percentage for finger occlusion was as high as 85%. Furthermore, finger occlusion was regarded as unhygienic and at times inconvenient. Conversation was inhibited if the hands were dirty or if both hands were occupied in activities such as driving, dancing, sport or eating. Various devices to replace finger occlusion have been tried in the last 10–15 years, but none has proved entirely satisfactory. The VoiceBak prosthesis (see Figure 13.7) was expensive, mechanically complex, bulky and difficult to maintain. The tracheostoma valve developed by Blom et al. required the application of adhesives, in a potentially wet field around the stoma; furthermore, this gave way under back pressure of speech, leading to air leakage. All these disadvantages have been rectified in the Singh plastic tracheostoma valve (Figure 13.15).

The Singh tracheostoma valve has a rib on its inner end to fit the corresponding groove in the stoma button or fistula valve. The flap (0.35 mm thick) hinges on the front of its floor, and rests on a screw to allow adjustments of the open position. Clockwise rotation of the screw raises the flap and increases the sensitivity of the valve; anticlockwise rotation of the screw lowers the flap and decreases the sensitivity of the valve. The sensitivity of the valve depends upon the position of the flap. Depending on the respiratory needs the patient can adjust the position of the flap by turning the screw.

The *Singh tracheostoma button* (Figure 13.16) can be of various sizes (12, 14, 16, 18, 20). Its inner end has a grooved flange which maintains the button in position. Its external end has a wide flange to prevent it from accidentally slipping into the trachea during insertion, and a corresponding groove on its inner surface to 'snap-fit' with the rib on the tracheostoma valve. The tracheostoma valve fits snugly into the stoma button and the whole system is airtight.

Depending upon the size of the patient's tracheostoma a suitable stoma button is selected, and inserted with the wide outer flange resting against the skin of the neck. The patient inserts the tracheostoma valve into the stoma button, so that the rib on the tracheostoma valve snaps into the groove on the stoma button. The position of the flap is then adjusted by rotating the screw until the flap remains open during quiet breathing and routine physical activity (Figure 13.17). When the patient speaks, the slightly increased pressure of exhaled air closes the tracheostoma valve (Figure 13.18) and diverts the air through the fistula for speech. It automatically reopens when the patient stops speaking. During coughing and strenuous physical exertion the tracheostoma valve can be removed temporarily leaving the stoma button/fistula valve in situ.

The tracheostoma valve has been used by 12 patients over a period of 7 years. All the patients found the valve easy to use, and experienced no discomfort. All of them were able to insert the valve in a few seconds, and all except one could speak immediately without any prior training. One patient needed some training in relaxation and confidence in manoeuvring the screw, clockwise or anticlockwise, depending on the needs of respiration and speech. The tracheostoma valve was worn continuously by all the patients for the whole day, on average 10–12 hours. None of them experienced any air leakage or extrusion of the tracheostoma valve. During sleep the tracheostoma valve was removed and the tracheostoma button/fistula valve retained in situ.

Vocal efficiency was assessed using the following parameters: intelligibility (%), the ratio of phonation time to total time (%), maximum phonation time, relative intensity, fundamental frequency range and distribution, voice quality, pressure studies and psychological status. Most of these quantifications and qualifications were done in the well-equipped, fully computerized voice research laboratory at St John's Hospital. The intelligibility was obtained by asking the speaker to read a standard text passage into a tape recorder. The recording was then transcribed by both trained listeners and untrained listeners. The rate of speech was calculated from the phonation time to the total time taken to read the passage. A measure of voice intensity with a sound level meter is essential when quantifying the vocal performance of the patients. Tracheal pressure is recorded matching that intensity. The results of the vocal efficiency measurements are encouraging. The quality of speech with finger occlusion and with the tracheostoma valve is the same, although the patients report that their speech seems clearer and more natural than when using finger occlusion. As the patients realized that they could use both their hands while speaking, so they regained their self-confidence and felt more acceptable socially. This was a great help to them psychologically and helped to raise their morale. The initially encouraging results demand a wider assessment in the future.

Future developments

The stigma of a permanent tracheostoma, as an indicator of cancer of the larynx, has not so far been eliminated. Previous attempts to decannulate laryngectomy patients have been unsuccessful (Arslan and Serafini, 1972). Recently Laccourreye et al. (1990) described a partial laryngeal procedure without the need for a tracheostoma. It is too early to comment on this procedure, as studies are at present under way to assess the efficacy of this technique.

An attempt by Kluyskens and Ringoir (1970) to transplant a cadeveric larynx failed, and the cancer recurred promptly at the stoma with generalized metastasis leading rapidly to the death of the patient. It is probably not rational to undertake further experimentation with laryngeal transplantation in humans. Until the problem of immunosuppression is solved we will have to find alternative ways to solve this problem of eliminating the stigma of the tracheostoma.

Although a solution does not seem near, it is hoped that our joint interest and efforts will eventually lead us to our goal. To avoid the social embarrassment of manual occlusion of the stoma, the tracheostoma valve has been useful in speech rehabilitation of patients using fistula speech as their mode of communication. The Singh tracheostoma valve has been used successfully by some of our patients since 1984, to achieve 'hands free' speech (Figure 13.19).

(a)

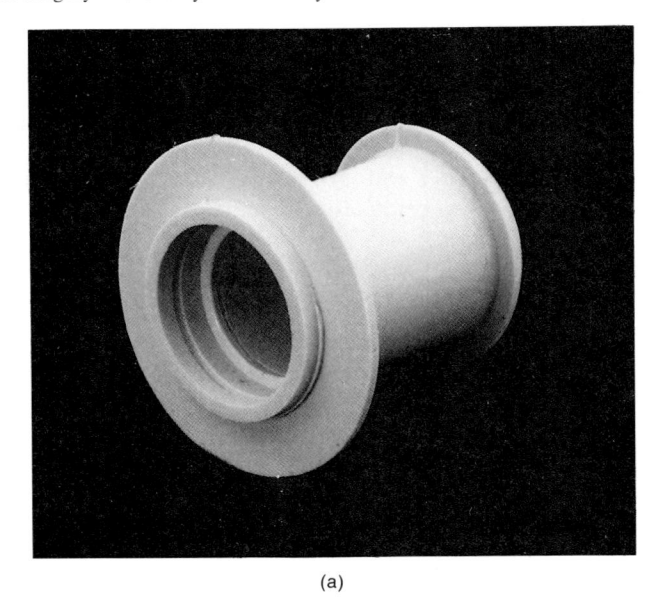

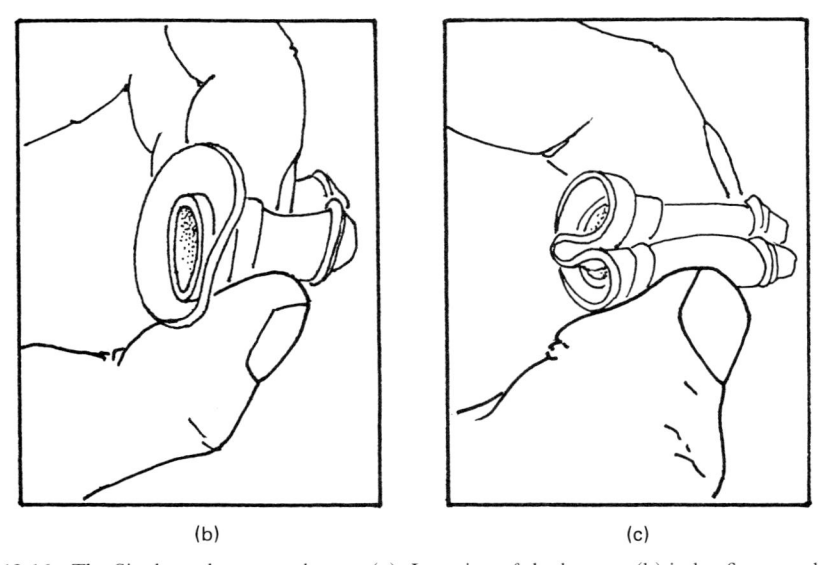

(b)　　　　　　　　　　　　　　(c)

Figure 13.16 The Singh tracheostoma button (a). Insertion of the button: (b) index finger makes a groove in the button; (c) the button folded between finger and thumb; (d) folded button inserted in tracheostoma; (e) released button pushed fully home with finger. Removal of button: (f) lower margin of button grasped and tilted upwards; (g) button almost completely removed. Cleaning the button (h)

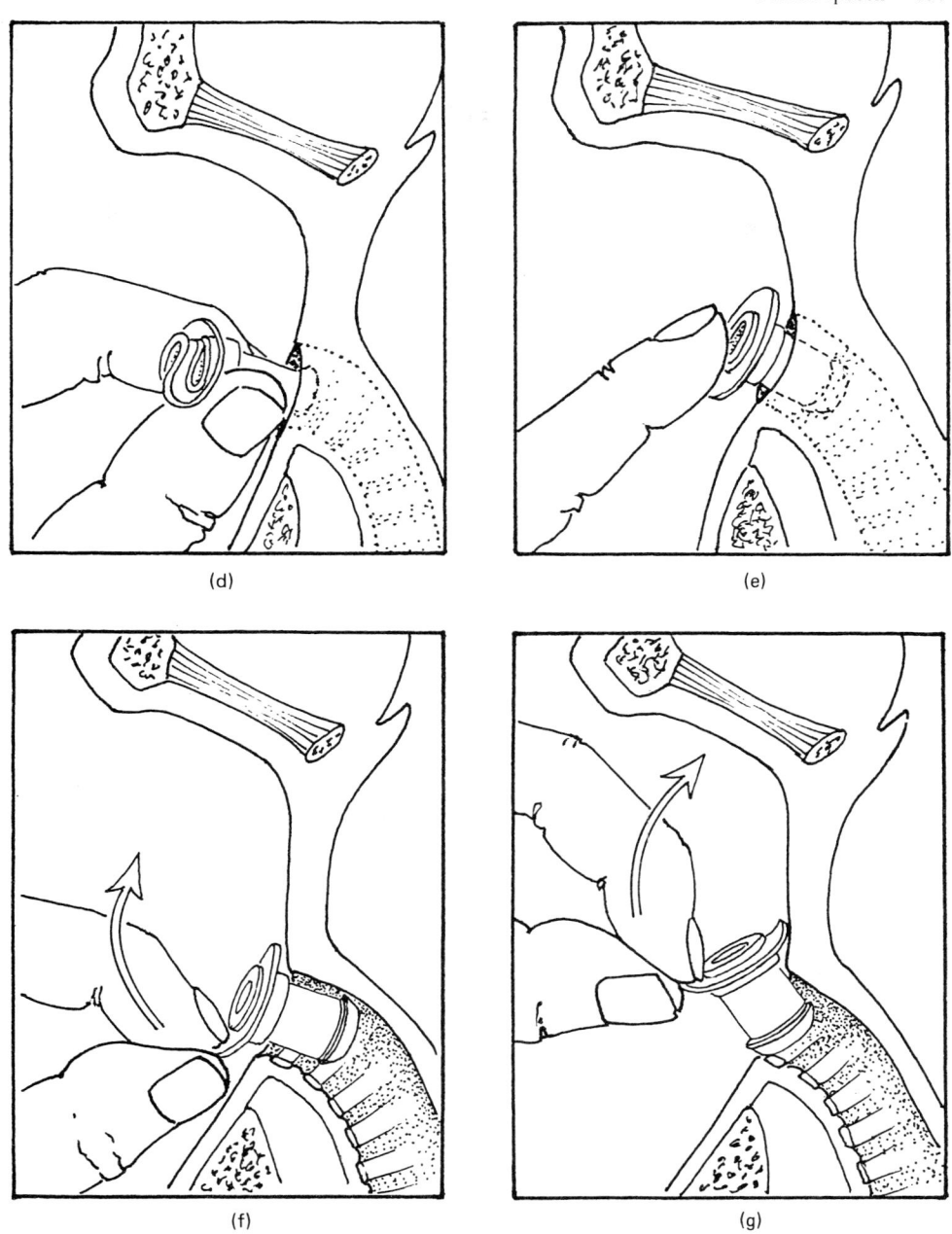

Fistula speech 197

(d)

(e)

(f)

(g)

(h)

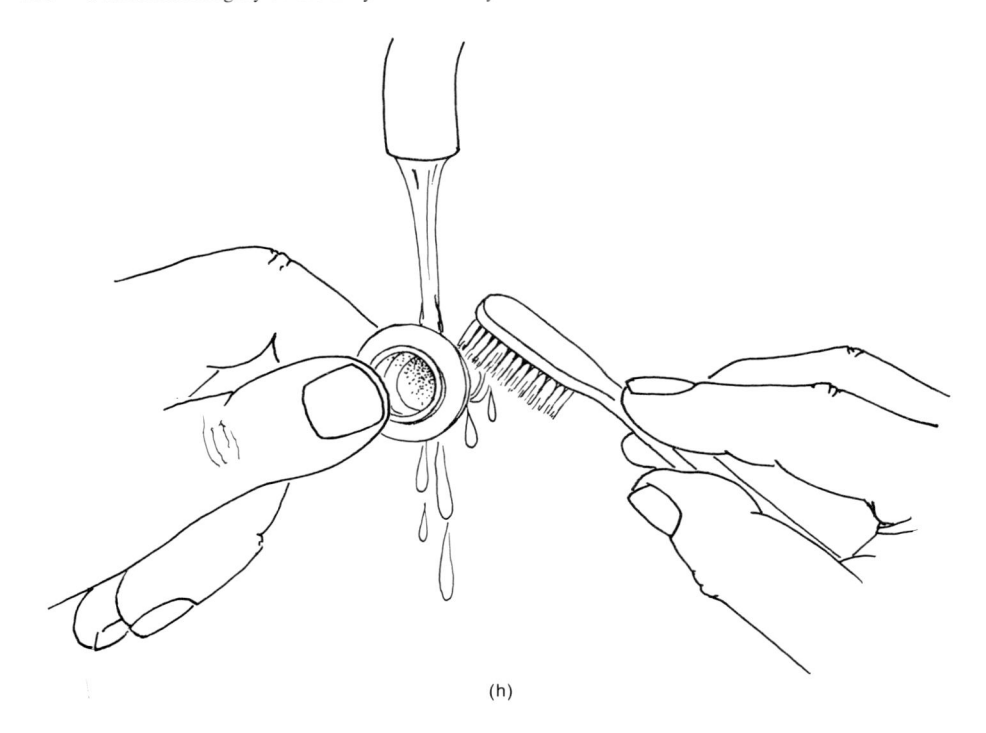

Fistula speech 199

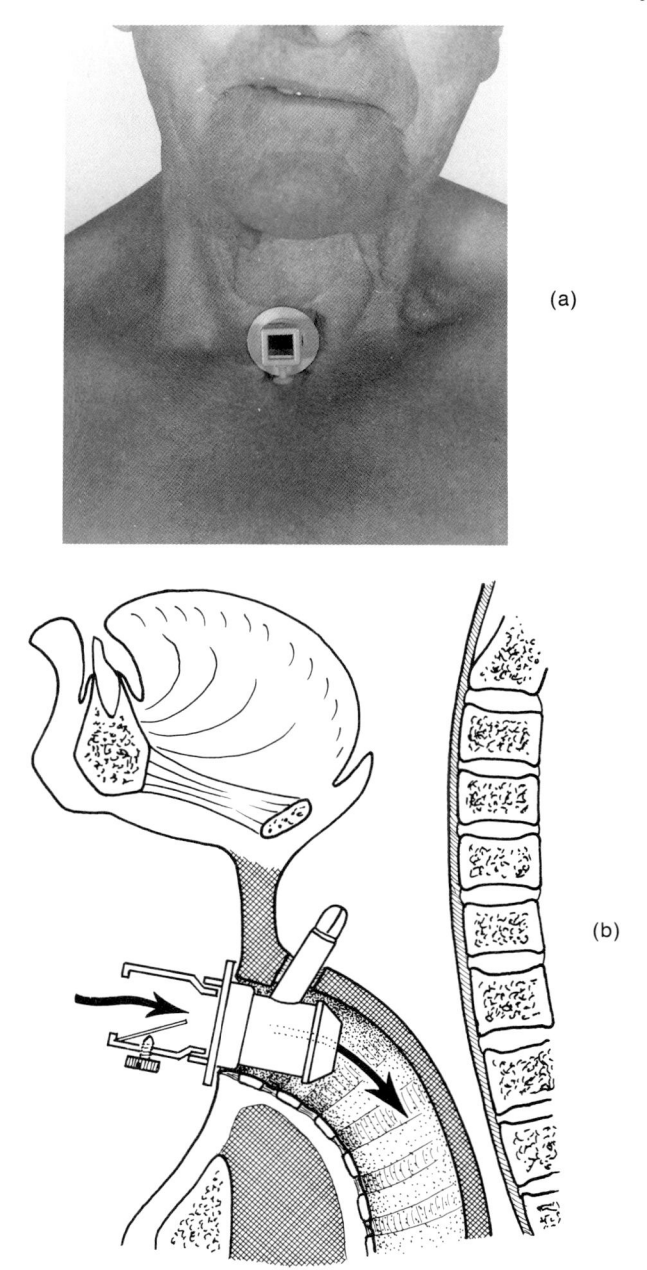

Figure 13.17 The tracheostoma valve during normal respiration (a); (b) section of the valve. During inspiration, the flap valve opens allowing air to pass into the trachea

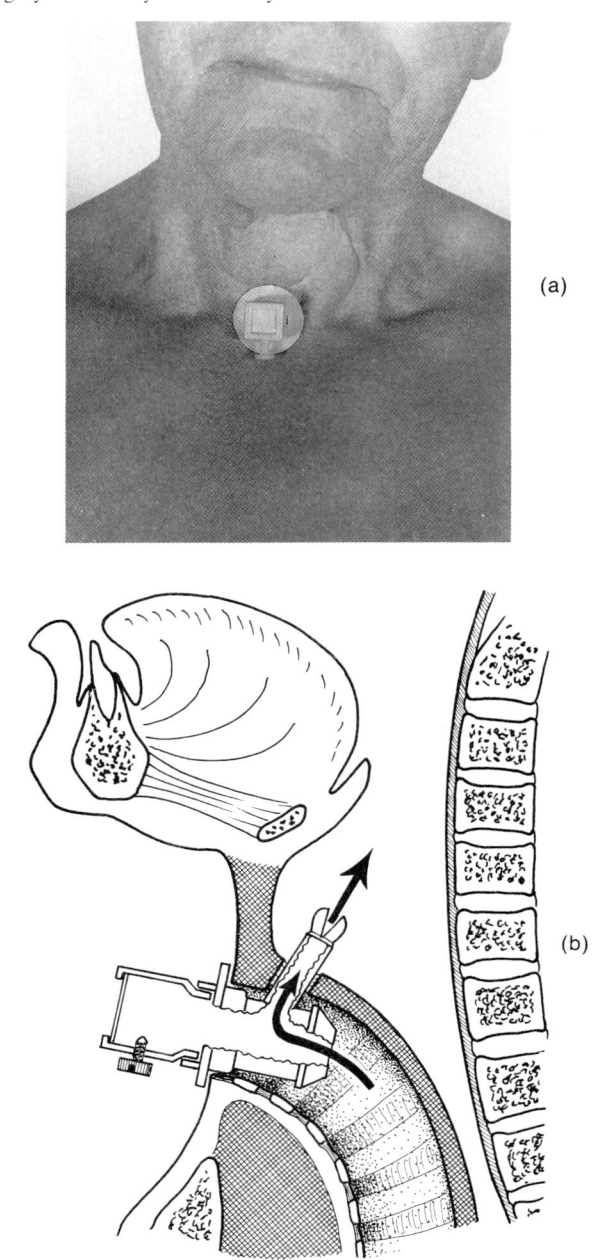

(a)

(b)

Figure 13.18 The tracheostoma valve during speech (a); (b) section of the valve. During speech, the flap valve closes causing air to flow through the fistula valve into the pharyngo-oesophagus

Fistula speech 201

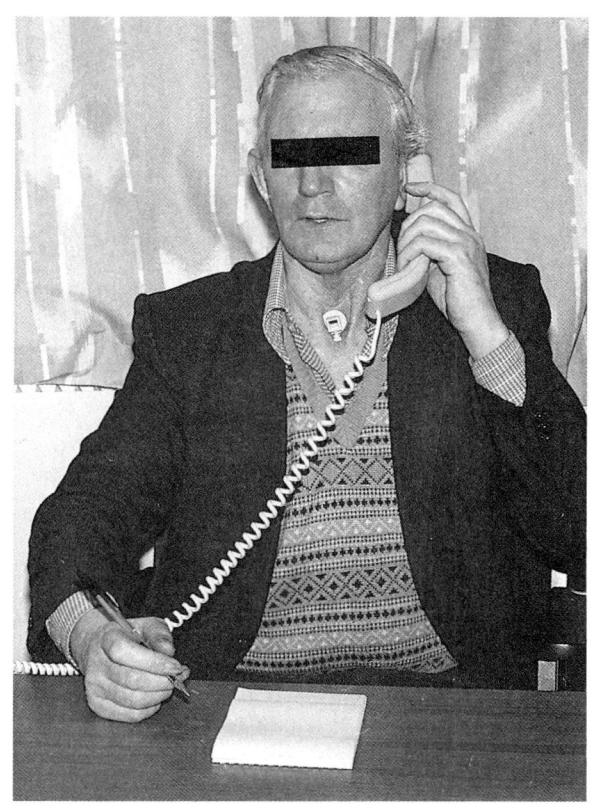

Figure 13.19 Neoglottal speaker during 'hands free' speech

References

Ainsworth W., Singh W. (1990). Analysis of fundamental frequency and temporal characteristics of neoglottal, oesophageal and normal speech. In *Proceedings of the Institute of Acoustics*, **12**, 12–32.
Amatsu M. (1980). A one stage surgical technique for post-laryngectomy voice rehabilitation. *Laryngoscope*, **90**, 1378–86.
Arslan M., Serafini I. (1972). Restoration of laryngeal function after total laryngectomy. *Laryngoscope*, **82**, 1349–60.
Asai R. (1960). Laryngoplasty. *J. Japan Bronchoesophagol. Soc.*, **12**, 1–3.
Asai R. (1972). Laryngoplasty after total laryngectomy. *Arch. Otolaryngol.*, **95**, 114–19.
Barria R.R. (1985). Oesophageal speech. In *New Dimensions in Otolaryngology — Head and Neck Surgery* (Myers E. ed.) Amsterdam: Elsevier, pp. 405–10.
Blom E.D., Singer M.I., Hamaker R.C. (1982). Tracheostoma valve for post laryngectomy voice rehabilitation. *Ann. Otol. Rhinol. Laryngol.*, **91**, 576–8.
Briani A.A. (1952). Riabilitazione fonetica di larigectomizzati a mezzo della corrente aerea espiratoria polmonare. *Arch. Ital. Otol.*, **63**, 469.
Calcaterra T.C., Jafek B.W. (1971). Tracheo-oesophageal shunt for speech rehabilitation after total laryngectomy. *Arch. Otolaryngol.*, **94**, 124–8.
Conley J.J. (1959). Vocal rehabilitation by autogenous vein graft. *Ann. Otol. Rhinol. Laryngol.*, **68**, 990–5.
Conley J.J., De Amesti F., Pierce M.K. (1958). A new surgical technique for the vocal rehabilitation of the laryngectomized patient. *Ann. Otol. Rhinol. Laryngol.*, **67**, 655–64.
Dworkin P.J., Sparker A. (1980). Surgical vocal rehabilitation following total laryngectomy. *Clin. Otolaryngol.*, **5**, 339–50.
Gatti W.M., Lucchinetti M., Thinaklal R. (1981). Creation of the phonatory neoglottis. *Acta Otolaryngol.*, **91**, 305–12.
Gluckman J.L., Donegan J.O., Singh J. (1981). Limitations of the Blom–Singer technique for voice restoration. *Ann. Otol. Rhinol. Laryngol.*, **90**, 495–7.
Gussenbauer C. (1874). Uber die erste durch Th. Billroth an Menchen ausgefuhrte Kehlkopf-Exstirpation und die Anwendung eines Künstlichen Kehkopfes. *Verh. Deutsch Ges. Chir.*, **17**, 343–56.
Guttman M.R. (1935). Tracheo-hypopharyngeal fistulization. A new procedure for speech reproduction in the laryngectomized patients. *Trans. Am. Laryngol. Rhinol. Otol. Soc.*, **41**, 219–26.
Hamaker R.C., Singer M.I., Blom E.D. (1985). Primary voice restoration at laryngectomy. *Arch. Otolaryngol.*, **111**, 182.
Kluyskens P., Ringoir S. (1970). Follow up of a human transplantation. *Laryngoscope*, **80**, 1244–50.
Komorn R.M. (1974). Vocal rehabilitation in the laryngectomized patient with a tracheo-oesophageal shunt. *Ann. Otol. Rhinol. Laryngol.*, **83**, 445–51.
Laccourreye H., Laccourreye O., Weinstein G., et al. (1990). Supracricoid laryngectomy with cricohyoidopexy: a partial laryngeal procedure for selected supraglottic and transglottic carcinomas. *Laryngoscope*, **100**, 735–41.
Leipzig B. (1980). Neoglottic reconstruction following total laryngectomy. *Ann. Otol. Rhinol. Laryngol.*, **89**, 534–7.
Li S.L. (1985). Functional tracheo-oesophageal shunt for vocal rehabilitation after laryngectomy. *Laryngoscope*, **95**, 1267–71.
Mahieu H.F., Schutte H.K., Annyas A.A. (1989). Rehabilitation of the laryngectomee. In *Proceedings of the International Voice Symposium*, Edinburgh (Singh W., ed.) pp. 102–4.
Maniglia A.J., Lundy D.A., Casiano R.C., Swim S.C. (1989). Speech restoration and complications of primary versus secondary tracheo-oesophageal puncture following total laryngectomy. *Laryngoscope*, **99**, 489–91.
McGrail J.S., Oldfield D.L. (1971). One-stage operation for vocal rehabilitation at laryngectomy. *Trans. Am. Acad. Ophthalmol. Otolaryngol.*, **75**, 510.
Miller A.H. (1967). First experiences with the Asai technique for vocal rehabilitation after total laryngectomy. *Ann. Otol. Rhinol. Laryngol.*, **76**, 829–33.
Miller A.H. (1971). Four years experience with the Asai technique for vocal rehabilitation for the laryngectomized patient. *J. Laryngol. Otol.*, **85**, 567–76.
Montgomery W.W. (1972). Postlaryngectomy vocal rehabilitation. *Arch. Otolaryngol.*, **95**, 76–83.
Montgomery W.W., Toohil R.J. (1968). Voice rehabilitation after laryngectomy. *Arch. Otolaryngol.*, **88**, 499–506.

Nijdam H.F., Annyas A.A., Schutte H.K., Leeuer H. (1982). A new prosthesis for voice rehabilitation after laryngectomy. *Arch. Otolaryngol.*, **237**, 27–33.
Panje W.R. (1981). Prosthetic vocal rehabilitation following laryngectomy — the voice button. *Ann. Otol. Rhinol. Laryngol.*, **90**, 116–20.
Park R. (1886). A case of total extirpation of the larynx. *Ann. Surg.*, **3**, 28–38.
Pearson B.W. (1981). Sub-total laryngectomy. *Laryngoscope*, **91**, 1904–11.
Robbins J., Fisher H.B., Blom E.D., Singer M.I. (1984). A comparative study of normal, oesophageal and tracheo-oesophageal speech production. *J. Speech Hear. Disord.*, **49**, 202–10.
Ryan W.J. (1979). How people communicate after laryngectomy. Paper presented at ASHA Convention, Atlanta, Ga. (quoted by Zanoff et al., 1990).
Saito H., Yoshida S., Saito T. (1989). Simple mucodermal tracheo-oesophageal shunt method for voice restoration. *Arch. Otolaryngol.*, **115**, 494–6.
Scottish Cancer Registration Scheme (1981). *Cancer Registration and Survival Statistics in Scotland 1963–1977*. Edinburgh: Common Services Agency.
Scuri M., quoted by Briani A.A. (1959). Récupération sociale des laryngectomisés par une méthode operatoire personnelle. *L'Evolution Méd.*, **3**, 17–25.
Singer M.I., Blom E.D. (1980). An endoscopic technique for restoration of voice after laryngectomy. *Ann. Otol. Rhinol. Laryngol.*, **89**, 529–33.
Singh W. (1985). New tracheostoma flap valve for surgical speech reconstruction. In *New Dimensions in Otorhinolaryngology — Head and Neck Surgery* (Myers E.D., ed.) Amsterdam: Elsevier, pp. 480–1.
Singh W. (1987). Tracheostoma valve for speech rehabilitation in laryngectomees. *J. Laryngol. Otol.*, **101**, 809–14.
Singh W. (1988a). A simple surgical technique and a new prosthesis for voice rehabilitation after laryngectomy. *J. Laryngol. Otol.*, **102**, 332–4.
Singh W. (1988b). Valvula fonatoria de Singh. In *Recuperacion de la Voz en los Laryngectomizados* (Algaba J., ed.) Madrid: Garsi, pp. 331–3.
Singh W. (1989). Near-total laryngectomy. In *Proceedings of the International Voice Symposium*, Edinburgh (Singh W., ed.), pp. 53–8.
Singh W. (1990). Singh tracheostoma valve. In *Proceedings of the XXIst International Congress of the International Association of Logopedics and Phoniatrics*, Prague, pp. 435–7.
Singh W. (1991). Preservation of voice in laryngectomy. *Acta Phoniatrica Latina*, **13**, 302–4.
Singh W., Hardcastle P. (1985). Near total laryngectomy with myo-mucosal valved neoglottis. *J. Laryngol. Otol.*, **99**, 581–8.
Singh W., Kaur A. (1987). Laryngeal carcinoma in a six-year-old, with a review of the literature. *J. Laryngol. Otol.*, **101**, 957–8.
Snidcor J.C., Curry E.T. (1959). Temporal and pitch aspects of superior oesophageal speech. *Ann. Otol. Rhinol. Laryngol.*, **68**, 623–36.
Staffieri M. (1976). La chirirgia riabilitiva della voce dopo laringectomia totale. In *Associazione Otologi Ospedalieri Italiani XXIX Congresso Nazionale*, Bologna, 5, p. 222.
Taub S., Spiro H.R. (1972). Vocal rehabilitation of laryngectomees. *Am. J. Surg.*, **124**, 87–90.
Weinberg B., Moon J. (1984). Aerodynamic properties of four tracheo-oesophageal puncture prostheses. *Arch. Otolaryngol.*, **110**, 673–5.
Wenig B.L., Mullooly V., Levy J., Abramson A.L. (1989). Voice restoration following laryngectomy: the role of primary versus secondary tracheo-oesophageal puncture. *Ann. Otol. Rhinol. Laryngol.*, **98**, 70–3.
Wetmore S.J., Johns M.E., Baker S.R. (1981a). The Singer–Blom voice restoration procedure. *Arch. Otolaryngol.*, **107**, 674–6.
Wetmore S.J., Krueger K., Wesson K. (1981b). The Singer–Blom speech rehabilitation procedure. *Laryngoscope*, **91**, 1109–17.
Zanoff D.J., Wold D., Montague J.C. Jnr, et al. (1990). Tracheoesophageal speech: with and without tracheostoma valve. *Laryngoscope*, **100**, 498–502.
Zwitman D., Calcaterra T. (1973). Phonation using the tracheo-oesophageal shunt. *J. Speech Hear. Disord.*, **38**, 369–73.

Index

Adenocarcinoma, 16
Adenoid cystic carcinoma, 16
Amyloidosis, laryngeal, 13
Anemometer, hot-wire, 21
Angiomatous lesions, laser surgery, 155
Arytenoid cartilage, anatomy, 5
Asai three-stage tracheopharyngeal shunt, 176, 178–80
Aspiration, 127
Atresia, laryngeal, 12

Benign tumours see Tumours, benign
Blom-Singer voice prostheses, 177–80, 190, 194
Blood supply, laryngeal, 7
Bowel transfers, 106, 107

Cancer see Malignant disease
Carcinoma in situ, 15
Carcinoma see Malignant disease
Cartilage, anatomy
   arytenoid, 5
   cricoid, 3
   thyroid, 4
Chondroma, 14
Chondrosarcoma, 16
Colon transfer, 106
Computers, role of see under Voice problems
Congenital abnormalities, 12
Conley's tracheo-oesophageal shunt, 175, 176
Cooper-Rand artificial larynx, 171, 172
Cricoid cartilage, anatomy, 3
Crisopharyngeal myotomy, 138
C_x displays, 42–8

Cysts
   laryngeal, 12
   voluminous, laser surgery, 154

Deltopectoral flap, 103
Developmental abnormalities, 12
Digitization, voice, 60
D_x displays, 42–8, 73–9
Dysphagia, 127
Dysplasia, 15

Effort closure, larynx, 12
EGG see Electroglottography
Electroglottography, 36, 56–8, 139, 141
Electrolaryngography, 35–50, 71–82, 139, 141
   D_x displays, 42–8, 73–9
   F_x displays, 34–50, 79–82
   L_x displays, 34–50, 72
Electromyography, 58
Electrostroboscopy, 55, 87–9
Epiglottis, anatomy, 5
Extrinsic muscles, anatomy, 6

FIGS see Functional intraoral Glasgow scale
Fistula speech, 111, 112, 171–203
   future developments, 195
   historical perspective, 173–7
   procedures, 177–82
   prostheses see Voice prostheses
   Singh system see Singh speech system
   subglottal pressure see Subglottal pressure
Frequency, definition, 34
   fundamental see Fundamental frequency

Functional intraoral Glasgow scale, 111
Fundamental frequency, 64–5, 73–82
F_x displays, 34–50, 79–82

Gastric pull-up, 106
Glasgow scale, functional intraoral, 111
Glottis, 123–4
   efficiency in voice production, 20
   glottal pulse shape estimation, 65
   malignant disease see under Malignant disease
   stenosis, 152, 153
Granulomas, pharyngeal, 154
Gussenbauer voice prosthesis, 173, 174
Guttman tracheohypopharyngeal fistula, 175

Haemangioma, 14
Hot-wire anemometer, 21
Hyoid bone, anatomy, 5
Hypoglottic stenosis, 152, 153

Infection
   in near-total laryngectomy, 127
   laryngeal, 13, 14
Inflammatory conditions, laryngeal, 13
Infraglottis see Subglottis
Intensity, definition, 34
International Phonetic Association, sound groups, 31
Intrinsic muscles, 10, 11

Jejunum transfer, 106

Keratoses, laser surgery, 149, 155

Laryngeal atresia, 12
Laryngeal cysts, 12
Laryngeal papillomatosis, 148
Laryngeal spaces, 8, 119
   paraglottic space, 8, 119
   pre-epiglottic space, 8, 119
   Reinke's space, 8, 13, 118
      oedema, 13, 148
Laryngeal surgery, 97–100
   future techniques, 100
   history, 97–8
   laser surgery, 147–54
      glottic cancer, 149–51
      keratosis, 149
      laryngotracheal stenosis, 152
      malignant disease, 149–51
      nodules, 147
      papillomatosis, 148
      polyps, 147, 148
      Reinke's oedema, 148
      supraglottic cancer, 149
   vocal cord paralysis, 151
   present techniques, 98–100
   see also Laryngectomy
Laryngeal webs, 12
Laryngectomy
   aerodynamics after, 27
      typical values, 28
   fistula speech see Fistula speech
   near-total see Near-total laryngectomy
   nursing see Nursing care
   oesophageal speech see Oesophageal speech
   parsimonious see Near-total laryngectomy
   quality of life after, 169
   subglottal pressure see Subglottal pressure
   supraglottic, 120
   see also Pharyngo-oesophageal reconstruction
Laryngoceles, 12
Laryngograph see Electrolaryngography
Larynx
   anatomy, 3–8
   artificial, 171–3
      Cooper-Rand, 171, 172
      Servox, 171, 172
      Tokyo, 171, 173
   embryonic development, 3
   physiology, 9–12
   spaces see Laryngeal spaces
   submucosal compartments, 118–25
   surgical pathology, 12–6
   voice production, 18
Laser surgery see under Laryngeal and Pharyngeal surgery
Latissimus dorsi flap, 106
Leukoplakia, 14
L_x displays, 34–50, 72
Lymphatic drainage, laryngeal, 7

Malignant disease, 15
   adenocarcinoma, 16
   adenoic cystic carcinoma, 16
   chondrosarcoma, 16
   glottal, 123, 125, 128
   laser surgery see under Laryngeal and Pharyngeal surgery
   near-total laryngectomy, 116–25
   pharyngo-oesophageal reconstruction, 102
   piriform sinus, 124, 128
   premalignancy see Premalignant conditions
   spindle cell carcinoma, 16
   squamous cell carcinoma, 15

subglottic, 124, 125, 128
supraglottic, 120, 125, 128
transglottic, 121–3, 125, 128
verrucous carcinoma, 16
see also Tumours
Maximal phonation time, 21
Muscles, laryngeal *see* Extrinsic *and* Intrinsic muscles
Myocutaneous flaps *see* Skin flaps
Myotomy, crisopharyngeal, 138

Near-total laryngectomy, 116–45
  complications, 126
    aspiration, 127
    dysphagia, 127
    infection, 127
    nerve injury, 126
    stenosis, 126
  contraindications, 126
  crisopharyngeal myotomy, 138
  future developments, 144
  history, 116
  indications, 125
  neoglottal speech *see* Neoglottal speech
  neoglottis, 137
  nursing *see* Nursing care
  operative technique, 129–39
  principle, 117
  procedure, 127–39
  results and comments, 144
  subglottal pressure *see* Subglottal pressure
  submucosal compartments, 118–25
  terminology, 117
  voice production, 139–41
Neoglottal speech
  electrolaryngography *see* Electrolaryngography
  research, 70–94
  subglottal pressure *see* Subglottal pressure
  voice analysis, 141
Neoglottis
  in near-total laryngectomy, 137
  speech *see* Neoglottal speech
  Staffieri and Serafini technique, 177, 183
Nerve supply, laryngeal, 7
Nodules, laryngeal, 147
Nursing care, 157–62
  postoperative assessment
    early, 160
    rehabilitation, 160
  preoperative assessment
    admission to hospital, 158
    clinical investigation, 158

    initial consultation, 157
    preparation for theatre, 150
    psychological support, 158

Oesophageal speech, 165–70, 171
  aerodynamics, 165
  obstacles to, 167
  practice, 166–9

Papillomas
  laryngeal, 14, 148
  pharyngeal, 154
Paraglottic space, 8, 119, 120
Parsimonious laryngectomy *see* Near-total laryngectomy
Pectoralis major flap, 103
Periodicity, definition, 34
Perturbation analysis, 65
Pharyngeal surgery, 97–100
  laser surgery, 154–5
    angiomatous lesions, 155
    chronic tonsillitis, 154
    granulomas, 154
    keratosis, 155
    malignant disease, 155
    papillomas, 154
    premalignant lesions, 155
    voluminous cysts, 154
  future techniques, 100
  history, 97
  present techniques, 98–100
Pharyngo-oesophageal reconstruction, 101–5
  distant, 109
  examination under anaesthesia, 102
  indications, 102
  local, 103
  preoperative assessment, 101
  radiological investigations, 102
  rehabilitation, 109–13
    speech *see* Speech rehabilitation
    swallowing, 110
  techniques, 102–9
Phonation *see* Voice
Phone level, 31
Phoneme level, 31
Phonetography, voice research, 82
Physiology, larynx, 9–12
Piriform sinus, 124
Pneumotachograph, 21
Polyps, 12, 147
Pre-epiglottic space, 8, 119
Premalignant conditions, 14
  carcinoma in situ, 15
  dysplasia, 15

Index   207

laser surgery *see* Laryngeal *and* Pharyngeal surgery
leukoplakia, 14

Q_x displays, 48, 49

Radial forearm flap, 107
Rehabilitation, 109–13
  speech *see* Speech rehabilitation
  swallowing, 110
  nursing *see* Nursing care
Reinke's oedema, 13, 148
Reinke's space, 8, 13, 118
Respiratory system, voice production, 9, 18

SAMPA sound groups, 31
Sarcoidosis, laryngeal, 13
Scleroma, laryngeal, 14
Servox artificial larynx, 171, 172
Singh speech system, 182–201
  fistula dummy, 182, 185, 190
  fistula valve, 182, 185, 190
  tracheo-oesophageal fistula, 184–90
  tracheostoma button, 194, 196
  tracheostoma valve, 137, 192–5, 199–200
Skin flaps, 103, 107
Sonography, 58
Sound groups
  International Phonetic Association convention, 31
  SAMPA, 31
S_p displays, 34–50
Spectogram, speech, 36
Spectral analysis, 62–3
Spectrography, voice research, 86–7
Speech
  alaryngeal, research, 70–94
  analysis, 31–51
    electrolaryngography *see* Electrolaryngography
    limitations, 71
    role of computers *see under* Voice problems
  fistula *see* Fistula speech
  frequency, definition, 34
  intensity, definition, 34
  neoglottal *see* Neoglottal speech
  normal, 31–51
  oesophageal *see* Oesophageal speech
  pathological *see* Voice problems
  periodicity, definition, 34
  prostheses *see* Voice prostheses
  rehabilitation *see* Speech rehabilitation
  segmental descriptions, 31–4
  signals, 34–7
  sound groups *see* Sound groups
  spectogram, 36
  turbulence, definition, 34
  vowels and consonants, 32–4
  see also Voice
Speech colour transformation, 58
Speech rehabilitation, 111–3
  air injection, 111
  artificial larynx, 111
  fistula speech *see* Fistula speech
  nursing, 160
  oesophageal speech *see* Oesophageal speech
  role of computers, 67
Spindle cell carcinoma, 16
Squamous cell carcinoma, 15
Squamous cell papilloma, 14
Stenosis
  glottic, 12, 152, 153
  hypoglottic, 152, 153
  laryngotracheal, 152–4
  laser surgery, 152–4
  in near-total laryngectomy, 126
  in pharyngo-oesophageal reconstruction, 110
  subglottic, 12
  supraglottic, 152, 153
  tracheal, 152, 153
Sternocleidomastoid flap, 106
Stomach transfer, 106
Stroboscopy, 55, 86–9
Subglottal pressure, 11, 19, 89, 142
  measurement, 22
  normative values, 25
Subglottis, 124
  malignant disease *see under* Malignant disease
  stenosis, 12
Supraglottis, 118, 119–21
  malignant disease *see under* Malignant disease
  stenosis, 152, 153
Swallowing
  rehabilitation, 110
  larynx function in, 10

Thyroid cartilage, anatomy, 4
Tissue transfer, free, 106
Tokyo artificial larynx, 171, 173
Tonsillitis, chronic, laser surgery, 154
Tracheal stenosis, 152, 153
Tracheohyoidopexy, Arslan and Serafini technique, 176, 183
Tracheohypopharyngeal fistula, Guttman, 175

Tracheo-oesophageal fistula
  Amatsu's technique, 177, 184
  Conley's, 175, 176
  Singh *see under* Singh speech system
Tracheopharyngeal shunt, Asai three-stage technique, 176, 178–81
Tracheostoma valve, 111
  Singh, 137, 192–5, 199–200
Trapezius flap, 106
Tuberculosis, laryngeal, 13
Tumours
  benign, 14
  glottal, 123, 125, 128
  laser surgery *see under* Laryngeal and Pharyngeal surgery
  near-total laryngectomy, 116–45
  piriform sinus, 125, 128
  premalignant *see* Premalignant conditions
  subglottic, 124, 125
  supraglottic, 120, 125, 128
  transglottic, 121–3, 125, 128
  see also Malignant disease
Turbulence, definition, 34

Ventricle of larynx, 118, 121–3
Verrucous carcinoma, 16
Videostroboscopy, 88
Vocal cords
  nodules, 12
  paralysis, 151
  polyps, 12
  true, 118
Voice
  aerodynamics, 18–30
    after laryngectomy, 27
  air flow, 19
  efficiency, 20
    normative values, 25
  electroglottography, 36, 56–8, 139, 141
  electrolaryngography *see* Electrolaryngography
  electromyography, 58
  electrostroboscopy, 55, 87–9
  frequency *see* Frequency
  glottal efficiency, 20
  laryngographic aspects, 37–40
  larynx in, 10, 18
  maximal phonation time, 21
  mean air flow rate measurement, 21
    hot-wire anemometer, 21
    maximal phonation time, 21
    normative values, 25
    phonation volume, 21
    pneumotachograph, 21
  phonetography, 82
  problems *see* Voice problems
  quality, 40–50
  research, 70–94
  respiratory system in, 18
  sonography, 58
  sound spectrography, 86–7
  speech colour transformation, 58
  subglottal pressure, 19
  videostroboscopy, 88
  voice range profiles, 55
  see also Speech
Voice field measurement *see* Phonetography
Voice problems, 31–51
  aids to diagnosis, 55–9
  role of computers, 60–9
    aid to diagnosis, 66
    digitization, 60
    fundamental frequency estimation, 63–5
    glottal pulse shape estimation, 65
    perturbation analysis, 65
    spectral analysis, 62
    waveform analysis, 61
  see also Speech *and* Voice
Voice prostheses, 112, 177–82
  biflanged silicone, 180
  biflanged voice button, 180
  Blom-Singer, 177–80, 190, 194
  Groningen, 180
  Gussenbauer, 173, 174
  VoiceBak, 176, 182, 194
VoiceBak prosthesis, 176, 182, 194
Voluminous cysts, laser surgery, 154

Waveform analysis, 60–2
Webs, laryngeal, 12
Wegener's granulomatosis, laryngeal, 13